Challenging Cases in Allergy and Immunology

Massoud Mahmoudi
Editor

Challenging Cases in Allergy and Immunology

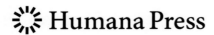 Humana Press

Editor
Massoud Mahmoudi D.O, Ph.D. RM (NRM), FACOI, FAOCAI, FASCMS,
    FACP, FCCP, FAAAAI
Assistant Clinical Professor of Medicine
University of California San Francisco
San Francisco, California
Chairman, Department of Medicine
Community Hospital of Los Gatos
Los Gatos, California
USA

ISBN 978-1-60327-442-5   e-ISBN 978-1-60327-443-2
DOI 10.1007/978-1-60327-443-2
Springer Dordrecht Heidelberg London New York

Library of Congress Control Number: 2009928233

Cover Illustration: Fig. 17.3. Duodenal biopsy demonstrating duodenal mucosa with diffuse chronic enteritis with near complete villous atrophy and glandular elongation. There are diffuse infiltrates of lymphocytes and plasma cells. These finding are consistent with the diagnosis of autoimmune enteritis. Photograph courtesy of Beverly B. Dahms

Printed on acid-free paper

Springer is part of Springer Science+Business Media (www.springer.com)

To the memory of my father,
Mohammad H. Mahmoudi, and
to my mother, Zohreh, my wife Lily,
and my son, Sam, for their continuous
support and encouragement.

Preface

Sometimes we need to put down our stethoscopes, place our pens on the table, take a seat, and think deeply about a case. If all our patients were classic textbook examples, we would have easy jobs and be more productive every day. In reality, that is not the case. A challenging clinical case is somewhat like driving very fast on the freeway and then hitting a traffic jam due to an accident, forcing you to slow down quickly.

The benefits to slowing down and thinking deeply are considerable, and that, I hope, will be the result of reading these excellent cases. I have been fortunate to gather over 30 national and international experts in the field of allergy/immunology, rheumatology, and pulmonology to prepare this unique resource of challenging cases. This is a small yet comprehensive collection comprised of the thoughts and expertise of various leading educators and clinicians.

This book consists of 20 chapters covering all aspects of allergy and immunology in a case-study format. Indeed, the content covers not only the common allergic diseases such as allergic rhinitis, asthma, and food allergy but also areas in immune regulation, autoimmunity, and immunodeficiencies. Each chapter presents two or more challenging cases from one to several expert contributors. To make this product a more comprehensive medium for education, we have added five to ten multiple-choice questions and answers at the end of each chapter.

The cases presented are intended to stimulate the thought processes of all health providers involved in treating patients with allergic and immunologic diseases. All allergists/immunologists, fellows in training, primary care physicians, residents, medical students, nurse practitioners, physician assistants, and other allied health providers will find this collection a valuable resource. While the book is an independent source of information, it may also be combined with my other textbook *Allergy and Asthma: Practical Diagnosis and Management* for better cross-referencing of the subjects.

I am indebted to Richard Lansing, Executive Editor at Springer/Humana Press, for accepting my proposal and for guiding me with his thoughtful advice throughout the preparation of this manuscript. I also thank Amanda Quinn for her editorial assistance, as well as the entire editorial and production team at Springer/Humana Press for their wonderful effort in preparation of this work.

I would appreciate hearing your comments and suggestions for use in what I hope will be a second edition of this title in the years to come. Please contact me at allergycure@sbcglobal.net.

Los Gatos, CA   Massoud Mahmoudi

Contents

Contributors

Pedro Avila, M.D.
Associate Professor, Division of Allergy-Immunology, Department of Medicine, Northwestern University's Feinberg School of Medicine, Chicago, IL, USA

James L. Baldwin, M.D.
Associate Professor, Division of Allergy and Immunology, University of Michigan, Ann Arbor,
MI, USA

H. Michael Belmont, M.D.
Associate Professor of Medicine, Lupus Clinic, Bellevue Hospital, NYU-Hospital for Joint Diseases, Division of Rheumatology, Department of Medicine, New York University, School of Medicine, New York, NY, USA

Jonathan Bernstein, M.D.
Professor of Clinical Medicine, Division of Immunology, Department of Internal Medicine, College of Medicine, University of Cincinnati, Cincinnati, OH, USA

I. Leonard Bernstein, M.D.
Clinical Professor emeritus, Division of Immunology, Department of Internal Medicine, College of Medicine, University of Cincinnati, Cincinnati, OH, USA

Leonard Bielory, M.D.
Professor of Medicine, Pediatrics, and Ophthalmology, Department of Medicine, Pediatrics, and Ophthalmology, UMDNJ-New Jersey Medical School, Asthma and Allergy Research Center, Newark, NJ, USA

Marcy Bolster, M.D.
Professor, Rheumatology Fellowship Training Program, Division of Rheumatology, Department of Medicine, Medical University of South Carolina, Charleston,
SC, USA

Timothy J. Craig, D.O
Professor of Medicine and Pediatrics, Division of Allergy, Department of Medicine, Penn State University, Hershey,
PA, USA

Oscar L. Frick, M.D.
Professor Emeritus, Pediatric Allergy Clinic, University of California,
San Francisco, CA, USA

Marianne Frieri, M.D., Ph.D., F.A.C.A.A.I., F.A.A.A.A.I.
Chief of Allergy and Immunology, Department of Medicine,
Nassau University Medical Center, New York, NY, USA
State University of New York, Stony Brook, NY, USA

Patricia C. Fulkerson, M.D., Ph.D.
Department of Pediatrics, College of Medicine, University of Cincinnati,
Cincinnati, OH, USA

Hellen Hollingsworth, M.D.
Associate Professor, Department of Pulmonary, Critical Care, Allergy and
Immunology, Boston University Medical Center, Boston, MA, USA

Peter Jensen, M.D.
Chief, Division of Infectious Diseases, Division of Infectious Diseases,
San Francisco Veteran Affairs Medical Center, University of California,
San Francisco, San Francisco, CA, USA

Alexander Kapp, M.D., Ph.D.
Professor and Chairman, Department of Dermatology and Allergology,
Hannover Medical University, Hannover, Germany

Nicholas J. Kenyon, M.D.
Associate Professor of Medicne, Division of Pulmonary and Critical Care
Medicine, Department of Internal Medicine, University of California,
Davis Health System, Asthma Network (UCAN™), Davis, CA, USA

Anna Kovalszki, M.D.
Fellow, Division of Allergy and Immunology, University of Michigan,
Ann Arbor, MI, USA

Dennis K. Ledford, M.D.
Professor of Medicine and Pediatrics, University of South Florida
College of Medicine, James A. Haley V. A. Hospital, Tampa, FL, USA

David Lim, M.D.
Clinical Instructor and Postdoctoral Fellow, Division of Infectious Diseases,
J. David Gladstone Institute of Virology and Immunology, University of California,
San Francisco, San Francisco, CA, USA

Samuel Louie, M.D.
Professor, Division of Pulmonary and Critical Care Medicine,
Department of Internal Medicine, University of California,
Davis Health System, Asthma Network (UCAN™), Davis, CA, USA

Aymeric Louit, M.B.B.S.
Fellow, Division of Allergy-Immunology, Department of Medicine,
Northwestern University's Feinberg School of Medicine, Chicago, IL, USA

Massoud Mahmoudi, D.O., Ph.D., R.M. (N.R.M.), F.A.C.O.I., F.A.O.C.A.I., F.A.S.C.M.S., F.A.C.P., F.C.C.P., F.A.A.A.A.I.
Assistant Clinical Professor of Medicine, University of California
San Francisco, San Francisco, CA, USA
Department of Medicine, Community Hospital of Los Gatos, Los Gatos, CA, USA
Department of Medicine, UMDNJ, School of Osteopathic Medicine, Stratford, NJ, USA
Division of Allergy and Immunology, Department of Pediatrics, Stanford
University, School of Medicine, Stanford, CA, USA
Department of Medicine, San Francisco College of Osteopathic Medicine, Touro
University, Mere Island, CA, USA

Howard Maibach, M.D.
Professor, Department of Dermatology, University of California San Francisco,
San Francisco, CA, USA

Amy L. Marks, D.O.
Attending Physician, Department of Pediatrics, Richmond Medical Center,
Richmond Heights, OH, USA, University Hospital of Cleveland,
Cleveland, OH, USA

Kris G. McGrath, M.D.
Associate Professor of Medicine, Northwestern University,
Feinberg School of Medicine, Chicago, IL, USA
Allergy and Immunology, Saint Joseph Hospital, Chicago, IL, USA

Tracy Prematta, M.D.
Fellow, Division of Allergy, Department of Medicine, Penn State University,
Hershey, PA, USA

Ron Purcell, M.D.
Fellow, Division of Allergy and Immunology, University of South Florida College
of Medicine, James A. Haley V. A. Hospital, Tampa, FL, USA

Marc Rothenberg, M.D., Ph.D.
Director and Endowed Chair, Division of Allergy and Immunology,
Cincinnati Children's Hospital Medical Center,
University of Cincinnati College of Medicine, Cincinnati, OH, USA

Michael Sachivo, M.D.
Division of Pulmonary and Critical Care Medicine, Division of Pulmonary and
Critical Care Medicine, Department of Internal Medicine, University of California,
Davis Health System, Asthma Network (UCAN™), Davis, CA, USA

Haig Tcheurekdjian, M.D.
Assistant Clinical Professor, Department of Medicine and Pediatrics,
Case Western Reserve University, Cleveland, OH, USA
Allergy/Immunology Associates, Inc., Cleveland, OH, USA

Kelly Haw-Yuen Thong, M.D., M.S.
Fellow, Department of Dermatology, University of California San Francisco,
San Francisco, CA, USA

Jennifer Toth, M.D.
Fellow, Division of Allergy, Department of Medicine,
Penn State University, Hershey,
PA, USA

Brttina Wedi, M.D., Ph.D.
Professor, Department of Dermatology and Allergology,
Hannover Medical University, Hannover, Germany

Philip Wexler, M.D.
Fellow, Allergy and Immunology, Boston University Medical Center,
Boston, MA, USA

Satoshi Yoshida, M.D., Ph.D.
Vice President, Department of Medicine, Sakuragaoka Chuo Hospital,
Yamato, Japan

Amir Zeki, M.D.
Fellow, Division of Pulmonary and Critical Carte Medicine,
Department of Medicine, University of California, Davis Health System,
Asthma Network (UCAN™), Davis, CA, USA

Chapter 1
Rhinitis

Dennis K. Ledford and Ron Purcell

Abstract Rhinitis is a common problem encountered daily by most health professionals. Although allergy is the most common cause of rhinitis, the clinician should be aware of the complex differential diagnosis and the variety of allergens that may be responsible for the symptoms. The clinical challenge is magnified by the lack of specific symptoms in the various forms of rhinitis and by the number of potential allergens not routinely tested. Thus, an accurate assessment and effective treatment plan requires attention to details of the history and physical examination. These two cases are intended to illustrate these points.

Keywords Rhinitis • Allergic rhinitis • Sarcoidosis

Case 1

History of Present Illness

Mr. GA is a 52-year-old African American male who was born in Antigua and who moved to the USA as a young adult. His primary complaint is nasal congestion and sinus pressure.

He experienced no significant problems with allergic disease, eczema, food allergy, or asthma as a child. He works for a university in Florida serving in various custodial positions. This work requires some exposure to chemicals, primarily chlorinated products and detergents. He began to notice nasal congestion that started approximately at the age of 45 years. The congestion was bilateral and associated with a modest degree of nasal discharge that was generally thick, but not discolored. There was no seasonal pattern and he did not experience severe itching or sneezing

D.K. Ledford (✉) and R. Purcell
University of South Florida College of Medicine, James A. Haley V. A. Hospital,
13000 Bruce B. Downs Blvd., VAR 111D, Tampa, FL 33612, USA
e-mail: dledford@health.usf.edu

M. Mahmoudi (ed.), *Challenging Cases in Allergy and Immunology*,
DOI: 10.1007/978-1-60327-443-2_1,
© Humana Press, a part of Springer Science+Business Media, LLC 2009

paroxysms. He was evaluated by his family physician who tried therapy with oral antihistamines without benefit. Oral decongestants helped slightly but he had mild hypertension that required treatment and the oral decongestant was not continued. Topical decongestant sprays with oxymetazoline did provide relief and he began to use this therapy more regularly. Three years after onset of the nasal congestion, he was evaluated by an allergist/immunologist who documented a mild degree of allergic sensitivity and initiated allergen immunotherapy, which made little difference in his symptoms, and immunotherapy was discontinued after 8 months. He was also treated with intranasal corticosteroids, which initially provided some relief, but he eventually resumed the use of the oxymetazoline. The nasal congestion became more persistent, and he noticed worsening when he was at work, particularly when he used spray cleansers and floor stripper. Perfume inhalation or alcohol ingestion did not make the congestion worse. Other complaints included fatigue and an inter-mittent, nonproductive cough. He had a series of laboratory tests performed and was referred for consultation.

Past Medical History, Family History, Personal History, and Review of Systems

Past history was negative for asthma, wheezing, or shortness of breath. His blood pressure had been controlled with an oral thiazide diuretic and an angiotensin converting enzyme (ACE) inhibitor. Family history was negative for documented allergy or asthma but was positive for hypertension. His home environment did not include passive cigarette exposure or indoor pets. His home had central air conditioning. He did not smoke cigarettes and only drank ethanol during holidays. He had smoked marijuana in the past but never used intranasal cocaine or intravenous recreational drugs. He occasionally traveled to Antigua to visit family and felt that the symptoms improved in that location. Review of systems was primarily positive for a decrease in energy and fatigue with some difficulty in sleeping due to nasal congestion.

Physical Examination

Exam revealed a slightly overweight black male who was in no distress and did not have a prominent nasal voice. He did exhibit frequent nasal sniffing. Positive findings included violaceous, waxy skin lesions on his cheeks and around the nasolabial folds (Fig. 1.1). Nasal findings included marked congestion with an erythematous mucosal appearance but no bleeding or crusting. His conjunctivae were slightly injected. No lymphadenopathy was palpable; his chest was clear of crackles or wheeze and the remainder of his examination was normal. Spirometry demonstrated a mild restrictive defect. His laboratory showed a hemoglobin of 12 g/dl (normal 13–15 g/dl), a WBC of 9,800 with 7% eosinophils, 10% lymphocytes, and 62% polymorphonuclear cells.

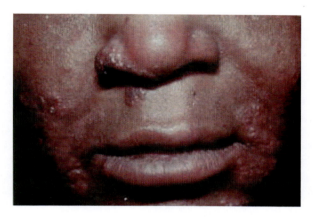

Fig. 1.1 Picture of facial lesions of sarcoidosis is presented. Papules that are relatively asympto-matic are demonstrated, with clustering in proximity of the nasolabial folds and around the mouth. The finding of noncaseating granulomas on biopsy confirmed that the lesions are dermatologic sarcoidosis, termed lupus pernio. The skin lesions on the nasolabial folds correlate with nasal mucosal sarcoidosis, which was responsible for our patient's nasal symptoms. Conjunctival mucosa may also be affected by sarcoidosis but is not specifically associated with the skin papules demonstrated in this figure

When Presented with This Data What Is Your Diagnosis?

The differential diagnosis includes perennial or persistent allergic rhinitis, nonallergic rhinitis, mixed rhinitis (allergic and nonallergic rhinitis), anatomical obstruction from nasal polyps or lymphoid hyperplasia and sinusitis. A primary nasal malignancy, such as a squamous cell carcinoma or inverted papilloma or esthesiochemodectoma, is in the differential diagnosis but seems highly unlikely with an 8-year history of symptoms. Irritant or allergic rhinitis from his work environment is a consideration, but exposure was only to irritants and the contribution to symptoms did not seem significant. Certainly a component of rhinitis medicamentosa from the use of topical nasal decongestants and oral antihypertensives is likely.

Additional Assessment

Percutaneous or prick allergy skin tests and selected intradermal tests showed minimal allergic sensitivity to perennial allergens. Nasal smear showed primarily neutrophils. Treatment was initiated with intranasal budesonide 64 mcg (two puffs) in each nostril twice a day, and he was advised to discontinue the oxymeta-zoline. He returned in 10 days reporting that the nasal congestion was insufferable and he had to restart the oxymetazoline. Nasal exam revealed turbinate edema with a striking mucosal erythema but no bleeding. The skin lesions were unchanged.

Oral corticosteroid therapy was initiated for suspected rhinitis medicamentosa from regular use of oxymetazoline. He was treated with 20 mg of prednisone twice daily for 3 days and once daily for 3 days. On the last 2 days of the prednisone treatment, intranasal fluticasone was initiated at 220 mcg in each nostril twice daily. This was delivered by adapting an asthma inhaler for nasal use. He returned in 1 week reporting marked improvement. The violaceous skin lesions on his cheeks had improved and the nasal congestion was less, although the mucosal erythema was little changed. The oxymetazoline was not restarted and he maintained the high-dose nasal corticosteroid therapy, but his congestion gradually worsened over the next 4 weeks. Fiberoptic rhinoscopy showed diffuse erythema of the nasal mucosa with slight adenoid enlargement but no evidence of laryngeal reflux, nasal malignancy, or purulent sinusitis. Sinus imaging showed only mucosal thickening. Total IgE was low normal and IgG was increased with normal IgA and IgM. A diagnostic test was performed.

What Is Our Diagnosis and Why?

The initial diagnosis was perennial nonallergic rhinitis with rhinitis medicamentosa. The drugs associated with rhinitis mediamentosa are listed in Table 1.1. Although ACE inhibitors may cause nasal congestion, beta and alpha blockers are the most common therapy to aggravate congestion, and he did not use these treatments. However, the regular use of the oxymetazoline would be expected to cause rebound congestion. Of note, however, is the fact the congestion was bothering him prior to using the oxymetazoline and, in the authors' experience, this is often the case with individuals who utilize nasal decongestants. That is, they have a nasal problem that preceded their use of topical decongestants and probably is the primary reason they started the decongestants. After the failure of the standard dose of nasal corticosteroid therapy, oral corticosteroids were used to "break the cycle" of decongestant use and were initially successful. However, the relapse while using high-dose nasal corticosteroids suggests that the patient is nonadherent with nasal spray, is using nasal cocaine, or is suffering from another cause of rhinitis in addition to the use of nasal decongestants. The response to oral corticosteroids that could not be maintained with nasal treatment and the unusual facial rash suggested the possibility of an alternative cause of nasal congestion. The diagnostic test performed was a skin biopsy of the face, which demonstrated noncaseating granulomas consistent with sarcoidosis, and the skin lesions were diagnosed as lupus pernio. This cutaneous manifestation of sarcoidosis is associated with nasal and upper airway involvement.

The treatment plan was revised and utilized: very high dose nasal corticosteroid, fluticasone 440 mcg in each nostril twice daily. Nasal decongestant spray was also used. Other therapies, including nasal antihistamines and oral leukotriene antagonists, provided little additional relief. Oral corticosteroids were used for severe

Table 1.1   Rhinitis syndromes

Allergic rhinitis
  Seasonal or intermittent allergic rhinitis
  Perennial or persistent allergic rhinitis
Nonallergic rhinitis
Atrophic Rhinitis
  Idiopathic
  Kertaoconjuncitivitis sicca (Sjögren's syndrome)
  Radiation therapy
  Postsurgical (middle turbinectomy)
Drug-induced rhinitis
  Rhinitis medicamentosa [Topical treatments (e.g., oxymetazoline, cocaine)]
  Systemic treatments [e.g., beta blockers, alpha antagonists, angiotensin-converting enzyme
    inhibitors, aspirin or NSAIDs (in subjects with sensitivity), phosphodiesterase 5-selec-
    tive inhibitors, anticholinergics, phentolamine]
  Infectious rhinitis
  Viral
  Mycobacterial
  Rhinitis associated with bacterial sinusitis
  Ozena (Klebsiella, Staphylococcus, Streptococcus, Proteus)
Nonallergic rhinitis with eosinophilia (NARES)
Occupational rhinitis
  Allergic
  Irritant
Rhinitis associated with local malignancy or disease or anatomical abnormalities
  Adenoid hyperplasia
  Angiofibroma
  Conchal bullosa
  CSF leak
  Esthesioneuroblastoma
  Inverted papilloma
  Lethal midline granulomas
  Lymphoma
  Nasal polyposis
  Partial submucosal cleft palate
  Severe septal deviation
  Squamous cell carcinoma
Rhinitis associated with systemic diseases
  Autoimmune diseases
  Sarcoidosis
  Sjögren's syndrome
  Syphillis
  Vasculitis (Wegener's granulomatosis, Churg Strauss vasculitis)
Vasomotor rhinitis

exacerbations, typically following irritant inhalant exposure, respiratory infection, or travel. The nasal symptoms diminished over the next 18–24 months, and the dose of nasal corticosteroid was reduced with minimal to moderate symptoms.

Discussion

Rhinitis is defined by a set of symptoms, which include congestion, anterior or posterior nasal discharge, sneezing, and itching (1). The most specific symptoms for allergy are the last two, which are typical of acute allergic rhinitis. Congestion and nasal discharge are unspecific and associated with a variety of nasal syndromes (Table 1.1). The most common form of rhinitis is allergic rhinitis, which is divided into two subcategories based upon allergic sensitivity and pattern of symptoms: perennial or persistent allergic rhinitis and seasonal or intermittent allergic rhinitis (2). Nonallergic rhinitis is composed of a series of conditions, which share nasal symptoms in common but have disparate pathophysiologies. Some of the nonallergic rhinitis syndromes do not have inflammation consistently identified in the nasal mucosa, suggesting that the term rhinitis may be incorrect. Nevertheless, rhinitis is used to describe all of these conditions.

Allergic rhinitis is diagnosed with appropriate symptoms, specific IgE to allergens which correlate with symptoms and physical findings consistent with allergic rhinitis. Generally the family history is positive for atopic disease and the onset is usually prior to the age of 30 years. The challenge is that the remaining subjects are "lumped," by default, into the heterogeneous group of conditions termed nonallergic rhinitis. The optimal treatment of these nonallergic patients is achieved if the diagnosis is accurate. Finally, up to 50–60% of allergic rhinitis subjects also have a nonallergic component to their disease. This overlap of conditions and complicated differential diagnosis often limit the effectiveness of therapy. In the authors' experience, nasal symptoms generally are attributed to allergy or "sinus" and if allergic treatment and antibiotics are ineffective, the treatment is changed to different allergy therapies or different antibiotics rather than considering other diagnoses. The authors think that fiberoptic rhinoscopy is an essential part of the diagnostic strategy and ideally should be a skill of the diagnostician. The clinician should resist the temptation to diagnose allergic rhinitis with low-level sensitivity and the lack of other features of allergy but rather seek out alternative explanations. Occupational rhinitis is one of the considerations in this regard. Most patients who complain of worsening of rhinitis at work suffer from chronic rhinitis unrelated to work, so such work symptoms are generally unspecific aggravation of chronic rhinitis. Exceptions include allergic rhinitis in individuals who work in industries with allergen exposure.

Sarcoidosis is a multisystem disease of unknown etiology and is associated with respiratory involvement in the lung (3, 4). The disease is characterized by tissue accumulation of T lymphocytes, usually with a CD4+ predominance, and mononuclear phagocytes, with formation of noncaseating granulomas. The lungs are involved in more than 90% of affected individuals. Other tissues with pathology may include the skin, eyes, lymph nodes, liver, and kidneys (Table 1.2). The presence of lupus pernio, or the waxy skin lesions about the nose, is a strong predictor of nasal involvement with sarcoidosis (Fig. 1.1). The mucosal inflammation associated with sarcoidosis is characterized by erythema and some nasal bleeding. Thus, the differential includes Wegener's granulomatosis, nasal lymphoma, squamous cell carcinoma of the nose, and midline granuloma. Nasal polyposis is generally associated

Table 1.2 Systemic involvement in sarcoidosis

Type of abnormality or organ affected	Percent affected
Lung	95%
Skin other than erythema nodosum	16%
Lymph nodes	15%
Eye	12%
Liver	12%
Erythema nodosum	8%
Spleen	7%
Central or peripheral nervous system	5%
Bone marrow	4%
Calcium homeostasis	4%
Upper airway	3%
Heart	2%
Kidney	1%
Bone and joints	<1%
Muscle	<1%

with a pale nasal mucosa, distinguishing nasal polyposis from these other conditions. As with other inflammatory conditions of the nasal mucosa, the primary complaint in nasal sarcoidosis tends to be congestion, watery rhinorrhea, and sneezing. However, the more common perennial allergic rhinitis is also characterized by nasal congestion and less frequent itching and sneezing. Finally other causes of nonallergic rhinitis are in the differential diagnosis.

This patient's chest radiograph did not demonstrate significant lymphadenopathy or infiltrates. However, sarcoidosis may involve the upper airway without lung involvement. Conjunctival injection is a manifestation in the eye that could be confused with allergic conjunctivitis and the nasal symptoms are usually congestion. Sinus imaging may be abnormal, suggesting pyogenic infection, when sarcoidosis involves the sinus mucosa.

The diagnosis of nasal sarcoidosis lead to a treatment regimen of very high dose nasal corticosteroids and a patient grateful for an explanation. There is no dose response with corticosteroids in allergic disease, but nonallergic conditions usually require, in the authors' experience, an increased dose of corticosteroid for optimal response. Using off-label doses of topical therapy is often the result. This may lead to concerns related to potential side effects, lack of coverage for the purchase of multiple nasal canisters each month, and telephone calls from pharmacists or pharmacy benefits managers advising the clinician that the dose being utilized is "excessive". Unfortunately, there is no body of evidence-based medicine that supports this concept of using "ultrahigh dose" corticosteroid therapy. If oral corticosteroid treatment improves the nasal symptoms but topical treatment is not effective or less effective, a clinical trial of greater dosages of nasal corticosteroids seems justified. Proof of safety of these doses is not available, but it is likely that topical treatment with dosages greater than recommended for rhinitis is still safer than oral or systemic corticosteroid therapy. The use of other treatment options, such as oral antihistamines or montelukast, is not likely to be effective in cases unresponsive to conventional doses of intranasal corticosteroids. Topical azelastine is indicated for vasomotor or perennial nonallergic rhinitis, and topical ipratroprium is effective for rhinorrhea, particularly watery rhinorrhea, in most nasal syndromes.

Case 2

History of Present Illness

MB is a 28-year-old male with a 6-month history of nasal congestion, rhinorrhea, and occasional sneezing paroxysms. The current problem started in late summer. The symptoms occur primarily at home but also worsen during lawn work, grocery shopping, spraying of insecticides and fertilizer on his lawn, and during work. The nasal discharge is clear and copious. The congestion is sufficiently severe to affect his sleep and that of his spouse. He has a past history of childhood eczema and springtime rhinitis but no asthma. The seasonal rhinitis has remained relatively constant during the past 5 years. He works as an auto mechanic and has regular contact with volatile organic hydrocarbons. He occasionally must do some arc welding when repairing automobile frames and does have exposure to metal dust. He has not hobbies with organic dust contact. His wife smokes but primarily outside of the home. He only smokes cigars on weekends. They have two children and have had a dog as their only mammalian pet since they were married 8 years ago. The dog is inside and sleeps on the bed. Their mattress is 8-years old and they use feather pillows.

Past Medical History, Family History, and Review of Systems

He has had no surgery on his nose or sinuses. Family history is positive for his sister having asthma and hay fever, and his son has eczema and chronic ear infections. Review of symptoms is negative for headache, fever, gastroesophageal reflux, wheezing, or shortness of breath. He does complain of a cough.

Physical Examination

The patient appears as a healthy appears male in no distress. Vital signs were BP 116/78, pulse 78/min, and respirations 12/min. Conjunctivae are slightly injected; nasal mucosa is pale and swollen with clear nasal discharge and minimal, mucoid postnasal drainage. Tonsils are slightly enlarged. Tympanic membranes are clear. Chest examination reveals no rhonchi or wheeze with good air exchange. The skin is slightly dry but there is no active rash.

When Presented with This Data What Is Your Diagnosis?

The clinical presentation is most consistent with perennial or persistent rhinitis. An allergic mechanism seems likely with nasal pallor, clear nasal discharge, and positive personal and family history of allergy. However, there is no apparent allergic trigger by history. The clinician might suspect an indoor allergen such as dog, dust mite, cockroach, or indoor molds such as *Penicillium*, *Aspergillus*, or *Curvularia* species. Occupational allergic rhinitis seems unlikely with work activities described but a component of nonallergic or irritant rhinitis would need to be considered with exposure to welding, metal dust, and organic hydrocarbons (Table 1.1). Bacterial sinusitis seems less likely with the mucous appearing clear.

Additional Assessment

Allergy skin testing by the percutaneous or prick methodology demonstrated 1–2+ wheal and flare response to dust mite and cat with a 3+ reaction to oak, bayberry, and cypress trees. Dog testing was negative. A nasal smear when not exposed to spring seasonal pollens showed a predominance of eosinophils. A topical nasal corticosteroid was prescribed, and the patient reported remarkable improvement in symptoms. Repeat examination demonstrated reduced turbinate edema, normal mucosal color, and no evidence of nasal polyps. Additional history revealed that the patient had two iguanas in a large dry aquarium in his bedroom. Cleaning the enclosures aggravated his symptoms.

What Is Your Diagnosis and Why?

MB has a chronic history of springtime allergic rhinitis with consistent allergy test results demonstrating tree allergy. His recent increase in symptoms suggested a perennial or nonseasonal allergic trigger but the history and skin tests did not initially demonstrate the apparent cause. This introduces the broad differential of rhinitis syndromes (Table 1.1); however, allergic rhinitis still seemed most likely because of the nasal pallor on examination, clear nasal discharge, nasal eosinophilia, atopic family history, and gratifying response to topical corticosteroid. History is paramount in identifying allergy, and the additional history of having iguanas in his home suggested allergic rhinitis due to "exotic animal allergy" (5). Elimination of the iguanas from the bedroom resulted in a gradual reduction of symptoms and the nasal corticosteroid therapy was modified to an intermittent regimen.

Discussion

Individuals with known or suspected allergic rhinitis may develop additional symptoms from new allergens if sufficient exposure results in sensitivity. Clinicians rely on their experience and knowledge of the common airborne allergens in their community to determine which allergens to use for testing. The increasingly complex indoor environment is modified by the personal choices of our patients. The attraction of having unusual animals as pets may result in symptoms from triggers that are generally not considered and from allergens difficult to test. These include a variety of birds such as macaws and cockatiels, Madagascar hissing cockroach (which may not

Table 1.3 Alternative allergen sources

Arthropods
  Mites
    Blomia tropicalis (dust mite)
    Euroglyphus maynei (dust mite)
    Lepidoglyphus destructor (storage mite)
  Insect
    Flea
    Madagascar hissing cockroach
Birds
  Cockatiel
  Conure
  Finch
  Macaw
  Parakeet
  Parrot
  Pigeon
Other mammals
  Ferret
  Pig
  Predatory cats
  Rabbit
  Raccoon
  Sugar glider
  Primates
    Lemur
    Howler monkey
    Macaque
    Spider monkey
    Squirrel monkey
    Tamarin
Reptiles
  Iguana
  Rodents
    Gerbil
    Guinea pig
    Hamster
    Mouse
    Rat

cross-react with other cockroach allergens), an assortment of rodents, sugar gliders, rabbits, ferrets, predatory cats, pigs, iguanas, and primates (Table 1.3) (5). Although reptiles are generally not considered allergenic, the iguana sheds skin in small,respirable flakes rather than contiguous pieces as with snakes. The resulting iguana epidermal debris contains proteins that may be inhaled, may be recognized by human IgE, and may resultin upper respiratory symptoms. In addition, skin rashes from salivary contact and asthma have been described from iguanas being in homes. Therefore, the clinician must take a thorough history of domestic, occupational, and recreational allergen exposure before accepting a diagnosis of nonallergic rhinitis or considering systemic diseases that are associated with rhinitis. Some of the more unusual allergens do not have testing reagents available, but university resource centers may be able to prepare a skin test solution or perform an in vitro assay for suspected allergens. Clinicians must be wary not to discount the possibility of allergic rhinitis until all possible allergens have been explored. This is a challenge when the testing reagents are not available and some allergen sources, such as alternative dust mite species, are not visible. The allergist sometimes must be a detective.

Nonallergic rhinitis is usually the diagnosis if allergy is not confirmed (6). Nasal eosinophilia is a strong indicator of allergy, although nasal polyps, hyperplastic rhinosinusitis, fungal hypersensitivity sinusitis, nonallergic rhinitis with eosinophilia (NARES), and aspirin-exacerbated respiratory disease are usually associated with nasal eosinophilia as well. Response to symptomatic treatment is generally more definitive with allergy, but there are many rhinitis syndromes that respond to topical or oral treatments (1). The clinician should be wary of too quickly ascribing the label of nonallergic rhinitis until all allergen triggers are considered. There is also evidence that up to 50% of patients with allergic rhinitis have some nonallergic features (1).

Conclusions

Rhinitis is a common condition with multiple etiologies, usually allergic or nonallergic rhinitis. The diagnosis and treatment is often straightforward but clinicians must maintain vigilance to consider alternative causes when rhinitis presents with unusual features or does not respond to appropriate therapy. The possibilities of unusual allergens and rhinitis associated with systemic diseases should always be in the differential diagnosis of nasal symptoms.

Questions

1. The pathology of sarcoidosis is characterized by:

   (a) Granulomas localized in the walls of blood vessels
   (b) Necrotizing granulomas in the mucosa

(c) CD4+ T cell mucosal inflammation

(d) Thickening of the mucosal subbasement membrane

Answer: (c)

The airway inflammation associated with sarcoidosis is characterized by pre-dominance of CD4+ T lymphocytes. The lymphocyte balance in the peripheral blood typically has a decrease in the CD4+ T lymphocytes, suggesting that the CD4+ lymphocytes have migrated into the tissue leaving a relative increase in the CD8+ lymphocytes. The tissue inflammation of sarcoidosis is characterized by noncaseating, nonnecrotizing granulomas that are not selectively in the blood vessels.

2. The presence of which of the following skin manifestations has the strongest relationship with sarcoidosis affecting the nasal airway?

   (a) Lupus profundus
   (b) Lupus pernio
   (c) Discoid lupus
   (d) Erythema nodosum

Answer: (b)

The facial rash presenting with waxy lesions around the nasal vestibule is described as lupus pernio but has no relationship with SLE. Discoid lupus and lupus profondus are rashes associated with cutaneous or systemic SLE. Erythema nodosum is typical of acute sarcoidosis (Lofgren's syndrome), which generally occurs in women and resolves after the initial exacerbation.

3. The rhinitis symptom that is the most specific for allergic rhinitis is:

   (a) Congestion
   (b) Sneezing paroxysms
   (c) Rhinorrhea
   (d) Postnasal drip

Answer: (b)

All of the symptoms listed are reported by patients with rhinitis. Congestion is the most common reason for patients to seek medical care but congestion is more universal among the rhinitis syndromes and is therefore less specific for allergic rhinitis. Sneezing paroxysms (four or more in succession) and severe itching are the most typical symptoms of allergic rhinitis. These symptoms are more typical of seasonal or acute allergic rhinitis than perennial or persistent allergic rhinitis.

4. Which of the following causes of nasal symptoms is associated with eosinophils in the nasal secretions?

   (a) Sjögren's syndrome
   (b) Fungal hypersensitivity sinusitis
   (c) Vasomotor rhinitis
   (d) Cystic fibrosis

Answer: (b)
Nasal eosinophilia is associated with nasal polyps other than those in cystic fibrosis, allergic rhinitis, NARES, aspirin-exacerbated respiratory disease, and fungal hypersensitivity sinusitis. Typically subjects with Sjögren's syndrome or cystic fibrosis would show neutrophils in the nasal mucous. Vasomotor rhinitis secretions are usually acellular.

5. What is the most common nasal tumor?

   (a) Inverted papilloma
   (b) Squamous cell carcinoma
   (c) Adenocarcinoma
   (d) Angiofibroma

Answer: (b)
Inverted papillomas are locally invasive and may appear as a nasal polyp. Squamous cell carcinomas are associated with cigarette smokers and are the most common malignancy in the nasal airway. Angiofibromas are highly vascular tumors that generally occur in adolescent males. Adenocarcinomas are relatively uncommon and usually arise from minor salivary gland tissue.

References

1. Wallace DV, Dykewicz MS, Bernstein DI et al. The diagnosis and management of rhinitis: an updated practice parameter. J Allergy Clin Immunol 2008;**122**:S1–S84.
2. Bousquet J, Van Cauweberge P, Khaltaev N. Allergic rhinitis and its impact on asthma. J Allergy Clin Immunol 2001;**108**:S147–S334.
3. Baughman RP, Lower EE, du Bois RM. Sarcoidosis. Lancet 2003;**361**:1111–1116.
4. Agostini C, Adami F, Semenzato G. New pathogenic insights into sarcoid granulomas. Curr Opin Rheumatol 2000;**12**:71–78.
5. Phillips JF, Lockey RF. Exotic pet allergy. J Allergy Clin Immunol 2009;**123**(2):513–515.
6. Salib RJ, Harries PG, Nair SB, Howarth PH. Mechanisms and mediators of nasal symptoms in non-allergic rhinitis. Clin Exp Allergy 2008;**38**(3):393–404.

Chapter 2
Chronic Rhinosinusitis

Philip Wexler and Helen Hollingsworth

Abstract Rhinosinusitis describes a group of inflammatory conditions of the nasal mucosa and paranasal sinuses that affect 31 million people in the USA each year. When the term chronic rhinosinusitis (CRS) is used, it implies that the condition has persisted for more than 12 weeks despite medical therapy. The diagnosis of CRS requires the presence of at least two of the following over a 12-week period: anterior and posterior mucopurulent drainage; nasal obstruction; facial pain, pressure, and/ or fullness; and a decreased sense of smell; nasal polyposis may or may not be present. Allergic rhinitis and asthma may be present concurrently in patients with CRS. Tobacco smoke and environmental irritants are known to exacerbate symptoms. Typically, CRS does not cause altered vision, proptosis, periorbital edema, ophthalmoplegia, focal neurologic signs, severe headache, fever, meningeal signs, or signs of systemic illness or vasculitis. The presence of these warning signs should prompt an immediate work-up for an alternative diagnosis. Treatment follows a multipronged approach including avoidance of allergens and irritants, saline lavage, chronic intranasal glucocorticoids, anti-inflammatory treatment with systemic glucocorticoids if symptoms are severe, and consideration of an initial empiric course of antibiotics.

Keywords Chronic rhinosinusitis • Allergic rhinitis • Acute rhinosinusitis • Nasal polyposis • Allergic fungal rhinosinusitis • Aspirin-exacerbated respiratory disease • Churg Strauss syndrome • Wegener's granulomatosis

Case 1

A 58-year-old woman with a past medical history of asthma, atopic dermatitis, and hypertension presents with complaints of year-round nasal congestion, postnasal drip, nasal discharge, and decreased sense of smell. These symptoms have bothered

P. Wexler and H. Hollingsworth (✉)
Department of Pulmonary, Critical Care, Allergy and Immunology,
Boston University Medical Center, Boston, MA, USA
e-mail: hholling@bu.edu

M. Mahmoudi (ed.), *Challenging Cases in Allergy and Immunology,*
DOI: 10.1007/978-1-60327-443-2_2,
© Humana Press, a part of Springer Science+Business Media, LLC 2009

her for about 5 years, but have worsened in the past 2 years. She has tried intranasal glucocorticoid spray and oral nonsedating antihistamines without improvement. A recent course of prednisone improved her nasal obstruction and drainage but not her sense of smell. Nasal congestion is severe enough to interrupt her sleep. She denies headaches, fevers, chills, night sweats, or weight loss.

She feels that her asthma is well controlled and that she rarely needs to use albuterol. She does not report any rhinorrhea, increased nasal congestion, wheezing, or shortness of breath after ingestion of aspirin or NSAIDs.

She has no pets at home but does have mite-proof mattress and pillow covers. She works in a clean office environment and has not noted any variation in her symptoms whether she is at work or at home.

Her medications include triamterene/hydrochlorothiazide, topical triamcinolone ointment, hydroxyzine 25 mg at bedtime, montelukast 10 mg daily, fluticasone/salmeterol 250/50, one puff twice a day, and albuterol as needed.

Physical examination reveals a decreased light reflex on the right tympanic membrane, bilaterally diminished nasal airflow, mucosal edema over the turbinates, and gelatinous, gray intranasal tissue, consistent with nasal polyps. The conjunctiva is not injected. Lungs are clear. Skin exam shows moderate xerosis and keratosis pilaris.

Spirometry is normal.

With the Presented Data What Is Your Working Diagnosis?

The history of allergic dermatitis and asthma would be consistent with atopy; however, it seems unlikely that her symptoms are entirely explained by allergic rhinitis because her nasal symptoms developed after age 50. The nasal exam and associated anosmia make chronic rhinosinusitis (CRS) and nasal polyposis more likely. The description of her workplace and lack of temporal association with her symptoms make occupational rhinitis less likely.

Differential Diagnosis

The differential diagnosis of perennial rhinitis symptoms includes perennial allergic rhinitis, CRS with or without nasal polyposis, nonallergic rhinitis including vasomotor rhinitis (irritant triggered, cold air, and exercise), gustatory rhinitis, infectious rhinitis, NARES (nonallergic rhinitis with eosinophilia syndrome), drug-induced including rhinitis medicamentosa (e.g., oral contraceptives, antihypertensives), aspirin/nonsteroidal anti-inflammatory drugs [i.e., aspirin-exacerbated respiratory disease (AERD)], or atrophic rhinitis.

Work-Up

The presence of perennial nasal symptoms is an indication for allergy skin testing, which in this case shows positive reactions to cat and dog dander on prick testing and positive intradermal tests to ragweed, the mold hormodendrum, and both dust mites (*Dermatophagoides farinae* and *Dermatophagoides pteronyssinus*). The skin test to aspergillus is negative. The total IgE is 283 IU/mL (normal 10–179 IU/mL).

Sinus CT scan is obtained because of the severity of her nasal symptoms and lack of response to empiric medications for allergic rhinitis. On the CT scan, all of the paranasal sinuses are either opacified or have moderate mucosal thickening (Fig. 2.1a–c). The left maxillary sinus contains hyperdense material, and a slight expansile change is noted in the ethmoid sinuses. Polypoid lesions are noted around the turbinates leading to almost complete obstruction of the nasal cavities.

The hyperdense or flocculent material in the maxillary sinus and the suggestion of expansion within the ethmoid sinus raise the possibility of allergic fungal sinusitis; however, the negative aspergillus skin test provides evidence against allergic aspergillus sinusitis. Serum total IgE and aspergillus-specific IgE and IgG are generally elevated in allergic aspergillus sinusitis, but not to the degree of allergic bronchopulmonary aspergillosis.

What Is Your Diagnosis and Why?

The diagnosis is CRS with nasal polyposis. This is based on the history, physical examination, sinus CT scan, and diagnostic tests.

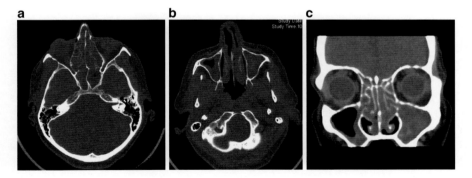

Fig. 2.1 (**a–c**) Sinus CT images show almost complete opacification of the left maxillary, ethmoid, and sphenoid sinuses; a slight expansile change is noted in the ethmoid sinuses (**a**); polypoid lesions along and around the turbinates with moderate mucosal thickening in the right maxillary sinus and hyperdense material in the left maxillary sinus (**b**); near complete filling of the nasal passages and ostiomeatal complexes (**c**)

Management

Evaluation by otolaryngology leads to a recommendation for functional endoscopic sinus surgery (FESS) for removal of nasal polyps, sinus drainage, and culture of the sinus contents for fungus. At the time of surgery, multiple polyps are noted in the nasal cavities, and polypoid debris was noted in the ethmoid sinus and both maxillary sinuses. Fungal culture is negative. After surgery, the patient notes a dramatic improvement in nasal airflow and a partial return of her sense of smell. She remains on intranasal glucocorticoids in addition to her usual asthma medications.

Discussion

Rhinosinusitis describes a grouping of inflammatory conditions of the nasal mucosa and paranasal sinuses that affect 31 million people in the USA each year (1, 2). The term CRS implies that the condition has persisted for more than 12 weeks despite medical therapy. The etiology of acute rhinosinusitis is usually infectious, while CRS may result from a wide array of etiologies. CRS has been noted to have significant effects on quality of life. Allergic rhinitis and asthma are frequent concurrent diagnoses in patients with CRS. Tobacco smoke and environmental irritants are known to exacerbate symptoms.

The diagnosis of CRS requires the presence of at least two of the following over a 12-week period: anterior and posterior mucopurulent drainage; nasal obstruction; facial pain, pressure, and/or fullness; and a decreased sense of smell (1). In addition to a complete history and physical examination, documentation of nasal airway inflammation in the decongested nose, including presence or absence of discolored mucus, or edema of the middle meatus or ethmoid sinuses, and inspection for nasal polyps is a requirement for diagnosis and further classification. Typically, CRS does not cause double or reduced vision, proptosis, periorbital edema, ophthalmoplegia, focal neurologic signs, severe headache, fever, other signs of vasculitis, meningeal signs, or signs of systemic illness. The presence of these warning signs should prompt an immediate work-up for an alternative diagnosis.

There are three major subtypes of CRS including allergic fungal rhinosinusitis (AFRS), CRS with nasal polyposis, and CRS without nasal polyposis. CRS without nasal polyposis is more prevalent than CRS with nasal polyposis and AFRS combined. The three subtypes may be distinguished from each other based on the history and physical exam. A sinus CT, while not necessary to distinguish these three subtypes, may help confirm the diagnosis and assist in defining the severity of the disease (e.g., bony erosions in AFRS). Once the diagnosis of CRS has been made, certain potential contributing conditions should be considered, including allergic rhinitis, primary ciliary dyskinesia, cystic fibrosis (particularly in younger patients with nasal polyposis), and immunodeficiency. In addition, a small number of systemic illnesses can cause rhinosinusitis, such as sarcoidosis, Churg Strauss vasculitis, and Wegener's granulomatosis; these should be evaluated in patients with symptoms suggesting systemic illness.

CRS without nasal polyposis is the most common type of CRS. It is defined as CRS (the presence of 12 weeks of 2 of the 4 cardinal symptoms named earlier, despite medical therapy) that lacks nasal polyps and allergic mucin. A sinus CT cannot definitively confirm the presence or absence of nasal polyps. However, the CT may help in confirming the inflammatory nature of this condition in the setting of a nonrevealing history and physical (1). Histologically, there are basement membrane thickening, goblet cell hyperplasia, limited submucosal edema, prominent fibrosis, and mononuclear cellular infiltration (1). The inflammation in CRS without nasal polyps is typically neutrophilic and less eosinophilic. Cytokines that are elevated in the nasal mucosa include IL-1, IL-6, IL-8, TNF-α, GM-CSF, ICAM-1, and myeloperoxidase (1).

CRS with nasal polyposis is defined by the presence of bilateral nasal polyps on the middle meatus on direct visualization or endoscopy, in the past or at present (1). Nasal polyps appear yellow-gray to white and are pearlescent with gelatinous inflammatory material. They are relatively avascular structures and are distinguished from the pink swollen nasal turbinates by their color and by the fact that they are not tender to touch. Histologically, there is frequent epithelial damage, basement membrane thickening, and edematous and fibrotic stromal tissue (1). Nasal polyps demonstrate increased eosinophils with similar histology to the inflamed sino-nasal mucosa (3). In contrast to CRS without nasal polyps, the inflammation of CRS with nasal polyps is characterized by elevation in the mediators IL-5 and eotaxin (1). Unilateral polyps should raise suspicion of a sinonasal tumor and require an imaging study (1).

Controversy continues in the medical literature as to the utility of subclassification of CRS with or without nasal polyposis (1). Although similar in histology, they are not identical pathophysiologic processes. The immunologic basis of the conditions also appears discordant. Subjects who have CRS with nasal polyposis are more likely to have peripheral blood eosinophilia, asthma, and aspirin sensitivity.

AFRS is a type of CRS in which the patient has "allergic mucin," a thick, purulent, inspissated mucus that contains fungal hyphae with degranulating eosinophils. The diagnosis is usually confirmed on endoscopy where the allergic mucin is documented. AFRS is a result of fungal colonization, not invasive fungal disease. Untreated AFRS may lead to sinus opacification and local bony demineralization/erosion of the sinus walls. Fungal-specific IgE (skin or blood testing) and a mucosal biopsy demonstrating absence of invasive fungal disease are requirements for the diagnosis of AFRS (1).

CRS with or without nasal polyposis typically does not respond completely to therapy and often needs to be treated for protracted periods of time (4). The goals of treatment are to improve quality of life by alleviating symptoms and to prevent disease progression. Treatment follows a multipronged approach including avoidance of allergens and irritants, saline lavage, chronic intranasal glucocorticoids, initial anti-inflammatory treatment with systemic glucocorticoids if symptoms are severe, and consideration of an initial empiric course of antibiotics. Saline washes are useful in all forms of CRS and should be performed daily prior to the use of other topical medical therapies. Saline washes remove draining particulate matter and secretions and may remove allergens or irritants from the nasal and sinus passages. Washes can be performed routinely, one or more times per day.

Intranasal glucocorticoids act by suppressing inflammation and are well tolerated and are considered the mainstay of maintenance therapy for CRS with or without nasal polyposis (4, 5). In general, the metered dose aqueous sprays are sufficient when used in the upper end of the dose range. Some authors recommend the use of intranasal instillation of liquid budesonide once or twice a day, but controlled trials are lacking (5). In cases of severe, refractory inflammation and edema, and nasal obstruction, a brief course of systemic glucocorticoids (5–14 days) may be considered (4).

In acute rhinosinusitis, antimicrobials are a mainstay of therapy. In contrast, their use in CRS is less well-defined; some authors recommend an empiric initial 3–4-week course of antibiotics timed with a brief course of systemic glucocorticoids in patients with CRS without nasal polyps (5). In CRS with or without nasal polyps, patients may have disease flares related to bacterial superinfection and need treatment for acute rhinosinusitis. A protracted course of macrolides may serve as an anti-inflammatory therapy in addition to intranasal glucocorticoids, but this has not been well studied (4). Scientific data to support antifungal therapy, either topical or systemic, for CRS are lacking.

The antileukotriene agent, montelukast, has been shown to be effective in treating some patients with CRS with nasal polyposis, aspirin sensitivity, and asthma (AERD) (6). In addition, aspirin desensitization has been reported to markedly improve symptoms and reduce polyp regrowth in AERD patients. Aspirin desensitization needs to be performed in specialized centers with experienced personnel. The required dose of aspirin is 325–650 mg twice a day, which may cause significant gastrointestinal side effects, thus limiting treatment.

In CRS with nasal polyposis, FESS is often needed to debulk severe polyposis and restore sinus ventilation and drainage. General indications include polyp tissue completely obstructing nares, recurrent sinus infections, evidence of expansion in sinuses, and concern about AFRS. Medical therapy is necessary after polypectomy, as the polyps tend to reaccumulate over time. AFRS requires a surgical procedure to diagnose allergic mucin, remove inspissated mucus, and improve sinus ventilation and drainage. Postoperatively, subjects with AFRS should be treated with oral and intranasal glucocorticoids for a protracted period of time; when oral glucocorticoids are tapered and stopped, intranasal glucocorticoids are continued (7).

Case 2

A 17-year-old male presents with symptoms of persistent upper respiratory tract infection for 3 months. His symptoms include daily fevers up to 102°F, headache, fatigue, loss of appetite, a 15-lb weight loss, dry cough, rhinorrhea, nasal obstruction, "severe" pain at the bridge of his nose, epistaxis, and crusting of his nasal passages. He has been unsuccessfully treated with multiple courses of antibiotics, antihistamines, nasal lavages, and other over-the-counter nasal preparations. He did have significant improvement while taking a solumedrol dose pack. His symptoms returned upon completion of the glucocorticoids.

He has no significant past medical history. He is in his last year of high school and works part time in a restaurant. He denies tobacco, alcohol, or drug use. He is not sexually active. He has no known drug allergies. He has not had hemoptysis, dyspnea, rash, joint pains, ocular or auditory problems, or central or peripheral nervous system problems.

On exam, he is a well-developed young male with normal vital signs including pulse oximetry. He has a saddle-nose deformity, but no rash. His ocular exam is normal. His external ears, canals, and tympanic membranes are normal. His nasal passages have significant crusting, hyperemia, and significant tenderness over the bridge of his nose, frontal and maxillary sinuses. He has good dentition, no tongue lesions, and no pharyngeal exudates or swelling. Enlarged cervical lymph nodes are noted. His cardiopulmonary and abdominal exams are normal. There is no evidence of arthritis.

With the Presented Data What Is Your Working Diagnosis?

His chronic, progressive, severe symptoms, including headache and "severe facial pain," his saddle nose deformity, weight loss, and daily fevers are concerning for rhinitis associated with inflammatory-immunologic disorders.

Differential Diagnosis

Rhinosinusitis associated with inflammatory-immunologic disorders may be due to granulomatous infections (bacterial, mycobacterial, and fungal), Wegener's granulomatosis, sarcoidosis, midline granuloma, Churg-Strauss, relapsing polychondritis, and amyloidosis.

Work-Up

Blood work reveals a normal creatinine and a positive antineutrophil cytoplasmic antibody (ANCA) test by immunofluorescence with a cytoplasmic (C) pattern. His urinalysis is normal and without hematuria. A CT scan of his sinuses demonstrates significant nasal mucosal swelling and sinus opacification, predominantly in his maxillary sinuses, with the left one worse than the right (Fig. 2.2a). Chest X-ray demonstrates a large right upper lobe cavitary mass, which is confirmed by chest CT (Fig. 2.2b). A nasal biopsy demonstrates granulomatous inflammation. Fiberoptic

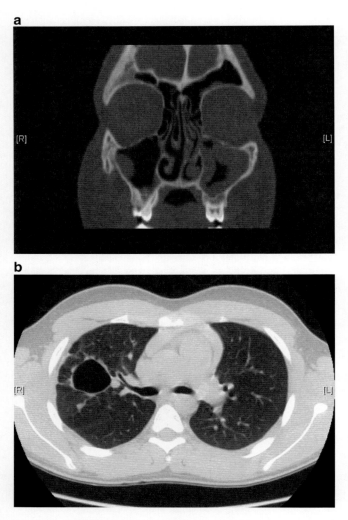

Fig. 2.2 (**a**) Sinus CT coronal image from case 2 shows scattered nodular mucosal thickening in both maxillary sinuses (left greater than right) and the left frontal sinus. A right concha bullosa and septal deviation to the left are also noted; (**b**) Chest CT image from case 2 shows right upper lobe cavitary lesion and three smaller nodular lesions, one of which is adjacent and medial to the cavity

bronchoscopy with bronchoalveolar lavage in the right upper lobe reveals no blood; bacterial, mycobacterial, and fungal cultures are negative.

What Is Your Diagnosis and Why?

The diagnosis is limited to Wegener's granulomatosis, based on his presentation, biopsy results, and positive c-ANCA.

Management

The patient responds to high-dose systemic glucocorticoids, methotrexate, and sulfamethoxazole-trimethoprim 400/80 mg by mouth once daily. His fevers resolve; nasal airflow improves; the right upper lobe cavity closes and the pulmonary nodules shrink. Prednisone is slowly tapered and he remains asymptomatic on methotrexate therapy for the next 2 years.

Discussion

There are numerous warning signs of patients with CRS that alert the practitioner that symptoms of CRS need further evaluation. These include double or reduced vision, proptosis, periorbital edema, ophthalmoplegia, focal neurologic signs, severe headache, fever, meningeal signs, and signs of systemic illness or vasculitis. The presence of these signs indicates that an alternative diagnosis should be considered and evaluated promptly.

Wegener's granulomatosis (WG) is a multifocal inflammatory illness that affects the upper and lower airway and kidneys preferentially (8). The diagnosis of WG requires the presence of two of the following four criteria (9):

1. Nasal or oral inflammation: development of painful or painless oral ulcers or purulent or bloody nasal discharge
2. Abnormal chest radiograph: chest radiograph showing the presence of nodules, fixed infiltrates, or cavities
3. Urinary sediment: microhematuria (>5 red blood cells per high-power field) or red cell casts in urine sediment
4. Granulomatous inflammation on biopsy: histologic changes showing granulomatous inflammation within the wall of an artery or in the perivascular or extravascular area (artery or arteriole)

There have been numerous definitions of limited form of WG, but expert consensus defines the condition as a "manifestation of WG that poses no immediate threat to either the patient's life or the function of a vital organ" (10). The Wegener's Granulomatous Etanercept Trial defines limited WG as meeting the following four criteria (10):

1. The patient has no red blood cell casts in the urine.
2. If hematuria is present (but no red blood cell casts), the serum creatinine is 1.4 mg/dl, and there must be no evidence of a rise in creatinine 25% above the patient's baseline level.
3. Pulmonary involvement must be circumscribed, such that the room air PO_2 is 70 mmHg or the room air O_2 saturation by pulse oximetry is 92%. Pulmonary hemorrhage may be treated as a limited disease provided there is no evidence of progression of the process. In the absence of data on progression, pulmonary hemorrhage may be treated as a severe disease at the discretion of the physician.

4. No disease may exist within any other critical organ (e.g., the gastrointestinal tract, eyes, central nervous system) that, without the immediate institution of maximal therapy (i.e., pulse methylprednisolone and daily oral cyclophosphamide), threatens the function of that organ and/or the patient's life.

Limited WG is more prevalent in females, and the mean age at onset is younger for patients presenting with the limited versus the severe form (9).

Systemic anti-inflammatory medications are the treatment for WG. The limited form of WG can be treated with systemic glucocorticoids and methotrexate. Systemic WG is usually treated with cyclophosphamide and systemic glucocorticoids. Plasma exchange remains an option for treatment in many subsets of patients with WG. Referral to a WG specialist is crucial.

Questions

1. CRS is likely to be associated with which of the following?

    (a) Decreased sense of smell
    (b) A 6-week history of nasal congestion, mucopurulent nasal drainage, and facial pressure
    (c) Occupational exposure to latex
    (d) Serum antineutrophil cytoplasmic antibodies

2. A 16-year-old boy presents with nasal polyposis, chronic nasal congestion, and also purulent nasal discharge and sputum. The nasal polyps were first noted about a year ago. CT scan confirms pansinusitis. Which of the following statements about this patient is correct?

    (a) Both of his parents probably have similar disease manifestations.
    (b) Tissue removed from his sinuses is likely to have characteristics of allergic mucin.
    (c) A sweat chloride test should be obtained.
    (d) He should be started on IVIG once every 4 weeks.

3. A 40-year-old man presents with a 5-month history of nasal congestion, facial pressure, and anosmia. He has no occupational exposure to inhalant allergens. Allergy skin testing is negative. He denies any problems with ingestion of ibuprofen, which he takes several times a month. A nasal biopsy would be most likely to show which of the following patterns?

    (a) Eosinophilic inflammation
    (b) Elevated TNF-alpha, GM-CSF, and myeloperoxidase
    (c) Perivascular lymphocytes without granuloma formation
    (d) Elevation of IL-5 and eotaxin

4. A 35-year-old woman presents with nasal congestion not responding to intranasal glucocorticoid or oral antihistamine. She reports a nonproductive cough and

some shortness of breath on climbing stairs. She has lost about 15 lb in the past 2 months and notes awakening during the night, feeling feverish. Around her nose and on her back, she has nonpruritic pinkish brown papules about 2–3 mm in diameter. Which of the following statements is correct?

(a) A prolonged course of antibiotics is likely to be helpful.
(b) Skin biopsy of a back lesion is likely to show noncaseating granulomata.
(c) She should start an emollient regimen on her face, using ammonium lactate cream.
(d) A serum ANCA is likely to be positive in a cANCA pattern.

5. A 55-year-old attorney presents with nasal congestion and faint bulges along both sides of the nose. He has a past history of asthma that is becoming more difficult to control. His sense of smell and taste are poor. Nasal exam reveals edema and grayish cystic structures that are not tender. Which of the following statements is correct?

(a) A prolonged course of antibiotics is likely to cure his symptoms.
(b) Allergy skin testing to aspirin is most likely positive.
(c) A 3-day aspirin desensitization is often curative in this condition.
(d) After nasal polypectomy, ongoing therapy with intranasal glucocorticoids is needed.

6. A 55-year-old male smoker presents with nasal congestion. He reports being unable to breathe through his right nostril. He denies rhinitis. He reports pain on the right side of his face. On exam he has obstruction of the right nasal passage by what appears to be a nasal polyp. What should be done next?

(a) Sinus CT to evaluate the unilateral obstruction.
(b) Prescribe a course of intranasal glucocorticoids and nasal saline washes.
(c) Refer for FESS.
(d) Spirometry before and after bronchodilators and allergy skin testing to aspirin.

7. A 34-year-old woman presents with 6 weeks of nasal congestion, facial pressure, nasal crusting, and purulence. She has not improved with intranasal glucocorticoids and a 3-week course of antibiotics. Which of the following choices would be most appropriate?

(a) RAST testing to fruits and vegetables
(b) Sinus CT scan
(c) A trial of an antihistamine and an antileukotriene agent
(d) Aspirin desensitization

8. A patient with a thick, dark green and brown nasal discharge and persistent maxillary sinus opacification on sinus CT undergoes FESS; allergic mucin is sampled from the right middle meatus. A mucosal biopsy does not show invasive fungus. An aspergillus skin test is positive. What should occur next?

(a) Begin a 4-week course of intravenous amphotericin.
(b) Chest CT.

(c) Topical antifungal therapy to the nasal passages.

(d) Surgical drainage followed by systemic and topical glucocorticoids.

9. Which of the following statements about Wegener's granulomatosis is correct?

(a) An ANCA is always negative in limited Wegener's.

(b) Limited Wegener's is limited to the upper airways.

(c) In limited Wegener's a combination of systemic glucocorticoids and methotrexate will often control the disease.

(d) Asthma, nasal polyps, and eosinophilia are often seen in association with Wegener's.

10. In the evaluation of patients with CRS without polyps, which of the following would be most appropriate?

(a) Nasal saline lavage and an initial course of amoxicillin-clavulanate and prednisone

(b) Intranasal fungal cultures

(c) Amphotericin B nasal lavage

(d) Patch testing to a panel of fungal species

Correct answers: 1. (a), 2. (c), 3. (b), 4. (b), 5. (d), 6. (a), 7. (b), 8. (d), 9. (c), 10. (a)

References

1. Meltzer, EO, Hamilos, DL, Hadley, JA, et al. (2004) Rhinosinusitis: establishing definitions for clinical research and patient care. *J Allergy Clin Immunol* **114**, 155–212.
2. International Rhinosinusitis Advisory Board. (1997) Infectious rhinosinusitis in adults: classification, etiology and management. *Ear Nose Throat J* **76**, 5–22.
3. Hamilos, DL. (1996) Nasal polyps as immunoreactive tissue. *Allergy Asthma Proc* **17**, 293–6.
4. Scadding, GK, Durham, SR, Mirakian, R, et al. (2008) BSACI guidelines for the management of rhinosinusitis and nasal polyposis. *Clin Exp Allergy* **38**, 260–75.
5. Hamilos, DL. (2007) Approach to the evaluation and medical management of chronic rhinosinusitis. *Clin Allergy Immunol* **20**, 299–320.
6. Micheletto, C, Tognella, S, Visconti, M, Pomari, C, Trevisan, F, Dal Negro, RW. (2004) Montelukast 10 mg improves nasal function and nasal response to aspirin in ASA-sensitive asthmatics: a controlled study vs placebo. *Allergy* **59**, 289–94.
7. Schubert, MS, Goetz, DW. (1998) Evaluation and treatment of allergic fungal sinusitis. II. Treatment and follow-up. *J Allergy Clin Immunol* **102**, 395–402.
8. Stone, JH. (2003) Limited versus severe Wegener's granulomatosis: baseline data on patients in the Wegener's granulomatosis etanercept trial. *Arthritis Rheum* **48**, 2299–309.
9. Leavitt, RY, Fauci, AS, Bloch, DA, Michel, BA, Hunder, GG, Arend, WP, Calabrese, LH, Fries, JF, Lie, JT, Lightfoot, RW, Jr, et al. (1990) The American College of Rheumatology 1990 criteria for the classification of Wegener's granulomatosis. *Arthritis Rheum* **33**, 1101–7.
10. The WGET Research Group. (2002) Design of the Wegener's Granulomatosis Etanercept Trial (WGET). *Control Clin Trials* **23**, 450–68.

Chapter 3
Allergic Diseases of the Eye

Sara Axelrod and Leonard Bielory

Abstract The eye is a common target of inflammatory responses induced by local and systemic immunological hypersensitivity reactions. Inflammatory ocular conditions resulting from immune responses are highly prominent because of the eyes' considerable vascularization and the sensitivity of the vessels in the conjunctiva embedded in a transparent medium. Cases related to the presentation and management of the spectrum of allergic conjunctivitis are discussed later.

Keywords Atopic keratoconjunctivitis • Seasonal allergic conjunctivitis • Perennial allergic conjunctivitis • Vernal keratoconjunctivitis • Giant papillary conjunctivitis

Case 1

A 42-year-old male presents with a recent increase in ocular irritation, in both of his eyes. His past medical history is significant for mild persistent asthma, controlled with a short-acting beta-agonist and an inhaled corticosteroid. The patient presents with bilateral itching, burning, and tearing, with a stringy mucous discharge. He also notes photophobia and new onset of blurred vision. He states that "the itch" is extremely bothersome, and he chronically rubs his eyes. He also notes that his eyes are constantly "gritty" and is constantly blinking. Additionally the patient mentions that as a teenager he experienced similar symptoms that were milder but had resolved without intervention.

On physical examination, one notes thickening of both lids with redness, fissuring, and swelling. There is increased redness and swelling around both eyes and cheeks, with

S. Axelrod and L. Bielory (✉)
Division of Allergy, Immunology, and Rheumatology, Departments of Medicine, Pediatrics, and Ophthalmology, University of Medicine and Dentistry of New Jersey, New Jersey Medical School, Newark, NJ, USA
e-mail: Bielory@umdnj.edu

M. Mahmoudi (ed.), *Challenging Cases in Allergy and Immunology,*
DOI: 10.1007/978-1-60327-443-2_3,
© Humana Press, a part of Springer Science+Business Media, LLC 2009

increased creases below his eyes, and a peculiar absence of the lateral eyebrows. The conjunctiva is noted to have diffuse fine areas of pinhead shaped and sized lesions of the upper and lower tarsal conjunctiva, diffuse multiple blood vessels, increased thickness of the clear portions of the conjunctiva, and a white stringy semisolid thread of white mucus in the inferior forniceal region of the conjunctiva. You also note small areas of loss of epithelium from the cornea with the application of fluorescein with some white lines running across the inside portions of the lower palbebral portion of the conjunctiva. Nasal mucosa is pale and boggy with a stringy nasal discharge and mucus covering the posterior oropharynx. The lung exam is significant for mild bilateral end expiratory wheezes with a prolonged expiratory phase of respiration; no nasal flaring or accessory muscle use is appreciated. Skin examination is significant for thickened, pigmented skin in the antecubital fossa. Family history is significant for a 7-year-old child with eczema.

Data

The patient's blood revealed a white blood cell count of 7,800 cells per mm^3, with 1,260 eosinophils per mm^3. The total serum IgE was 836 international units per ml. Delayed skin tests to candida and tuberculin did not reveal reactivity at 24 and 72 h. Further skin prick testing revealed normal, immediate responses to histamine and saline with minimal reaction to grass, pollen, and mixed trees. A scraping of the upper tarsal conjunctiva stained with giemsa revealed multiple eosinophils. Spirometry reveals an obstructive pattern with reversal after β-agonist administration. One notices that he is constantly rubbing both of his eyes.

Imaging Studies

See Figs. 3.1 and 3.2.

With the Presented Data What Is Your Working Diagnosis?

The patient's physical examination consisting of a pale and boggy nasal mucosa (allergic rhinitis), lichenified and pruritic skin (atopic dermatitis), an elevated serum IgE, and a conjunctival scraping with eosinophils is consistent with an atopic (allergic) disorder.

What is your specific "*differential diagnosis*" of his ocular complaints?

(a) Keratoconjunctivitis sicca
(b) Infectious conjunctivitis

Fig. 3.1 Atopic keratoconjunctivitis is associated with
increased injection of the
conjunctiva and atopic dermatitis affecting the periorbital skin

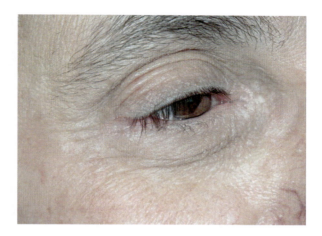

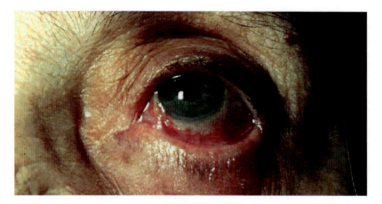

Fig. 3.2 Cicatricial changes (conjunctival fibrosis or scarring) result from chronic inflammation
seen in chronic forms of AKC. This may lead to alterations in conjunctival architecture, and symblepharon (adhesion) formation. As the patient looks up, there is loss of the "cul de sac." Periorbital
erythema is also evident

    (c) Seasonal allergic conjunctivitis (SAC)
    (d) Atopic keratoconjunctivitis (AKC)
    (e) Blepharitis
    (f) Tear dysfunction syndrome

What Is Your Diagnosis and Why?

This scenario describes a mixed diagnosis. This patient exhibits the appropriate
temporal pattern as well as physical findings consistent with AKC, including periorbital

eczema, photophobia, blurred vision, along with punctate keratitis and hyperemia. The symptoms are not associated with seasonal variation, which makes SAC less likely. He experiences a *gritty* sensation with an increase in blinking indicative of a tear film dysfunction; however, there is no mention of associated autoimmune disorders ruling out keratoconjunctivitis sicca. This yields the diagnosis of AKC with chronic blepharitis and tear film dysfunction.

Discussion

AKC is a severe form of allergic conjunctivitis, due to the chronic nature, potential corneal involvement, and impairment in vision. It is both a cell-mediated IgE-mast cell and lymphocytic cell-mediated immune reaction, with additional genetic and environmental factors. AKC occurs most frequently in adults with current or past atopic dermatitis, as well as other signs of atopy. It presents as a chronic inflammatory process, with possible sight-threatening consequences from corneal involvement. The symptoms often begin from the late teens to the early twenties. They may persist until the fourth or fifth decades of life. This disease affects males more commonly than females. AKC is the most severe allergic disorder involving the ocular surface, with the capacity to cause blindness. Most patients have a family history of atopy, including asthma, atopic dermatitis, or allergic rhinoconjunctivitis (1). Patients often suffer from atopic disorders, with more than 95% presenting with atopic dermatitis and 87% with a history of asthma (2). Clinically, patients present with bilateral itching, burning, tearing, and a stringy mucous discharge, with photophobia and blurred vision. Patients suffer keratinization of the lids, often with induration, fissuring, and swelling due to the atopic dermatitis (Fig. 3.1). Chronic blepharitis and staphylococcal infections may complicate the picture (1–3). The eczema involves the periorbital skin and cheeks, with erythema and edema resulting in single or double infraorbital creases known as Dennie-Morgan lines. Absence or thinning of the lateral eyebrow (de Hertoghe's sign) may occur in older patients, due to chronic eye rubbing (1, 2, 4). The conjunctiva present with bilateral hyperemia and injection affecting the inferior forniceal and palpebral conjunctiva. In severe forms, cicatricial conjunctivitis with subepithelial fibrosis and symblepharon can occur with shortening of the fornix, as a result of scarring (1, 2) (Fig. 3.2). The papillary hypertrophy may involve the limbus. Corneal scarring and neovascularization is common, with early signs including punctate keratitis and later, plaque formation with ulcerations. Other complications include cataracts and primary corneal ectasias such as keratoconus or retinal detachment, which may result from repeated eye rubbing and degeneration of the vitreous (1). Severe and permanent visual impairment can result. Some patients experience seasonal exacerbations, mainly in the winter or summer or following exposure to dust or foods (1, 2). Histologically, there are increased numbers of both naïve-Th (CD4/45RA+) and memory-Th (CD4/29+) type cells in the blood and tear samples of patients with AKC (2). Additionally, there are increased levels of IL-2, IL-3, IL-4, and IL-5 in AKC compared with normal tissue reflecting a reactive immune state associated with allergy. IL-4 levels correlate with the severity of atopic disease, and IL-5 levels correlate with the severity of the ocular disease (5).

Blepharitis is inflammation of the eyelid margins, which often causes conjunctivitis. *S. aureus* frequently colonizes patients with atopic dermatitis and also colonizes the eyelids of patients with AKC. The inflammatory trigger may be through toll-like receptors (6). Patients report persistent burning, itching, tearing, and a dry eye sensation. The symptoms worsen in the mornings. A crusting may develop in these patients causing the eyes to be stuck together in the mornings, which is misleading to some physicians as this suggests an infectious process. However, the discharge seen in infectious processes is more often green or yellow due to the neutrophilic myeloperoxidase involvement. Physical findings include dilated blood vessels, erythema, scales, collarettes of exudative material around the eyelash bases, and foamy exudates in the tear film. Management includes improving eyelid hygiene, as well as steroid ointments to the lid margin, to loosen the scale and exudates.

Tear film dysfunction is a form of the dry eye syndrome. Patients often present with a mildly injected eye, with excessive mucous production. Symptoms include a gritty, sandy feeling in the eyes, as well as itching and burning. The symptoms worsen throughout the day, as the limited portion of the aqueous tear film evaporates (6). Exacerbations occur in the winter as humidity is decreased. The use of medications with anticholinergic effects creates a decrease in lacrimation, which is a cause of the dry eye syndrome. Topical cyclosporine (Restasis®) is the only FDA approved treatment as of 2008.

Keratoconjunctivitis sicca is a dry eye syndrome resulting from inadequate tear production of the lacrimal gland, which is associated with autoimmune disorders such as rheumatoid arthritis, systemic lupus erythematosus, or Sjögren's syndrome. Patients may present with itching or burning with foreign body sensation. The conjunctiva is hyperemic with mucus strands. Diagnosis is made clinically or with the use of a Schirmer test, in which a strip of filter paper is placed at the edge of the eyelid to measure the rate of tear production over the course of 5 min. Management is often with artificial tears, avoiding dry environments, and use of humidifiers. In the aforementioned case, the patient has a component of a dry eye syndrome; however, he does not have any evidence of an associated autoimmune disorder.

Management and treatment of the aforementioned case includes alleviating symptoms and maintaining visual acuity. History is important to identify offending allergen, and cold compresses, artificial tears, and adequate lid hygiene may be useful. Systemic antihistamines provide relief; however, they may further increase dryness of the ocular surface. Additionally, mast cell stabilizers and nonsteroidal anti-inflammatory drugs (NSAIDs) may reduce inflammation. Topical steroids are effective in relieving symptoms when other therapeutic options have failed; however, extreme caution must be employed as they can result in various serious ocular complications such as infection, cataracts, as well as raised intraocular pressure. In severe cases where vision has been compromised from scarring, vascularization, or perforation of the cornea, transplantation may be considered; however, systemic immunosuppression may be needed to prevent failure and graft rejection (1).

Case 2

A 21-year-old woman presents with progressive worsening itch of both eyes, over the past 5 years. The itching occurs with increased tearing, some redness, burning, and a sensation of fullness in the eyelids. In addition, she experiences sensitivity to light when the intensity of her itch is most extreme. She lives and works in Michigan. Initially, the itch began in early May and ended in mid-June, and then again from late August through early October. Over the past 2 years, she notes the itching sensation to become year-round, with exacerbations in the spring and fall. She obtains some relief from over-the-counter diphenhydramine (25-mg tablets). However, because of drowsiness and some increased grittiness of her eyes late in the day, she is unable to take the diphenhydramine during the workweek. She uses no ocular or systemic medication and wears daily disposable contact lenses for the past 5 years. She has not suffered from eczema or other atopic skin disorders. The patient is currently taking oral contraceptive pills. Her mother and sister suffer from rhinitis during the spring and fall.

On examination, she is a well-developed, well-nourished, young woman, occasionally rubbing her eyes. She has darkened skin about the eyelids, of both eyes. She has conjunctival redness and swelling, with palpebral edema, of both eyes. A ropey discharge is evident. Nasal examination reveals pale and boggy mucosa, with clear mucus covering the posterior oropharynx. Lung examination reveals good air entry and is clear to auscultation and percussion bilaterally. No cutaneous eruptions, subcutaneous nodules, or lesions are observed. No adenopathy is noted.

Data

Spirometry is normal. Skin prick testing reveals significant positive reactions to the positive control, trees, weeds, dust, and mold, with normal reaction to saline. Total serum IgE is 630 international units per ml. Conjunctival scraping and a smear of the ropey discharge reveal eosinophils.

Imaging Studies

See Fig. 3.3.

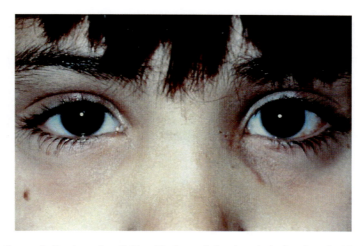

Fig. 3.3 Seasonal allergic conjunctivitis with chemosis (conjunctival edema), and with edematous eyelids, and the *allergic shiner*, darkening of the periorbital region

With the Presented Data What Is Your Working Diagnosis?

The temporal nature and characteristics of the patient's symptoms and the cutaneous reactivities to various aeroallergens (pollens) are consistent with an allergic process.

What is your specific *differential diagnosis* of her ocular complaints?

(a) SAC
(b) Perennial allergic conjunctivitis (PAC)
(c) Infectious conjunctivitis
(d) AKC
(e) Vernal keratoconjunctivitis (VKC)

What Is Your Diagnosis and Why?

This patient's symptoms initially occurred in the spring and fall seasons; however, more recently they have occurred year-round. This temporal pattern with her family history of atopy, as well as the results of her skin prick testing (positive results to both indoor and outdoor allergens), yields a diagnosis of SAC mixed with PAC. Infectious conjunctivitis is more likely to have a yellow-green discharge. VKC usually affects children, and the itch is severe. AKC presents as a chronic inflammatory process, with sight-threatening consequences from corneal involvement.

Discussion

The spectrum of conjunctivitis involves a vast range of clinical and immunological mechanisms including nonspecific, non-IgE/neutrophilic to specific, IgE-mediated/lymphocytic. Several disorders encompass both mechanisms (6). The acute IgE-mediated disorders include SAC and PAC; mixed lymphocyte and eosinophil-mediated disorders include VKC and AKC while lymphocyte-mediated disorders include giant papillary conjunctivitis (GPC). Neutrophil-mediated conjunctivitis is most commonly associated with bacterial infection (6).

Allergic conjunctivitis is a mast cell-mediated hypersensitivity reaction. It can present as an acute or chronic illness. It involves a benign inflammation of the conjunctiva, sparing the cornea. Symptoms include tearing, itching, and burning. Vasodilatation, which appears superficial and pink, accompanies itch. Chemosis, swelling of the conjunctiva, may occur.

In PAC, dust mites, animal dander, and feathers are the most common airborne allergens implicated, while in SAC it is grass pollen. Patients who have PAC and SAC are similar in age and sex, and both patient groups have the same prevalence of associated symptoms of asthma or eczema. PAC is similar to SAC in age, range, and length of history, although SAC is subjectively more severe. When patients who had PAC were compared with patients who had SAC, a history to exposure to house dust was more common (42% vs. 0%), as was the association of perennial rhinitis (75% vs. 12%) (7). Recent studies have estimated the prevalence of allergic conjunctivitis to be as high as 40% in the general population (8).

With seasonal or PAC, the history is essential to the diagnosis and treatment. The allergic response is characteristically elicited by ocular exposure to allergens, which causes cross-linkage of mast cell membrane-bound IgE, triggering mast cell degranulation, releasing allergic and inflammatory mediators (9).

Clinically patients present with bilateral ocular itching, tearing, redness, swelling, burning, sensitivity to light, and occasionally blurred vision. Conjunctival hyperemia and chemosis with palpebral edema are present. Oftentimes people develop "allergic shiners," which is darkening of the periorbital region from decreased venous return (Fig. 3.3). Contact lens use may lead physicians toward the diagnosis of GPC; however, daily disposal of contact lenses in fact removes allergens from the corneal surface and lens use is less commonly associated with GPC. However, contact lens use may increase a "dry eye" sensation similar to other patients with tear film dysfunction.

Tear film analysis in allergic patients reveals the presence of IgE antibody, histamine, and tryptase. Preformed mediators (histamine, tryptase, bradykinin) of inflammation are released immediately on allergen exposure, and the newly formed de novo mediators (leukotrienes, prostaglandins) are released within hours peaking in 8–24 h. The combined effects of these mediators yield the various signs and symptoms of allergic conjunctivitis including redness, itching, and watery discharge.

Work-up includes a thorough history to determine acuity of the process and relative associations or exposures. Family history is also significant, especially for allergic rhinitis, asthma, or other manifestations of atopy. Symptoms are usually bilateral. Management includes topical vasoconstrictors, antihistamines (or combination of the two), mast cell stabilizers, multiple action agents (antihistamines that have mast cell stabilizing and affect other proinflammatory mediators) or rarely, NSAIDs. The primary treatment is avoidance, but this becomes impractical with many airborne allergens such as pollen. Cold compresses and artificial tears are helpful in decreasing the intensity of nerve stimulus (pruritus) while lubricants dilute the allergen in the tear fluid as well as washes away the allergens and the various inflammatory mediators. Pharmacotherapy is directed at relieving symptoms while immunotherapy is focused on the downregulation of the allergic immune response and thus ameliorating the intensity of future exposures. It appears that mild symptoms of ocular allergy are even alleviated with the use topical intranasal steroids. If symptoms are severe, combination therapy may be required, combining topical ophthalmic medications and oral antihistamines. A "burst" of topical steroids (3–7 days) can be used in severe cases, but should be used with caution in patients well known to the practice to insure proper use and proper follow-up care. Immunotherapy is beneficial at decreasing future allergic symptoms by increasing the threshold to the allergens associated with the ocular as well as nasal signs and symptoms.

Questions

1. A 26-year mildly asthmatic patient whom you have been treating with immunotherapy for several years for allergic rhinoconjunctivitis associated with birch pollen, ragweed, and dust mite develops a progressive irritation in her right eye in the past 2 days. She does not complain of any change in her asthma or medication use. She does not complain of any nausea, vomiting, fever, or myalgia. She had a ropey white discharge from one eye initially. Now she has noticed that her eyelids appear to be stickier in the morning when she wakes up. She comes in for her routine visit for her "allergy shot" (immunotherapy) that coincides with the ragweed allergy season. On examination an opaque yellowish mucous strand is noted on the eyelid with moderate injection of the conjunctiva. The other eye had only mild injection.

Which of the following is *contraindicated*?

(a) Use of a topical mast cell-stabilizing agent
(b) Use of lubricants
(c) Use of cold compresses
(d) Use of a topical combined antibiotic and steroid agent
(e) Use of immunotherapy

This patient presents with an ongoing history of allergic conjunctivitis, involving both eyes. However, she now presents with a *unilateral* worsening of her eye disease, with an opaque yellowish mucous strand in one eye. Although she is in the midst of her ragweed season, the presence of unilateral worsening suggests a nonallergic and possibly an infectious etiology. The most common eye infection in this patient is a viral infection, which is not likely to improve with topical antibiotics, but many cases of viral conjunctivitis are subsequently followed by a bacterial infection and may be considered. A topical mast cell-stabilizing agent, an intranasal steroid, and continuation of her immunotherapy will help control her underlying allergic symptoms as she is entering her allergy season ("hay fever"), which is also associated with nasal symptoms in addition to the ocular symptoms. Lubricants and cold compresses may acutely relieve some of her right eye symptoms. The presence of the topical steroid combined with the antibiotic may exacerbate a viral (or chlamydial) infection and lead to severe site-threatening consequences and is thus contraindicated.

2. A 48-year-old patient presents with a recent increase in ocular irritation in both eyes. She has no significant medical history. She states that she has had eczema and food allergy to corn as a child that both resolved in her early teen years. She does not have any history of asthma and does not give any consistent history of seasonal allergies. In the early winter months for the past several years, she has noticed an increase in ocular symptoms of itching and grittiness with increased blinking, especially while working on the computer. The conjunctivae were mildly injected bilaterally. Further evaluation revealed that she had normal responses to histamine and saline with minimal reactions to grass pollen and mixed trees. Skin test results to indoor allergens (dust mite, cockroach, dog, and cat) are negative.

Which of the following is the most probable diagnosis?

   (a) SAC
   (b) AKC
   (c) GPC
   (d) Tear film dysfunction
   (e) VKC

This patient does not presently have features of a systemic allergic disorder. This makes the diagnoses of SAC, AKC, and VKC unlikely. The absence of a history of contact lens use, with only mild injected bilateral conjunctivae, in the absence of papillary hypertrophy makes the diagnosis of GPC unlikely. The patient notes her problem mostly in the dry early winter months, with itching and a gritty feeling in her eyes, particularly while working at the computer. These findings are consistent with the diagnosis of a tear film dysfunction.

3. Which of these treatments would be the long-term treatment?

   (a) Use of oral antihistamines (e.g., cetirizine or diphenhydramine)
   (b) Initiation of immunotherapy
   (c) Use of topical cyclosporine
   (d) Use of lid scrubs
   (e) Use of topical antibiotic

This patient suffers from dry eyes related to tear film dysfunction. Antihistamines, particularly cetirizine and diphenhydramine have demonstrated clinically relevant anticholinergic activity, which may worsen symptoms of dry eyes. Lid scrubs are used for inflammatory condition involving the eyelid (blepharitis) and is not present in this case. Although patients who suffer from tear film dysfunction have an underlying inflammatory basis for their disease, the problem in this case is not related to a specific IgE-mediated response. Therefore, immunotherapy will not likely improve her symptoms. As this is not an infectious disorder, the use of a topical antibiotic will not control her problem, and it may result in bacterial resistance and should be discouraged. The only immunomodulatory agent currently approved to treat the inflammation associated with tear film dysfunction is topical cyclosporine.

4. A 12-year-old boy is referred to you for chronic persistent red eyes. He first met his pediatrician 6 weeks ago after moving to your area from Morocco. The family history is significant for allergies, eczema, and asthma. The mother describes the child as having eye symptoms of severe ocular itching and, at times, burning in Morocco that started approximately 3 years ago, but it has been getting increasingly worse. The itching appears to have become constant. She also describes some seasonality in the spring months (April and May) that includes a runny nose and watery eyes. They have never owned any animals. It is now ragweed season, and he appears to still have mild to moderate injected conjunctiva with a white ropey filament in the lower fornices of both eyes, some clustered and enlarged papillae on the tarsal conjunctivae, minimally boggy nasal mucosa, with clear mucus covering the turbinates, and increased tearing at the time of the visit to you. Oral antihistamines have only been intermittently helpful and currently are not working. They have at times made his symptoms worse. Further evaluation revealed normal responses to histamine and saline with a mild reaction to grass pollen and none to mixed trees. Skin test results to indoor allergens (dust mite, cockroach, dog, cat) demonstrated minimal reactivity to cat.

Which of the following is the most probable diagnosis?

   (a) AKC
   (b) Viral conjunctivitis
   (c) GPC
   (d) VKC

Although this child has severe ocular pruritus, AKC is more common in older patients. The bilateral ocular involvement that has persisted over this length of time is not consistent with viral conjunctivitis. GPC is more commonly associated with a milder form of ocular pruritus than VKC, which has an incredibly intense ocular pruritus. The absence of contact lens use or a foreign body also makes the diagnosis of GPC unlikely. The age of onset, the severe itch with white ropey filament, and a Mediterranean origin suggest a diagnosis of VKC. In VKC, enlarged papillae up to 7–8 mm in diameter may form on the tarsal conjunctivae, which is a classic

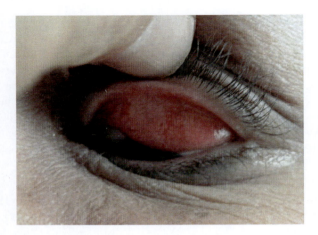

Fig. 3.4 Large papillae of the upper tarsus of vernal keratoconjunctivitis

hallmark of this disease, and form a "cobblestone appearance" (Fig. 3.4). VKC is commonly a disorder of children or young adults, most frequently occurring in warm/tropical climates. The most common symptoms include itching, burning, redness, photophobia, with a ropey mucus discharge in the conjunctival fornix (10).

5. Which of the following treatments is *not* indicated in the treatment of this patient?

  (a) Topical mast cell-stabilizing agent
  (b) Topical antihistamines
  (c) Cold compresses
  (d) Topical steroid agent
  (e) Immunotherapy

The mechanisms that lead to this disorder are unknown. However, the presence of large numbers of degranulated mast cells and eosinophils, with Th2 CD4+ lymphocytes is typical of VKC. As these patients are at risk for corneal involvement, which may affect their vision, treatment with agents that decrease this type of inflammation (topical mast cell-stabilizing agents, topical antihistamines, topical steroid agents) may be vision saving. Cold compresses may provide symptomatic relief. Although seasonal exacerbations exist (i.e., vernal being spring time) and patients may even have some immediate cutaneous reactivities to various "seasonal allergens" such as grass pollen, VKC is a perennial problem. Immunotherapy has not been shown to provide benefit.

Answers: Case 1: (a), (e), (f); Case 2: (d), (e); Question 1: (d); Question 2: (d); Question 3: (c); Question 4: (d); Question 5: (e)

References

1. Zhan, H., Smith, L., Calder V., Buckley R., Lightman S. (2003) Clinical and immunological features of atopic keratoconjunctivitis. *Int Ophthalmol Clin* **43**, 59–71.
2. Bielory L. (2000) Allergic and immunologic disorders of the eye, Part 2: Ocular allergy. *J Allergy Clin Immunol* **106**, 1019–32.
3. Calonge, M. (2000) Ocular allergies: Association with immune dermatitis. *Acta Ophthalmol Scand* **78**, 69–75.
4. Bielory, L., Friedlaender, M.H. (2008) Ocular allergy overview. *Immunol Allergy Clin North Am* **28**, 1–23.
5. Uchio, E., Ono, S., Ikezawa, Z., Ohno, S. (2000) Tear levels of interferon-gamma, interleukin (IL)-2, IL-4 and IL-5 in patients with vernal keratoconjunctivitis, atopic keratoconjunctivitis and allergic conjunctivitis. *Clin Exp Allergy* **30**, 103–9.
6. Bielory, L. (2007) Differential diagnoses of conjunctivitis for clinical allergist-immunologists. *Ann Allergy Asthma Immunol* **98**, 105–15.
7. Bielory, L., Friedlaender, M.H. (2008) Allergic conjunctivitis. *Immunol Allergy Clin North Am* **28**, 43–58.
8. Singh, K., Bielory, L. (2007) Ocular allergy: A national epidemiologic study. *J Allergy Clin Immunol* **119**, S154.
9. Ono, S.J., Abelson, M.B. (2005) Allergic conjunctivitis: Update on pathophysiology and prospects for future treatment. *J Allergy Clin Immunol* **115**, 118–22.
10. Jun, J., Bielory, L., Raizman, M.B. (2008) Vernal Conjunctivitis. *Immunol Allergy Clin North Am* **28**, 59–82.

Chapter 4
Urticaria and Angioedema

Bettina Wedi and Alexander Kapp

Abstract The different urticaria subtypes represent a common diagnostic and treatment challenge. In acute urticaria that is often induced by an acute infection and/or intake of NSAID such as acetylsalicylic acid, no further diagnostic procedures are recommended. In contrast, a targeted work-up and therapeutic management should be performed in spontaneous chronic urticaria, physical urticaria, and special urticaria types; this is because many of these subtypes are characterized by persistence for several years and have a profound impact on the quality of life. The management of chronic urticaria, two subtypes of physical urticaria, and a special subtype is presented by two characteristic case reports.

Keywords Chronic urticaria • Physical urticaria • Cold urticaria • Cholinergic urticaria • Angioedema • Management

Case 1

A 42-year-old man presents with a two-year history of nearly daily and often generalized wheals. The wheals are pruritic and red ranging from 1.0 centimeter to several centimeters in diameter. He reports frequent episodes of lip or eyelid swelling (every 2–3 week) and during the last year he had five episodes of tongue swelling. Two days before presentation he had to go to the emergency room because of generalized wheals and severe tongue swelling associated with tightness of the throat, although he had used his emergency drugs (liquid prednisolone, antihistamine syrup). Several months ago, he had to stop working as a postman because very often he had suffered from swellings of both palms and soles.

B. Wedi (✉) and A. Kapp
Department of Dermatology and Allergology, Hannover Medical School,
Ricklinger Str. 5, 30449, Hannover, Germany
e-mail: wedi.bettina@mh-hannover.de

M. Mahmoudi (ed.), *Challenging Cases in Allergy and Immunology*,
DOI: 10.1007/978-1-60327-443-2_4,
© Humana Press, a part of Springer Science+Business Media, LLC 2009

When telling his history he starts crying because he has severe difficulties to sleep, is anxious to develop life-threatening angioedema, and because his wife is very upset about his disease. He appears to be depressive. Inquiring about medication history reveals intake of aspirin 500 mg at least once in a week because of the painful swellings or headaches. His other medications include enalapril for hypertension for the past 5 years and allopurinol for high uric acid for 2 years. He denies family history of wheals or angioedema. Skin prick testing to aeroallergens and food had been negative and previous laboratory results that included complete blood count, urinalysis, and chemistry panel were also negative. His practitioner prescribed a single dose of a daily second-generation antihistamine and a nightly sedating H1-antihistamine, but throughout the day he has a hangover effect.

Physical examination reveals no angioedema but a giant wheal of several centimeters on the left dorsal thigh (Fig. 4.1) in addition to smaller wheals distributed over the body (Fig. 4.2). On enquiry, he reports that his child sat on this thigh some hours ago. There is a positive dermographism reaction. Everything else besides the skin is normal. Mean blood pressure is 140/80 mmHg.

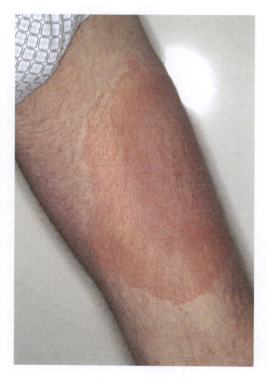

Fig. 4.1 Giant wheal on the left dorsal thigh after his child sat there several hours ago

Fig. 4.2 Small, confluent erythematous wheals on the volar arm

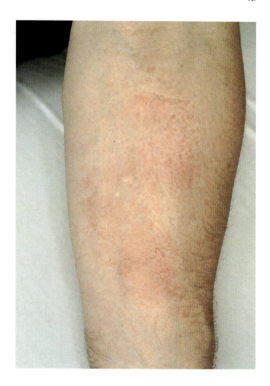

Data

Laboratory assessments to find a potential triggering factor are done (Table 4.1).

The following pathological findings are obtained:

^{13}C urea breath test for Helicobacter is positive. There is no evidence for other persistent bacterial infections or inflammatory process. Autologous serum skin test (ASST) is negative and C1-INH function is 100%.

To confirm delayed pressure urticaria standardized physical tests are performed, which reveal clear red pruritic swellings 6 h after 10-min application of weights, at the back, of 1,000 and 1,500 g/cm^{2,} whereas the result with 500 g/cm^2 weight is negative.

With the Presented Data What Is Your Working Diagnosis?

The patient's physical examination demonstrating spontaneous wheals distributed over the body and the history of nearly daily wheals for a period of 2 years are consistent with spontaneous chronic urticaria. As angioedema is associated with

Table 4.1 Recommended diagnostic work-up and first treatment approach for the different urticaria subtypes

Subtype	Group/definition	Diagnostic work-up	First treatment approach
Acute UR	*Spontaneous UR*/wheals < 6 weeks	Evaluation guided by history: Atopy? Drug history (ASA?), evidence of infection?	Symptomatic treatment: H1 antihistamines: regularly for 2–3 weeks (perhaps in increased dose up to fourfold) Glucocorticosteroids (0.5–1 mg/kg daily): in severe cases, only short term (up to 1 week)
Chronic UR	*Spontaneous UR*/wheals > 6 weeks	Infection diagnostics: differential blood count, CRP, Helicobacter 13C-urea breath test or histology or monoclonal stool antigen test, serology for streptococci, Yersinia; perhaps ENT/dental exam with imaging, perhaps parasite diagnostics	Avoidance of unspecific triggers: acetylsalicylic acid and other NSAIDs, mast cell-stimulating drugs, alcohol, overheating, tight clothing, in angioedema also ACE inhibitors (perhaps sartans also)
		Autoreactivity: autologous serum skin test, thyroid autoantibodies, perhaps determination of serum activity with cellular in vitro diagnostics	Specific treatment: of persistent infections (e.g., Helicobacter eradication), of autoimmune thyroiditis, diet in cases of nonallergic hypersensitivity toward additives proven by provocation
		Pseudoallergy: perhaps NSAID provocation or provocation with pseudoallergen-rich diet or additives after successful standardized preudoallergen-poor diet for 4 weeks	Symptomatic treatment: H1 antihistamines of the new generation, regularly, perhaps up to 4× daily (off-label use)
			Alternatives (always in addition to H1 antihistamines!): montelukast, (hydroxy)chloroquine, dapsone, oral low-dose glucocorticosteroids, cyclosporin A
Dermographic UR	*Physical UR*/mechanical shear forces	Testing of dermographism, infection diagnostics as in chronic UR	See chronic UR
Delayed pressure UR	*Physical UR*/ vertical pressure (latency of several hours)	Pressure testing, perhaps infection diagnostics as in CU	Prevention: H1 antihistamines of the new generation in increased dose (up to fourfold) regularly or as needed
			Alternatives (always in addition to H1 antihistamines): dapsone 100–150 mg daily (6 days per week) oral glucocorticosteroids below the Cushing threshold, methotrexate

Type	Subtype	Diagnostics	Therapy
Cold UR	Physical UR/Cold air/water/wind	Standardized cold testing; determine highest eliciting temperature; perhaps infection diagnostics as in CU, cryoglobulins, cryoagglutinins, cryofibrinogen, serology for borrelia, syphilis, perhaps HIV	Prevention: H1 antihistamines of the new generation (perhaps in increased dose up to fourfold) regularly or as needed. Alternatives: oral tetracyclines, intramuscular penicillin for 3→4 weeks (omalizumab)
Heat UR	Physical UR/local heat	Standardized heat testing; determine lowest eliciting temperature	Prevention: H1 antihistamines of the new generation in increased dose (up to fourfold) regularly or as needed. Alternatives: tolerance induction, (hydroxy)chloroquine
Solar UR	Physical UR/UV, visible light	Standardized photoprovocation with UV and visible light	Prevention: H1 antihistamines of the new generation in increased dose (up to fourfold) regularly or as needed. Alternatives: photohardening, (hydroxy)chloroquine
Vibratory UR/AOe	Physical UR/vibratory forces	Provocation with vibratory forces	Avoid trigger
Cholinergic UR	Special type/increase in body temperature	Ergometer exertion, perhaps infection diagnostics as in CU	Avoid trigger. Try prevention: H1 antihistamines of the new generation in increased dose (up to fourfold) regularly or as needed
Aquagenic UR	Special type/water contact (any temperature)	Testing with wet gauze at body temperature	
Contact UR	Special type/contact to urticariogenic substance	Open application test for 15 min, occlusive patch test with urticariogenic substance	
Exercise-induced UR	Special type/physical exercise	Ergometer exertion, perhaps additional food and/or ASA provocation	

UR Urticaria; AOe angioedema

more than half of the patients; this is in line with the diagnosis chronic urticaria. Frequent angioedema of the tongue is not so common in typical chronic urticaria with angioedema; this is more typical for ACE-induced angioedema. History, in fact, revealed regular intake of the ACE-inhibitor enalapril. C1-esterase-inhibitor function was 100%, therefore hereditary or acquired C1-INH-deficient angioedema is excluded.

Severe symmetric swellings of both palms and soles that resulted in inability to work are a typical feature of delayed pressure urticaria. In addition, the giant wheal on the dorsal left thigh that developed several hours after sitting of his child is consistent with the physical urticaria subtype that is clearly confirmed by delayed occurring deep wheals in the standardized pressure test.

History and work-up demonstrate *Helicobacter pylori* infection and nearly weekly intake of ASA as triggering factors. In addition, secondary psychosocial problems and perhaps even reactive depression developed.

Differential Diagnosis

Different urticaria subtypes are possible in this patient, such as spontaneous chronic urticaria and delayed pressure urticaria (a subtype of physical urticaria). In recurrent angioedema C1-esterase-inhibitor deficiency has to be considered. Regarding the age of the patient and negative family history, hereditary C1-esterase-inhibitor deficiency is unlikely but acquired C1-esterase-inhibitor deficiency associated with malignancy is a potential differential.

In view of the strong itch of the wheals differential diagnosis included scabies, arthropod reactions, urticarial stages of autoimmune bullous skin diseases such as bullous pemphigoid, and early stages of vasculitis and erythema multiforme.

The wheals are pruritic, therefore rare autoinflammatory syndromes such as Muckle-Well's syndrome, Hyper-IgD syndrome, chronic infantile neurological cutaneous and articular syndrome, or hematologic disorders such as Schnitzler's syndrome are unlikely; this is because they are characterized by nonpruritic urticaria-like skin lesions.

What Is Your Diagnosis and Why

In the scenario of spontaneous and itching wheal and flares persisting for more than 6 weeks, urticaria is defined as spontaneous chronic urticaria. More than half of the patients also have concurrent angioedema but those of the tongue are not so common; this sign together with drug intake history pointed to pharmacologically induced angioedema by ACE inhibitor. Physical urticaria may be associated with spontaneous chronic urticaria and this is the case in this patient as vertical pressure results in delayed swellings in the standardized physical pressure tests. In addition, health-related quality of life is significantly reduced due to intense pruritus, sleep-lessness, and fear to develop sudden and potential life-threatening angioedema. Therefore, reactive depression is assumed.

Discussion

It is estimated that at least 15–20% of the population will suffer one episode of wheals during their lifetime (1). Urticaria occurs most frequently between the ages of 20 and 40 and more commonly in women than in men. About 80% of urticaria is spontaneous, 10% is physical, and less than 10% is of a special type (Table 4.1), but two or rarely more subtypes can occur in the same patient (e.g., spontaneous chronic urticaria and dermographism or spontaneous chronic urticaria and delayed pressure urticaria). In these cases urticaria is long persisting and more often difficult to treat. Chronic urticaria usually persists on an average for 3–5 years but may be present even after 20 years. Comparably, most physical urticaria and special types persist for about 5 years. Quality of life is significantly impaired due to intense pruritus, sleep disturbances, and secondary psychosocial problems.

About two-third of spontaneous urticaria is acute (allergic or nonallergic), commonly seen in medical emergency service, and about one-third is chronic (nonallergic). In both types angioedema is associated in more than 50% of cases, often located at the lips, eye lids, or genitals, sometimes also at the tongue or larynx. Rarely angioedema without urticaria can be caused by C1-inhibitor deficiency (2), either of hereditary subtype (only 5% of all angioedema without urticaria) or acquired angioedema (very rare). However, most cases of angioedema are histamine-mediated like the wheals. Pharmacologically induced angioedema (Table 4.2) occurs in about 0.6% of patients receiving ACE inhibitor treatment (more rarely also sartans) and is more common in Afro-Americans. In most cases angioedema occurs within 3 months of starting the ACE inhibitor but occurrence after several years is also possible (3).

The presentation of urticaria is a distinctive pruritic skin rash fleeting in nature. The single lesions can vary in size from pinpoint sized edematous erythemas as in cholinergic urticaria to giant wheals, a single lesion that may cover almost an entire extremity. They also vary in shape, which may be round, oval, polycyclic when confluent, irregular, or with pseudopodia. The border may be reabsorbed giving the

Table 4.2 Non-C1 inhibitor-deficient angioedema

Subtype	Cause
Allergic	IgE-mediated (usually with urticaria)
Nonallergic	For example, NSAID-induced
Pharmacologic	ACE-inhibitor induced (class effect)
Infectious	For example, associated with *H. pylori* infection
Physical	Exposure to vibration, cold, and pressure
Idiopathic	No identifiable cause

appearance of incomplete rings. The single wheal usually is present for minutes to several hours but less than 24 h.

In physical urticaria, usually the wheals resolve within 2 h except in delayed pressure urticaria in which painful swellings develop 6–8 h after sustained pressure and persist for up to 2 days (1). Typical localizations are the palms and soles, buttocks, back, and skin under straps and belts. Systemic symptoms of malaise, arthralgia, myalgia, and leukocytosis can be associated. Delayed pressure urticaria is more common in middle-aged males and persists for an average of 6–9 years, often resulting in disability to work. It may be associated with chronic urticaria.

Urticaria is the clinical manifestation of a localized increase of permeability of capillaries and small venules in the dermal papilla whereas the swellings in angioedema are caused deeper in the subcutis.

Regarding the pathophysiology, urticaria and angioedema must be regarded as a symptom of mast cell and/or basophil activation and degranulation with histamine being the most important released mediator (1). An injection of histamine into the skin will produce a prototypic hive (as that used as a positive control in prick and intradermal skin testing). This "Triple Response of Lewis" demonstrates (a) *erythema* – the clinical expression of vasodilation, (b) *a wheal* – reflecting vascular leakage, and (c) *pruritus* – the result of activation of itch receptors in the epidermis. But histamine is probably not the sole inflammatory mediator causing wheals.

A variety of immunologic and nonimmunologic physical and chemical stimuli react with different cell membrane receptors of basophils and mast cells to activate them. Among these are, for example, bacterial substances, antigens, IgG autoantibodies against IgE, or the high-affinity IgE receptor. In physical urticaria, specific physical stimuli, such as pressure, temperature changes, ultraviolet light, vibration, and contact with water are recognized as "triggers" for mast-cell degranulation (Table 4.1). The connection between the physical stimulus and the release of mediators from mast cells is poorly understood.

The pathomechanisms of pharmacologic angioedema are accumulation of bradykinin caused by decreased bradykinin degradation by ACE inhibitors, angiotensin II receptor blockers (sartans), and vasopeptidase inhibitors.

Careful history and physical examination and directed laboratory evaluation remain the cornerstone in the evaluation of the condition. Potential triggering factors, a physical examination including a test for dermographism, laboratory investigations, and, if needed, additional specific procedures are recommended (for details see Table 4.1). Every attempt should be made to find an underlying etiology in each patient, because the identification and elimination of causal factors represent the best therapeutic approach. Several mechanisms can be active in a single patient.

IgE-mediated hypersensitivity is very rarely the cause of symptoms in chronic urticaria. Therefore, routine skin prick tests to inhalant and food allergens are of little value. To find autoreactive mechanisms an ASST should be performed (4), although the clinical relevance is far from being clear.

In vitro functional assays of serum-activity and/or autoantibodies against IgE or FcεRIα such as histamine release, leukotriene production, and increase in surface expression of basophil activation markers such as CD63 are not available for routine purposes. Since about 30% of chronic urticaria cases are also associated with thyroid antibodies, thyroid-function tests, including tests for antithyroglobulin and antimicrosomal antibodies, are recommended.

Complement determinations (C4, C1-esterase inhibitor function) are not indicated for patients who have wheals alone (since the values are normal), nor need they be done when angioedema accompanies chronic urticaria, since patients with a hereditary or acquired deficiency of C1 inhibitor usually do not have wheals.

Aspirin, NSAIDs, and other mast cell-activating drugs such as morphine, codeine, muscle relaxants, polymyxin, and dextran aggravate symptoms and evoke exacerbations. Rare, nonallergic hypersensitivity reactions to food additives should be proven by a double-blind, placebo-controlled challenge.

A skin biopsy is indicated in severe cases of chronic or persistent urticaria, particularly when urticaria vasculitis is considered.

Physical urticaria is diagnosed by thorough history, clinical examination, and provocation procedures using standardized physical tests (5). Diagnostics for delayed pressure urticaria are standardized pressure tests applying weights in amount of $0.5–1.5$ kg/cm^2 for 10 min in different areas (back, ventral, and dorsal thigh). Readings should be done at least after 30 min, 3 h, 6 h, and 24 h (5). Only definite raised wheals occurring after several hours indicate delayed pressure urticaria.

In chronic or physical urticaria subtypes the treatment goal is to maximize quality of life and ability to work or to attend school and to minimize drug-related side effects. Unspecific trigger factors should be avoided. Specific and sufficient treatment of identified persistent bacterial and parasitic infections can result in complete remission (Table 4.1).

Treatment approaches of the different urticaria subtypes are presented in Table 4.1.

Long-acting low-sedating antihistamines are the mainstay of symptomatic treatment in chronic urticaria and the only drugs approved for this condition. They can be given the highest grade of recommendation according to the criteria of evidence-based medicine (6–10). The primary choice is based on pharmacokinetic properties, side effects, comorbidity, and concomitant treatment (8). It is a common practice to exceed the licensed dose although available data are limited. The current European Guideline (10) recommends an increase up to fourfold the normal dose while considering the side effects (off-label!). Management is better achieved by taking antihistamines regularly, not just when the patient is symptomatic.

In delayed pressure urticaria, antihistamines, even in increased doses, often fail; nevertheless, they represent the mainstay of treatment. Some patients benefit from additional low-dose corticosteroids (e.g., 40–20-mg prednisone), others by treatment with dapsone (100–150 mg per day). Moreover, methotrexate (15 mg per week), montelukast, ketotifen plus nimesulide, sulfasalazine, or topical clobetasol propionate 0.5% ointment have been tried successfully (10).

In the earlier case 1, first intake of ASA should be stopped; acetaminophen is recommended instead, if needed. The patient should be referred to his family doctor to change the antihypertensive medication – if possible – to avoid ACE inhibitors and sartans. Helicobacter should be eradicated by triple treatment with amoxicillin, clarithromycine, and a proton pump inhibitor for 7 days.

Symptomatic treatment of urticaria is performed with a second-generation antihistamine in increased (off label!) dose up to four times daily, if needed. Moreover montelukast 1 × 10 mg is added (off-label!) because of the previous resistance to treatment with two antihistamines. Emergency medications including a liquid corticosteroid and epinephrine autoinjector are prescribed for immediate at-home treatment of severe angioedema of the tongue or larynx. Four to six weeks after Helicobacter treatment success should be controlled by a monoclonal stool antigen test or a second urea-breath test.

It is anticipated that the aforementioned management will improve the spontaneous chronic urticaria and associated angioedema but might not be successful in controlling delayed pressure urticaria. Therefore, dapson might be added later (off-label) 100 mg/day, 6 days a week, after lab results have demonstrated normal glucose-6-phosphate-dehydrogenase levels.

Case 2

A 22-year-old woman presents with a 1-year history of wheals and swellings occurring after contact to cold water or wind, particularly in winter but also in summer when swimming in cold water. She is avoiding cold exposure and does not receive special treatment. During the last month the symptoms got worse. She reports that when she was bicycling to school, she developed pruritic wheals on her trunk. She intends to start canoeing as a new hobby, but her mother wants to consult a doctor to find out whether canoeing is a potential risk for her condition.

Otherwise, the young woman is healthy and only suffers from itchy eyes, sneezing, and runny nose in summer. The family history is positive for atopic diseases (father: allergic rhinitis) but no family member develops symptoms after cold contact or exercising.

Data

Previous investigations of the general practitioner including complete blood count and blood chemistry were all normal. Physical examination is normal; there are no skin lesions. The dermographism reaction is white.

The standardized cold provocation test shows that 20°C is the highest temperature that elicited confluent and spreading wheals in the contact area 10 min after a cold arm bath (Fig. 4.3). Fifteen minutes after strong exercise on the ergometer the patient develops itchy pinpoint-headed erythematous wheals (Fig. 4.4) over the trunk, which disappear 30 min after stopping the exercise. The laboratory

Fig. 4.3 Cold urticaria. An arm bath at 20°C for 10 min resulted in itchy confluent wheals in the contact area. Finally the erythematous edema involved the whole contact area

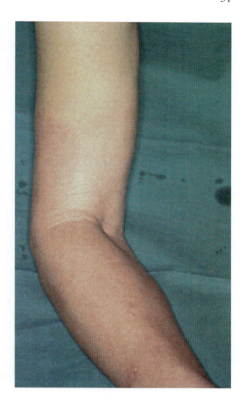

investigations including cryoglobulins, cryoagglutinins, cryofibrinogen, serology for borrelia, and syphilis (Table 4.1) do not reveal any abnormalities. Atopy prick test with common inhalant allergens confirms specific IgE-mediated sensitization to grass pollen.

With the Presented Data What Is Your Working Diagnosis?

History is consistent with cold urticaria as the patient develops wheals and swellings in contact areas to cold water or wind. This is confirmed by the demonstration of urticaria in the standardized cold provocation test.

Additionally she reports small wheals after bicycling. This implies cholinergic urticaria, which is confirmed by fleeting wheals that developed during the exercise test. The white dermographism together with the history of rhinitis in summer and the positive skin prick test results are consistent with seasonal allergic rhinitis to grass pollen.

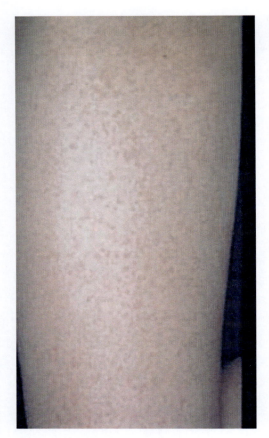

Fig. 4.4 Typically pinpoint-sized wheals after a 10-min exercise on a bicycle/ergometer

Differential Diagnosis

For differential diagnosis, familial cold autoinflammatory syndrome in which there are mutations of CIAS-1 encoding the pyrin-like protein (cryopyrin) as recently has been identified has to be considered. However, patient denies fever or arthralgia and family history is negative for cold-induced symptoms.

What Is Your Diagnosis and Why?

The development of wheals in cold contact areas is consistent with cold urticaria. This physical urticaria subtype can be associated with cholinergic urticaria, which was confirmed by the development of small wheals spread over the body after exercising. In addition, the positive skin prick to grass pollen together with a history of rhinitis during summer is consistent with intermittent (seasonal) allergic rhinitis due to IgE-mediated sensitization to grass pollen.

Discussion

Acquired cold urticaria and angioedema occur mainly in young adults within minutes after contact to cold objects, cold, cold water, cold air, and sometimes cold food/drinks (11). After warming they disappear within an hour. Coexistence of cold urticaria with cholinergic urticaria has to be considered. The average duration of both urticaria subtypes is 3–5 years. Generalized systemic, sometimes life-threatening reactions can follow lowering of the body temperature (e.g., after swimming in cold water). The relative drop in cutaneous temperature rather than the absolute temperature is the critical factor. For example, an overheated subject who plunges into a cool swimming pool on a hot day can develop generalized cold urticaria. Moreover, swellings of the oropharynx may follow a cold drink or eating cold food.

Cold urticaria may begin after an infection, drug therapy, or emotional stress. However, in over 90% of cases no trigger factor can be identified. Secondary cold urticaria accounts for about 5% of patients with cold urticaria and occurs in association with cryoglobulinemia, cryofibrinogenemia, and cold hemolysins, often secondary to viral infections such as syphilis, chronic hepatitis B or C, or autoimmune disorders. In cold urticaria standardized cold provocation tests should ideally define the highest eliciting temperature. Recently, low-voltage Peltier thermoelectric elements have been developed. Specific infectious diseases such as syphilis, borreliosis, hepatitis, infectious mononucleosis, and HIV infections but also unrecognized bacterial infections have been reported as triggering factors and need to be excluded (Table 4.1).

The known infectious diseases as well as unrecognized bacterial infections should be treated adequately. Low-sedating H1 antihistamines are the first line in treatment. In idiopathic cases, antibiotic treatment (e.g., with doxycycline or penicillin, i.m. or p.o.) is worthwhile trying. Other low-evidence alternatives are cyproheptadine, ketotifen, Montelukast (10), and as has been recently published, omalizumab. It is very important that patients learn to protect themselves from a sudden decrease in temperature.

Cholinergic urticaria results from the activation of cholinergic sympathetic autonomic-nerve fibers supplying eccrine sweat glands, after a period of exercise or a hot bath, or from a high fever, but also by emotional stress. The urticaria lesions in cholinergic urticaria are typically small sized (2–5-mm wheals, surrounded by an erythematous flare), resembling goose skin and last for about 20–60 min. The condition often remits spontaneously within several years and is almost exclusively seen in adolescents and young adults. The overall prevalence is about 11% (highest prevalence in the age group 26–28 years). A small subgroup is severely affected and may also suffer from systemic symptoms including angioedema, hypotension, wheezing, and gastrointestinal complaints, but most patients have mild symptoms and do not seek medical attention.

The diagnosis is suggested by history and confirmed by provocation of the typical small-sized wheals, e.g., by using an exercise bicycle for 10–15 min under strict observation (hypotension and other systemic symptoms may develop).

The mainstay of treatment is low-sedating H1-antihistamines (in increased dose) regularly and/or 60 min before typical triggering situations, but they often fail (10). It is difficult to achieve exercise tolerance. Optional medications to use are Ketotifen or Danazol, and as has been very recently published, omalizumab.

The initial management of the patient (case 2) should include a second-generation H1-antihistamine in single or, if needed, increased dose 30–60 min before expected exposure to cold or exercise. Furthermore, advice is given to avoid intense cold exposure and strong exercise. Canoeing is not recommended until the cold urticaria has disappeared because this might be too dangerous if the patient falls in cold water. Emergency drugs should be prescribed for severe exacerbations. If the pretreatment does not suppress the symptoms the aforementioned off-label options can be tried.

Questions

1. Which sentence is incorrect?

   (a) Urticaria is defined as chronic if wheals persist for a period longer than 6 weeks.
   (b) Delayed pressure urticaria is a subtype of physical urticaria.
   (c) Contact urticaria is a special type of urticaria.
   (d) Spontaneous chronic urticaria and physical urticaria can not coexist.
   (e) Different physical urticaria subtypes can coexist.

2. Which sentence is correct?

   (a) In delayed pressure urticaria wheals develop 20 min after vertical pressure.
   (b) In delayed pressure urticaria wheals develop 60 min after vertical pressure.
   (c) In delayed pressure urticaria wheals develop 4–8 h after vertical pressure.
   (d) Cholinergic urticaria is caused by an IgE-mediated sensitization to sweat.
   (e) The prevalence of cholinergic urticaria is most frequent in 40–50-year-old men.

3. Which sentence is incorrect? Chronic urticaria

   (a) Is a subtype of spontaneous urticaria
   (b) Significantly reduces quality of life
   (c) Usually persists for an average of 5 months
   (d) May be insufficiently treated with H1-antihistamines
   (e) Can be triggered by gastric *Helicobacter pylori* infection.

4. What is incorrect?

(a) First-line treatment of chronic urticaria consists of H1-antihistamines.
(b) In severe delayed pressure urticaria low-dose oral glucocorticosteroids or dapsone may be tried in addition to H1-antihistamines.
(c) First-line treatment of cholinergic urticaria consists of H2-antihistamines.
(d) Cyclosporine A can be a valuable second-line treatment in chronic urticaria.
(e) In cold urticaria antibiotic treatment, for example, with penicillin can be used.

5. Which diagnostic procedure is not routinely recommended in the management of chronic urticaria or physical urticaria subtypes?

(a) Test for dermographism
(b) Standardized physical tests
(c) Laboratory parameters guided by history
(d) Prick test with food allergens
(e) Autologous serum skin test

Answers: 1. (d), 2. (c), 3. (c), 4. (c), 5. (d)

References

1. Zuberbier T, Bindslev-Jensen C, Canonica W et al. EAACI/GALEN/EDF guideline: definition, classification and diagnosis of urticaria. Allergy 2006; 61(3):316–320.
2. Frank MM. Hereditary angioedema. J Allergy Clin Immunol 2008; 121(2 Suppl):S398–S401.
3. Kaplan AP, Greaves MW. Angioedema. J Am Acad Dermatol 2005; 53(3):373–388.
4. Grattan CE. Autoimmune urticaria. Immunol Allergy Clin North Am 2004; 24(2):163–181, v.
5. Kontou-Fili K, Borici-Mazi R, Kapp A, Matjevic LJ, Mitchel FB. Physical urticaria: classification and diagnostic guidelines. An EAACI position paper. Allergy 1997; 52:504–513.
6. Wedi B, Kapp A. Chronic urticaria: assessment of current treatment. Exp Rev Clin Immunol 2005; 1:459–473.
7. Wedi B, Kapp A. Urticaria and angioedema. In: Mahmoudi M, editor. Allergy: Practical Diagnosis and Management. New York: Mc Graw Hill; 2007, pp. 84–94.
8. Wedi B, Kapp A. Evidence-based therapy of chronic urticaria. J Dtsch Dermatol Ges 2007; 5(2):146–157.
9. Wedi B. Urticaria. J Deutsch Dermatol Ges 2008; 6(4):306–317.
10. Zuberbier T, Bindslev-Jensen C, Canonica W et al. EAACI/GALEN/EDF guideline: management of urticaria. Allergy 2006; 61(3):321–331.
11. Siebenhaar F, Weller K, Mlynek A et al. Acquired cold urticaria: clinical picture and update on diagnosis and treatment. Clin Exp Dermatol 2007; 32(3):241–245.

Chapter 5
Allergic Contact Dermatitis

Haw-Yueh Thong and Howard I. Maibach

Abstract Allergic contact dermatitis, an inflammatory skin disease characterized by erythema, edema, vesiculation, and scaling, is a delayed type hypersensitivity reaction following cutaneous exposure to allergenic chemicals.

Keywords Allergic contact dermatitis • Hair dye allergy • Quarternium-15 • Formaldehyde

Case 1

A 40-year-old housewife presented with recurrent, intermittently itchy and stinging rashes on the face. She first noticed the lesions approximately 1 year ago. She had since visited several doctors and received various treatments, but the skin condition had recurred. For each recurrence, her skin was red and scaling, with extreme itching and stinging that was barely tolerable. Each episode tended to last for a week and did not resolve by itself, mandating either topical or systemic corticosteroids. She denied any change in her skin care routine, which included skin cleansing with water followed by "hypoallergenic" skin care products. Because of the skin lesions she had refrained from using any kinds of makeup cosmetics or fragrances for months

The patient's medical history was unremarkable. She denied any occupational and environmental exposures to chemicals. She was not taking any medications and had no known drug allergies. Her family history was significant for hypertension and diabetes mellitus, but there was no family history of atopic dermatitis. She did not smoke or drink alcohol. The review of her systems was otherwise unremarkable

H.-Y. Thong and H.I. Maibach (✉)
Department of Dermatology, University of California,
School of Medicine, San Francisco, CA 94143, USA
e-mail: maibachh@derm.ucsf.edu

M. Mahmoudi (ed.), *Challenging Cases in Allergy and Immunology*,
DOI: 10.1007/978-1-60327-443-2_5,
© Humana Press, a part of Springer Science+Business Media, LLC 2009

The physical examination revealed ill-defined, erythematous patches on the forehead and cheeks with mild scaling. There were no vesicles, discharge, or crusting. Similar patches were also noted on the neck. The eyelids were spared. Her vital signs were within normal limits, and her other physical findings were unremarkable

With the Presented Data What Is your Working Diagnosis?

The recurrent nature of her condition, the poor response to various topical treatments (most likely corticosteroids), and the involvement of forehead and neck might suggest contact dermatitis.

Differential Diagnosis

Seborrheic dermatitis, irritant contact dermatitis (ICD), allergic contact dermatitis (ACD).

Work-Up

1. Detailed history is important in gathering more information once contact dermatitis is suspected. In this patient, detailed history suggests possibly temporal relationship to hair coloring performed monthly to every 6 weeks.
2. Patch testing is the next step to clarify the nature of her condition as suggested by the history. On patch testing, she has positive patch test reactions to paraphenylenediamine (PPD) and paratoluenediamine (PTD).

What Is Your Diagnosis and Why?

The diagnosis is ACD to hair dye. The recurrent and recalcitrant nature of her skin condition is suggestive of contact dermatitis. The location of the skin rash and the history of a temporal relationship between skin eruption and hair coloring strongly suggest ACD to hair dye. Patch testing is the golden standard for the diagnosis of ACD. Her patch test results confirmed the chemicals to which she is allergic to, that is, PPD and PTD, which are chemicals commonly found in hair dye.

Management and Follow-Up

The patient was instructed on ways to dye her hair carefully (avoid direct skin contact with hair dye). On follow-up, her skin lesion cleared completely after 1 year.

Case 2

A 34-year-old female business executive presents with recurrent facial dermatitis of duration of many months. She has visited several doctors and has been told to have seborrheic dermatitis. She has been treated with topical corticosteroids but the skin lesions have never been completely resolved. The patient denies any changes in her diet, cosmetics, medications, or soaps that could account for the dermatitis. Her skin care routine included cleansing with a mild cleanser, followed by hypoallergenic facial cream and then makeup.

The patient's medical history was unremarkable except for a history of allergic rhinitis. She denied any occupational and environmental exposures to chemicals. She denied any food or drug allergies. Her family history was unremarkable. She did not smoke or drink alcohol. The review of her systems was otherwise unremarkable.

On physical examination, there were patchy, low-grade erythema and scaling on the face, involving eyelid, forehead, cheeks, and chin. There were no vesicles, discharge, or crusting. Her vital signs were within normal limits, and her other physical findings were unremarkable.

With the Presented Data What Is Your Working Diagnosis?

The working diagnosis was endogenous and/or exogenous dermatitis. Given the covert nature of her eczema, the lack of history on exposures to chemicals, and the lack of temporal relationship with any event, the diagnosis may be challenging.

Differential Diagnosis

Seborrheic dermatitis, atopic dermatitis, ICD, ACD

Work-Up

1. As described earlier, detailed history is important for further information. In this patient, however, an exhaustive history has failed to document any temporal sequence between the use of cosmetics and onset of rash.
2. Patch testing is the next step to help clarifying the nature of her condition since ACD cannot be excluded. She was patch tested with routine series (to be discussed later) and her own products, and the patch testing revealed positive patch test reactions to formaldehyde and quaternium-15 (formaldehyde releasers) commonly used as preservatives in cosmetics and toiletries including fingernail polishers and

hardeners, antiperspirants, makeup, bubble bath, bath oils, shampoos, creams, mouthwashes, and deodorants.

What Is Your Diagnosis and Why?

The diagnosis is ACD to preservatives. Despite the lack of temporal relationship as described in case 1, the prolonged and overt nature of, and the distribution of, her skin rash is still suggestive of contact dermatitis. Patch testing is the best tool to clarify the presence of ACD. Her positive patch test results were clinically relevant as scrutinization of the labels of her skin care products revealed the presence of formaldehyde and quarternium-15.

Management and Follow-Up

Clinical interventions included teaching patients how to read cosmetic labels and the avoidance of preservatives. On follow-up, her skin condition cleared up in a year.

Discussion

Definition

Contact dermatitis, defined as inflammation of the skin invoked as a result of exposure to an exogenous agent, is generally divided into ICD and ACD. ACD is the clinical definition of an eczematous skin reaction that results from (specifically) delayed type IV hypersensitivity (DTH), which occurs at the site of skin contact with a typical small-molecule allergen (1).

Brief History

ACD was described by Joseph Jadassohn in 1895. He developed patch testing to identify the chemicals to which the patient was allergic. Sulzberger popularized patch testing in the USA in the 1930s. The TRUE Test (thin-layer rapid use epicu-taneous test) is currently the only allergen patch test that has received marketing approval from the US Food and Drug Administration (FDA). The Finn chamber, available since 1970s, has become the standard method for patch testing individuals to chemicals not found in the TRUE test. Commercially prepared allergens in either petrolatum or water are widely utilized.

Prevalence of ACD

ACD is a skin disease that affects around 1–4% of the global population at a considerable cost to society and industry. Studies on contact allergy in the general population have shown that the median prevalence of contact allergy to at least one allergen was 21.2% (range 12.5–40.6%), and the weighted average prevalence was 19.5%, based on data collected on all age groups and from all countries between 1966 and 2007. The most prevalent contact allergens were nickel (8.6%), thimerosal, and fragrance mix (1). The North American Contact Dermatitis Group (NACDG) reported the results of patch testing from January 1, 2001, to December 31, 2002 with an extended screening series of 65 allergens and found that the top ten allergens were nickel sulfate (16.7%), neomycin (11.6%), *Myroxylon pereirae* (balsam of Peru) (11.6%), fragrance mix (10.4%), thimerosal (10.2%), sodium gold thiosulfate (10.2%), quaternium-15 (9.3%), formaldehyde (8.4%), bacitracin (7.9%), and cobalt chloride (7.4%) (2).

New allergens may emerge due to the introduction of numerous new chemicals into the marketplace each year, some of which may eventually turn out to be allergenic under use condition. On the other hand, older allergenic chemicals employed in occupational settings will continue to be a constant source of ACD (3, 4).

Pathophysiology

Almost any chemical (including water) in sufficient concentration and under the right conditions can induce irritation, but typically only certain chemicals are allergens and only a small proportion of people become susceptible to them.

There are more than 3,700 suspected cutaneous allergens (5). The chemicals capable of inducing ACD are typically small (<500 dalton), uncharged, and fairly hydrophobic (5). ACD begins with a sensitization phase, in which molecules pass through the stratum corneum and are processed by Langerhans cells in the epidermis (6). Antigen-coupled Langerhans cells then leave the epidermis and migrate to the regional lymph nodes via the afferent lymphatics, where they present the antigen to naive CD4+ T cells. Only allergenic compounds are capable of inducing CD1a+ CD83+ Langerhans cell migration with partial maturation at subtoxic concentration. The responding T cells are then stimulated via a complex immunologic process to proliferate into memory and effector T cells, which are capable of inducing ACD after repeat exposure to the allergen. The initial sensitization typically takes 10–14 days from initial exposure to a strong contact allergen such as poison ivy, oak, and sumac. However, some individuals may develop specific sensitivity to allergens (e.g., chromate) following years of chronic low-grade exposure.

The elicitation of ACD typically occurs within 24–96 h after rechallenge of sensitized individuals and is typically presented as varying degree of erythema, edema, and vesiculation. CD4+ CCR10+ memory T cells persist in the dermis after ACD clinically resolves.

Clinical Manifestations

Onset

Individuals with presensitized ACD typically develop dermatitis (within a few days of exposure) in areas that were exposed directly to the allergen. Certain allergens (e.g., neomycin) penetrate intact skin poorly, and the onset of dermatitis may be delayed up to a week following exposure. Typically, a minimum of 10 days is required for individuals to develop specific sensitivity to a new contactant. Only potent allergens such as dinitrochlorobenzene (DNCB) sensitize and elicit with a single exposure.

Predisposing Factors

Mirshahpanah and Maibach (7) noted that eczematic skin is more prone to reactivity relative to healthy skin. However, there are numerous endogenous and exogenous factors that influence the development of ACD. Among these, age, gender, ethnicity, atopic constitution, environmental factors, and specific occupational risks have received the most attention in the literature.

Symptoms and Signs

The probability and severity of a reaction depend on the type of exposure and its duration. ACD may bear some similarities to irritant dermatitis but edema, erythema, and vesiculation are often prominent features. Acute ACD is characterized by pruritic papules and vesicles on an erythematous base, while chronic ACD may be manifested as lichenified pruritic plaques. Occasionally, ACD may affect the entire integument (i.e., erythroderma, exfoliative dermatitis). ACD can also complicate other dermatoses as a result of the application of numerous topical agents that then act as sensitizers (e.g., ACD to neomycin in stasis dermatitis), imposing diagnostic challenges to clinicians.

The initial site of dermatitis often provides the best clue regarding the potential cause of ACD. For example, the hands are noted to be the primary body part affected in many of the allergic occupational cases. Other common locations include facial, ear, and neck dermatitis in patients with ACD to chemicals used in hairdressing; and eyelid dermatitis suggestive of ACD to airborne allergens.

Diagnostic Procedures

History-Taking

A detailed history, both before and after patch testing, is crucial in evaluating individuals with ACD. Potential causes of ACD and the materials to which individuals are exposed should be patch tested. However, contact sensitivity cannot be reliably predicted from pretest historical information. Also, the sensitivity and specificity of patch testing are approximately 70%, with a 50% relevance for positive tests (8). Therefore, history is equally important after patch testing to determine whether the materials to which a patient is allergic are partly or wholly responsible for the current dermatitis.

Differential Diagnosis

The differential diagnosis of ACD includes common conditions such as ICD, superficial fungal infection, seborrheic dermatitis, and psoriasis (Table 5.1).

Acute ICD is sometimes easily diagnosed because of the significant erythema, vesicles, and/or bullae that develop in a sharply delineated area within minutes to hours after exposure. In contrast, chronic cumulative ICD may be clinically indistinguishable from ACD. There are no universally reliable clinical features to determine whether an eczema is ICD or ACD. The diagnosis of ICD is one of exclusion due to an absence of diagnostic test, whereas the diagnosis of ACD depends on proper diagnostic patch testing. Prior to patch testing, potassium hydroxide preparation and/or fungal culture to exclude tinea are often indicated for dermatitis of the hands and feet. Skin biopsy may be helpful in excluding other disorders, particularly tinea, psoriasis, cutaneous lymphoma, etc.

Table 5.1 Differential diagnosis of contact dermatitis

Exogenous	Endogenous
Irritant contact dermatitis (frictional, chemical, etc.)	Atopic dermatitis
Allergic contact dermatitis	Nummular dermatitis
	Pompholyx and/or dyshidrotic eczema
Contact urticaria	Hyperkeratotic palmar dermatitis
Tinea	Psoriasis
	Fingertip dermatitis

Patch Testing

Patch testing remains the "golden standard" for the diagnosis of ACD.

Patch testing is also highly recommended in patients suffering from various eczematous conditions considered (partly and entirely) endogenous (Atopica dermatitis, nummular dermatitis, seborrheic dermatitis, asteatotic eczema, stasis dermatitis, leg ulcers, dyshidrotic eczema, psoriasis) due to the fact that in many cases ACD may worsen underlying dermatitis, and the patch test results permit further avoidance of contact allergens in the management of eczematous conditions.

In patch testing, a preparation is applied to a patient's skin under an occlusive patch for 48 h and the skin is evaluated for evidence of erythema, edema, or more severe skin changes occurring 24, 48, or 72 h after removal of the patch. Allergenic materials are thereby identified by producing skin disease on a small scale. Patch testing must be performed by health care providers trained in the proper technique. Most dermatologists can perform patch testing using standard allergens, which can identify relevant allergies in as many as one-half of affected patients.

Individuals with suspected ACD without positive reactions with standard allergens or with chronic dermatitis or relapsing dermatitis, despite avoiding chemicals to which they are allergic (identified on routine patch testing), need additional patch testing with more extensive panels of chemicals. Testing to more allergens increases the accuracy of the diagnosis of ACD. Such extensive patch testing typically is available only in a limited number of dermatology offices and clinics.

Selection of allergens for patch testing requires consideration of the patient's history and access to appropriate environmental contactants. In such cases, aim testing, as opposed to more generalized testing, can be performed (Tables 5.2–5.4)

Positive patch test result mandates wide clinical interpretation. Recently, investigations have become more specific in discussing patch test frequency data. The term *allergic patch test reaction frequency* typically refers to patch test positivity numbers – without attempt to correct for clinical relevance – that is, the clinical disease of ACD, present or past. The number may include the result of false positives and nonreproducible positives from the Excited Skin Syndrome (a hyperirritable skin condition that occurs when multiple concomitant inflammatory skin conditions prevail and is often associated with multiple positive patch test reactions due to the strong positive responses that induce unspecific reactions in contiguous test sites). The fact that *contact allergy* implies true delayed hypersensitivity (a true allergic patch test response) but does not imply clinical relevance has been established. *False positive reactions* can be defined as positive patch test reactions occurring in

Table 5.2 Components of aimed testing

Level I	Routine series (Table 5.3)
Level II	Special series – hairdresser series, plant series, etc. (Table 5.4)
Level III	Patient's products that can be tested undiluted – moisturizers, lotions, etc.
Level IV	Patient's products – often only minimally characterized – Material Safety Data Sheets (MSDS)

Table 5.3 Routine series (North American Series, Dormer Laboratories, Inc., Toronto, ON, Canada)

Allergens	Concentration (%)
Benzocaine	5.0 petrolatum (pet)
2-Mercaptobenzothiazole (MBT)	1.0 pet
Colophony	20.0 pet
4-Phenylenediamine base	1.0 pet
Imidazolidinyl urea (Germall 115)	2.0 pet
Cinnamic aldehyde (Cinnamyl)	1.0 pet
Amerchol L 101	50.0 pet
Carba mix	3.0 pet
Neomycin sulfate	20.0 pet
Thiuram mix	1.0 pet
Formaldehyde	1.0 aqueous (aq)
Ethylenediamine dihydrochloride	1.0 pet
Epoxy resin	1.0 pet
Quaternium-15 (Dowicil 200)	2.0 pet
4-t-Butylphenolformaldehyde resin	1.0 pet
Mercapto mix	1.0 pet
N-isopropyl-N-phenyl-4-phenylenediamine	0.1 pet
Potassium dichromate	0.25 pet
Balsam Peru	25.0 pet
Nickelsulfate hexahydrate	2.5 pet
Diazolidinylurea (Germall II)	1.0 pet
DMDM hydantoin	1.0 pet
Bacitracin	20.0 pet
Mixed dialkyl thiourea	1.0 pet
Cl+ Me-isothiazolinone (Kathon CG, 100 ppm)	0.01 aq
Paraben mix	12.0 pet
Methyldibromoglutaronitrile (MDBGN)	0.5 pet
Fragrance mix	8.0 pet
Glutaraldehyde	0.5 pet
2-Bromo-2-nitropropane-1,3-diol (Bronopol)	0.5 pet
Sesquiterpene lactone mix	0.1 pet
Fragrance mix II	14.0 pet
Propylene glycol	30.0 aq
2-Hydroxy-4-methoxybenzophenone (Benzophenone 3)	3.0 pet
4-Chloro-3,5-xylenol (PCMX)	1.0 pet
Ethyleneurea, melamine formaldehyde mix	5.0 pet
Iodopropynyl butyl carbamate	0.2 pet
Disperse Blue 106/124 Mix	1.0 pet
Ethyl acrylate	0.1 pet
Glyceryl monothioglycolate (GMTG)	1.0 pet
Toluenesulfonamide formaldehyde resin	10.0 pet
Methyl methacrylate	2.0 pet
Cobalt (II) chloride hexahydrate	1.0 pet
Tixocortal-21-pivalate	0.1 pet
Budesonide	0.01 pet
Compositae mix	5.0 pet
Hydrocortisone-17-butyrate	1.0 pet
Dimethylol dihydroxyethyleneurea (Fix CPN)	4.5 aq
Cocamidopropylbetaine	1.0 aq
Triamcinolone acetonide	1.0 pet

Table 5.4 Special series

Extended routine series
Topical medicaments
Skin care/cosmetics
Antimicrobials
Acrylates
Dental/adhesives
Nails
Printing
Baking
Corticosteroids
Dental screen
Disinfectants
Epoxy
Fragrances and flavors
Hairdressing
Industrial biocides
Isocyanates
Leg ulcer
Medicament
Metals
Metals plus
Oil and cooling fluids
Opthalmics
Photography chemicals
Plants
Plastics and glues
Rubber
Shoe
Textile, color, and finish
Vehicles/emulsifiers
Photo allergens with/without ultraviolet light testing
Sunscreen with/without ultraviolet light testing
Environmentals/material safety data sheet chemicals
Immediate testing

the absence of contact allergy (9) and can be caused by technical errors, a misinterpretation of the test results, etc. False negative reactions can be defined as negative patch test reactions occurring in the presence of contact allergy, causes of which include insufficient penetration of allergen, too early reading or testing in an "anergy" phase, systemic treatment with corticosteroids, etc. (9).

The most important aspect in the interpretation of diagnostic test results is an assessment of the clinical relevance of positive patch test findings to the diagnosis. The investigator must establish that positive patch test results are consistent with a history of exposure to a particular chemical in a product and must exclude other possible environmental exposure conditions. Next, the location of the present dermatitis must correspond to the site of contact with the putative offending chemical. Finally, the patch test concentration must be nonirritating, as demonstrated by a dose-response effect when dilution of the putative allergen is employed. In essence, clinicians may follow defined algorithms to establish the relation (causality) between a positive patch test and the likelihood of clinical ACD (Table 5.5) (10).

Table 5.5 Algorithm to the diagnosis of clinically relevant ACD (10)

History of exposure
Appropriate morphology
Positive patch test to a nonirritating concentration of the putative allergen
Repeat patch test if excited skin syndrome is operative (more than one positive patch test)
Employ serial dilution patch testing to distinguish allergen from marginal irritant
Employ provocative use test (PUT) or repeat open application test (ROAT)[a]
Resolution of dermatitis

[a] For individuals who develop weak or 1+ positive reactions to a chemical, the provocative use test (PUT) or repeat open application test (ROAT) is useful in determining whether the reaction is significant. ROAT is most useful when an individual has a 1+ reaction to a chemical found in a leave-on consumer product

The evidence-based diagnosis of relevance can also be improved by requestioning the patient in the light of the test results, performing a worksite/home visit, seeking cross-reacting substances, considering concomitant/simultaneous sensitization and indirect/accidental/seasonal contact, obtaining information about environmental allergens from lists, textbooks, and the product's manufacturer, performing chemical analysis of products, and sequential testing with the allergens and the suspected products (testing with extract, ROAT, PUT, etc.) (10).

Management/Treatment

Clinical management of ACD includes symptomatic treatment (e.g., cold compresses for vesicular dermatitis, oral sedating antihistamines for pruritus) and/or topical or systemic corticosteroids. Topical corticosteroids are the mainstay of treatment, with the strength and potency of the topical corticosteroid appropriate to the body site. Systemic corticosteroids or other immunosuppressive medications (e.g., azathioprine) may be occasionally needed for widespread and severe chronic dermatitis, such as ACD, due to airborne allergens such as feverfew (Parthenium hysterophores). Topical immunomodulators may be prescribed for corticosteroid-resistant ACD or cases of ACD when they offer safety advantages over topical corticosteroids (e.g., for chronic ACD on eyelid to avoid steroid-induced glaucoma or cataracts).

In any case, the cause of ACD must be identified or else the patient is at increased risk for chronic or recurrent dermatitis. ACD to chemicals that are ubiquitous in the environment often carries a chronic and relapsing course.

Not all ACDs clear completely when the responsible contactant is apparently eliminated. There are patients who never recover for unclear reasons. Among the potential contributing factors are the possibilities that the repair capacity of skin can be overwhelmed, or that contact dermatitis (allergic or irritant) may enter a self-perpetuating and recurrent cycle by virtue of the fact that the ACD triggered an underlying propensity to endogenous eczema, or that individuals may develop new allergies. Efforts must be taken to clarify and verify the source of ACD and the presence of any endogenous factors. It is sometimes necessary to repeat patch testing in such cases.

To prevent recurrence of ACD, instruct patients thoroughly concerning allergen(s) and the types of products likely to contain allergen(s). The Contact Allergan Replacement Database (CARD) of the American Contact Dermatitis Society allows the physician to create a list of products free of allergens to which the patient is allergic (www.contactderm.org).

Conclusion

ACD is a frequent and vexing dermatologic problem. While the disease has probably plagued humans for millennia, its clinical recognition by patch testing is barely a century old. The management of ACD lies in identifying its cause correctly and thoroughly instructing the patient to avoid the responsible allergen(s). Legislation can be an effective tool in the prevention of contact dermatitis by mandating the labeling of cosmetics and household products. Occupational safety has a long tradition of setting different types of rules and limitations to prevent hazardous exposure, and some focus on hazardous skin exposure. The advent of experimental animal models and noninvasive bioengineering methods on human testing will provide useful information on the pathophysiology of ACD, which will help to refine our current practices in the management and prevention of ACD. General references for ACD are listed (4, 6, 9).

Questions

1. The proper management of ACD includes which of the following?

   (a) Use systemic corticosteroids as the first-line therapy for all types of ACD.
   (b) Topical corticosteroids are often not necessary because the clinical response is poor.
   (c) Instruct patients thoroughly concerning allergen(s) and the types of products likely to contain allergen(s).
   (d) Repeat patch testing for patients who do not recover despite the avoidance of allergen(s).

Answers: (c), (d)

2. Choose *one* correct answer:

   (a) It is always easy to distinguish ICD from ACD based on clinical presentation.
   (b) Patch testing is the golden standard for the diagnosis of ACD.
   (c) Provocative use test (PUT)/repeat open application test (ROAT) is the golden standard for the diagnosis of ICD.

(d) Skin biopsy is often necessary for the definite diagnosis of ACD.

Answer: (b)

3. Choose *one* correct answer:

   (a) Almost any chemical in sufficient concentration and under the right conditions can induce ACD.
   (b) Repeat patch test is not necessary if excited skin syndrome is operative.
   (c) Serial dilution patch testing is not necessary to distinguish allergen from marginal irritant.
   (d) PUT or ROAT have limited value in verifying the clinical relevance of positive patch test results.

Answer: (a)

4. The assessment to reach the diagnosis of clinically relevant ACD includes the following:

   (a) History of exposure
   (b) Appropriate morphology
   (c) Positive patch test to a nonirritating concentration of the putative allergen
   (d) Resolution of dermatitis
   (e) All of the above

Answer: (e)

5. Significant erythema, vesicles, and/or bullae that develop in a sharply delineated area within minutes to hours after exposure to a contactant are more likely to be

   (a) ACD
   (b) ICD
   (c) Seborrheic dermatitis
   (d) Atopic dermatitis

Answer: (b)

References

1. Thyssen, J.P., Linneberg, A., Menné, T., and Johansen, J.D. (2007) The epidemiology of contact allergy in the general population – Prevalence and main findings. *Contact Derm* **57**(5), 287–299.
2. Pratt, M.D., Belsito, D.V., Deleo, V.A., Fowler, J.F., Jr., Fransway, A.F., Maibach, H.I., Marks, J.G., Mathias, C.G., Rietschel, R.L., Sasseville, D., Sherertz, E.F., Storrs, F.J., Taylor, J.S., and Zug, K. (2004) North American Contact Dermatitis Group patch-test results, 2001–2002 study period. *Dermatitis* **15**(4), 176–183.
3. Nguyen, S.H., Dang, T.P., MacPherson, C., Maibach, H., and Maibach, H.I. (2008) Prevalence of patch test results from 1970 to 2002 in a multi-centre population in North America (NACDG). *Contact Derm* **58**(2), 101–106.

4. Kanerva, L., Elsner, P., Wahlberg, J.E., and Maibach, H.I., eds. (2000) Handbook of Occupational Dermatology. Berlin, Germany: Springer.
5. de Groot, A.C. (1994) Patch testing: Test Concentrations and Vehicles for 3700 Allergens, 2nd ed. Amsterdam, The Netherlands: Elsevier.
6. Rietschel, R.L. and Fowler, J.F., Jr. (2008) Fisher's Contact Dermatitis, 6th ed. Hamilton, ON: BC Decker.
7. Mirshahpanah, P. and Maibach, H.I. (2007) Relationship of patch test positivity in a general versus an eczema population. *Contact Derm* **56**(3), 125–130.
8. Nethercott, J.R. (1990) Practical problem in the use of patch testing in the evaluation of patients with contact dermatitis. *Curr Probl Dermatol* **2**, 97–123.
9. Lachapelle, J.-M. and Maibach, H.I., eds. (2003) Patch Testing and Prick Testing. A Practical Guide. Berlin, Germany: Springer.
10. Ale, S. and Maibach, H.I. (1995) Clinical relevance in allergic contact dermatitis. *Derm Beruf Umwelt* **43**, 119–121.

Chapter 6
Hypersensitivity Pneumonitis

Tracy Prematta, Jennifer Toth, and Timothy Craig

Abstract Hypersensitivity pneumonitis (HP), also known as extrinsic allergic alveolitis, encompasses a group of pulmonary disorders characterized by immune response to a variety of antigens derived from medications, chemicals, microorganisms, and plant and animal proteins. The first cases of HP were described in occupational or hobbyist settings, but HP secondary to home exposures is becoming more common. The clinical presentation has a wide range, from acute HP, which often presents as an acute febrile illness, to chronic HP, with insidious progression of dyspnea and systemic complaints. The development of HP requires TH1 cell, cytotoxic lymphocyte, and IgG immune responses. TH2 cells and IgE are not involved. The diagnosis of HP must be made clinically with consistent history and known appropriate antigen exposure. Supportive evidence can be gathered from serologic tests (including serum precipitans), radiographic evaluation, bronchoscopy with BAL, biopsy, and natural or direct antigen inhalation challenges. Although systemic corticosteroids may improve acute exacerbations, removal from the inciting antigen is paramount in the appropriate treatment of HP. Unfortunately, irreversible pulmonary fibrosis can develop in long-standing HP leading to significant morbidity and mortality, highlighting the need for early detection and antigen avoidance.

Keywords Allergic contract dermatitis • Hair dye allergy • Quarternium-15 • Fomaldehyde

Case 1

A normally healthy 13-year-old female was admitted to the hospital for evaluation of 3–4 months of progressive cough, dyspnea, anorexia, and weight loss. She had no significant illnesses prior to these symptoms, but had been treated with antibiotics multiple times for "bronchitis" in the preceding 3 months. The patient lived

T. Prematta (✉), J. Toth, and T. Craig

Division of Allergy, Department of Medicine, Penn State University, Hershey, PA, USA
e-mail: tprematta@hmc.psu.edu

M. Mahmoudi (ed.), *Challenging Cases in Allergy and Immunology*,
DOI: 10.1007/978-1-60327-443-2_6,
© Humana Press, a part of Springer Science+Business Media, LLC 2009

with her mother, father, and younger sister. She had a dog, cat, and two lovebirds. Their house was approximately 25-years old, and although there was no visible mold, it was noted that the basement had been flooded several times. There was no history of recent travel and no known exposures to tuberculosis (TB). She denied tobacco, alcohol, and illicit drug use. Immunizations were up to date. Family history was unremarkable.

She presented to her primary care physician's office again, and she was noted to be febrile, tachycardic, and tachypneic with oxygen saturations in the low 80s that improved to mid-90s with 2L nasal cannula. On physical exam, she had obvious dyspnea with supraclavicular retractions. On auscultation, she had audible bibasilar crackles. She was admitted to the hospital. Lab tests performed during her stay were significant for a white blood cell count (WBC) of 21,000 (normal level (nl) 4,800–10,800) with 75% neutrophils (nl 35–71%), 15% lymphocytes (nl 25–45%), and 10% eosinophils (nl 0–6%). A complete metabolic profile (CMP), lactate dehydrogenase (LDH), uric acid, urinalysis, and brain natriuretic peptide (BNP) were all normal. A PPD (purified protein derivative, screening test for exposure toTB) was also placed and found to be nonreactive. The initial chest X-ray (CXR) revealed bilateral interstitial infiltrates. An echocardiogram was also performed, which showed normal cardiac anatomy and function.

With the Presented Data What Is Your Working Diagnosis?

Given her initial presentation, a broad differential diagnosis was entertained including malignancy, congestive heart failure, pulmonary renal syndrome, cystic fibrosis, and α-1 antitrypsin deficiency. All these seemed unlikely with her unremarkable past medical and family history and test results. Infectious causes were also considered: tuberculosis was unlikely without a known exposure and nonreactive PPD; pertussis should have been improving; community-acquired pneumonia seemed the most likely given her fever, tachypnea, and abnormal chest radiograph, and it became the working diagnosis.

Additional History and Work-Up

The patient was treated for 5 days as an inpatient with IV levofloxacin and azithromycin for community-acquired pneumonia. She improved significantly and was able to be discharged to home. Within 6 h of returning home, however, her symptoms returned, so she was readmitted to the hospital and had additional work-up performed. Lab tests were remarkable for a positive rheumatoid factor (RF) and elevated IgG. The remainder of her lab tests, including IgA, IgM, IgE, antinuclear antibody (ANA), antineutrophil cytoplasmic antibody (ANCA), antiglomerular basement membrane antibody (anti-GBM), α-1 antitrypsin, and sweat chloride test, were all normal. High-resolution CT of the chest was significant for bilateral ground-glass opacities. A pulmonary function test (PFT) showed a restrictive pattern with decreased D_{LCO} (diffusing capacity of the lungs for carbon monoxide). Bronchoscopy with bronchoalveolar lavage (BAL) was also performed. Culture of BAL fluid yielded no growth, and flow cytometry revealed a lymphocytosis with a CD4+/CD8+ ratio of 0.6 (nl 0.5–6.4, based on values from healthy nonsmokers). Commercial peripheral blood HP panels were sent and were negative; however, serum precipitan testing to lovebirds was positive.

What Is Your Diagnosis and Why?

The patient was diagnosed with a hypersensitivity pneumonitis (HP) secondary to lovebird exposure. Her diagnosis was supported by the positive serum precipitan testing to lovebirds, as well the findings on CXR, CT scan, PFT, and clinical presentation. She was discharged to a family member's house and placed on an extended steroid taper for about 6 weeks. The lovebirds were removed and the home was extensively cleaned. She was able to return home, and at the completion of treatment, she was asymptomatic with normal spirometry.

Case 2

A 61-year-old Hispanic female presented for evaluation of pulmonary fibrosis. The symptoms first began 1½ years ago with fatigue, dyspnea, cough, dizziness, and headache. Overtime, the patient also developed an intermittent productive cough and a 35-lb weight loss, although her appetite had not decreased. Review of systems was otherwise negative. Past medical history was significant for hypothyroidism, for which she was being treated. She emigrated from Puerto Rico 16 years before, had no known exposure to TB, and had multiple PPDs placed, which were all negative. She had worked in a Beef Jerky Plant for the last 5 years, packing and disposing expired products. She had smoked 3–4 cigarettes per day for about 20 years, but quit over 20 years before. She had a parrot and lovebird at home, and lived by a neighbor who owned chickens. Family history was remarkable for multiple family members with asthma.

The patient was first evaluated by her primary care physician and noted to have decreased breath sounds with inspiratory and expiratory crackles. A chest radiograph was ordered and showed marked interstitial disease and honeycombing pattern in the periphery. Subsequently, she underwent a series of tests including a CT scan, bronchoscopy, and video-assisted thorascopic surgery (VATS) with lung biopsy. BAL fluid was negative for malignancy and infections. Cell count revealed 36.7% alveolar macrophages (nl 66.6–97%), 40.8% lymphocytes (nl 2–29.3%), and 22.5% neutrophils (nl 0–8.4%) (normal values based on healthy former smokers). Biopsy revealed organizing pneumonia with nonspecific interstitial pneumonitis (NSIP) versus usual interstitial pneumonia (UIP – formerly idiopathic pulmonary fibrosis).

Three months after her initial presentation, she was hospitalized with pneumonia and treated with levofloxacin. She was discharged to home on supplemental oxygen and was started on prednisone.

With the Presented Data, What Is Your Working Diagnosis?

At the time of presentation, the patient already had biopsy results consistent with NSIP versus UIP, but this did not rule out correctable causes of interstitial lung disease such as collagen vascular disease or HP. Thus, her working diagnosis became interstitial lung disease and she underwent further evaluation for a specific cause.

Additional Work-Up

PFT was performed and the patient was found to have a restrictive pattern with an FVC (forced vital capacity) of 1.06L (31% predicted), FEV1 (forced expiratory volume in 1 s) of 1.05 L (40% predicted), and a normal FEV1/FVC ratio (100%). She had no response to bronchodilators. Attempts at obtaining a D_{LCO} were unsuccessful. High-resolution CT showed diffuse interstitial thickening and mild bronchiectasis bilaterally, with honeycombing in the lung bases, and calcification in the right lung base, possible secondary to granulomas (Fig. 6.1). Complete blood count (CBC), CMP, ANA, ANCA, anti-GBM, and erythrocyte sedimentation rates (ESR) were all

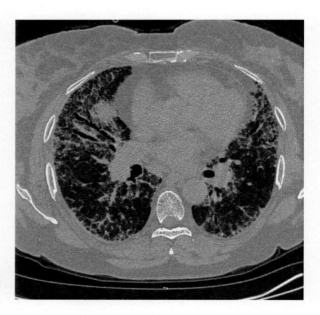

Fig. 6.1 Patient no. 2, high-resolution CT consistent with chronic HP

found to be normal. A commercial HP panel was sent and found to be negative. However, testing of IgG precipitans to parrot, lovebirds, and chicken was also ordered and was found to be strongly positive to both lovebirds and parrots.

What Is Your Diagnosis and Why?

This patient was diagnosed with end-stage HP secondary to lovebird and parrot exposure, supported by evidence of pulmonary fibrosis with positive serum precipitan testing. She was placed on prednisone and initially had a promising response. Unfortunately, her symptoms relapsed whenever prednisone was tapered, despite removing the birds and moving to her daughter's home. She also had persistent oxygen requirement and restrictive defects on PFT. After multiple attempts to wean prednisone, she was eventually referred for lung transplant.

Overview

Hypersensitivity pneumonitis (HP), also known as extrinsic allergic alveolitis, encompasses a group of pulmonary diseases caused by immune reactions to medications, low molecular weight chemicals, and organic compounds (derived from microorganisms and animal and plant products) in susceptible individuals. It was originally described as an occupational lung disease, with Farmer's lung being the classic example, but a growing number of cases caused by home exposures have been described. Diagnosis of HP requires a high degree of clinical suspicion followed by diagnostic testing. Identifying the causal agent can be challenging; however, it is critical in order to appropriately care for the patient, as the mainstay of treatment for HP is removal from the offending antigen.

Epidemiology

Given that HP is actually a group of disorders mediated by a large number of antigens, a true prevalence is difficult to determine. In addition, the clinical presentation can vary significantly, and exposed but asymptomatic individuals can have findings consistent with HP on serology testing without clinical disease. HP variability is also affected by the specific workplace environment, country, county, climate, and season. Finally, most of the epidemiologic studies that have been performed have looked at occupational causes of HP. Only one study, performed in the UK in 2007, has investigated a general population-based incidence. This study found the incidence of HP to be approximately 600 new cases per year with nearly equal rates in men and women (1).

Clinical Signs and Symptoms

The clinical presentation of HP can vary considerably, depending on the nature of the inciting antigen, the intensity of the exposure, and the individual's immune response (2). Generally, HP can present in an acute, subacute, or chronic way; however, these presentations can overlap considerably and the same individual may present with more than one presentation (Table 6.1).

Acute Presentation

The acute presentation of HP can often be mistaken for an acute pulmonary infection such as bronchitis, pneumonia, or a viral illness. Patients with the acute form will often present with fever, chills, nonproductive cough, dyspnea, myalgia, and fatigue. The onset of symptoms typically occurs within 4–8 h of exposure and will recur with repeated exposures, although the severity of symptoms can vary. The symptoms will usually spontaneously subside within 12 h of being removed from the antigen; however, they may sometimes last for several days. With repeated exposures, the individual may also develop progressive dyspnea, anorexia, and weight loss. Physical exam findings during an attack often include fever, dyspnea, and crackles on auscultation; wheezing is not usually present. If the individual is examined between attacks, the physical exam may be completely normal (2, 3).

Subacute Presentation

The subacute form of HP can be particularly difficult to diagnose as it can imitate a variety of other conditions. Although the patient may initially develop fever, cough, and malaise that can resemble bronchitis or pneumonia, the respiratory symptoms continue to progress over weeks to months. The cough may become productive, and at times, individuals will also have worsening fatigue, arthralgias, and myalgias. The slowly progressive course may also be accompanied by acute attacks of respiratory symptoms that may correspond to periods of particularly high

Table 6.1 Clinical presentation of HP

Stage	Symptoms	Physical exam
Acute	Fever, cough, dyspnea, myalgia, fatigue	Fever, dyspnea, crackles
Subacute	Cough, fatigue, myalgia, arthralgia, episodes of acute exacerbations	Low-grade fever (if present), Crackles ± wheezing and rhonchi
Chronic	Nonproductive cough, Progressive dyspnea, anorexia, weight loss	Diffuse bilateral crackles, possible digital clubbing

antigen exposure (4). Fever is not usually present on physical exam, although, when present, it is of low grade. On auscultation, crackles, along with wheezing and rhonchi, may be heard (3).

Chronic Presentation

Patients often present late in the chronic form of HP. They will usually report progressive dyspnea with or without exertion, nonproductive cough, malaise, anorexia, and weight loss. Unlike the other forms of HP, these patients do not have sudden severe episodes or fevers and may even have developed irreversible pulmonary fibrosis (4). On physical exam, they will typically be found to have diffuse bilateral crackles; wheezes or rhonchi are rare. Occasionally, they may have digital clubbing, which indicates a severe form of the disease (3).

Pathophysiology

The exact mechanisms involved in the pathophysiology of HP have not been fully delineated. It appears that both cellular and humoral immune responses are involved, with proliferation of both CD8+ cytotoxic lymphocytes and IgG being necessary for the development of disease. Recent evidence indicates that HP is a delayed-type hypersensitivity reaction, with a TH1 cell response being necessary to develop disease and a TH2 response being protective (5).

In the acute phase of HP, it is hypothesized that an inhaled antigen is deposited in the lower airway, where it is bound by a specific IgG antibody, leading to the initiation of complement and activation of macrophages. Activated macrophages, in turn, produce a variety of chemokines and cytokines that begin the inflammatory cascade. Leukocytes, predominantly neutrophils, are first attracted to the area, with the peak influx about 48 h after initial exposure (5). T lymphocytes as well as additional macrophages are attracted to the area within 48–72 h, associated with an increase in inflammatory mediators (5). IL-1 and TNF-α, pyrogens produced by macrophages, lead to the development of fever. Macrophages also generate IL-6 that contributes to the differentiation of B cells into plasma cells and the development of CD8+ cells into cytotoxic T lymphocytes. Finally, macrophages promote TH1 cells and the delayed-hypersensitivity response by producing IL-12 and macrophage inflammatory protein α1 (MIP-1α). IL-12 influences the differentiation of TH0 to TH1 cells (5). MIP-1α acts as a chemotactic factor for lymphocytes and macrophages and increases the differentiation of TH0 cells to TH1 lymphocytes (6).

In the next phase of HP, macrophages in the lung tissue develop into epithelioid and multinucleated giant cells, producing noncaseating granulomas that are surrounded by lymphoid follicles containing plasma cells. Interestingly, in mouse models, the activation of macrophages and development of granulomas are dependent on IFN-γ, produced by CD4+ TH1 lymphocytes. CD4+ TH1 lymphocytes also express CD40 on their surface, which is critical for the development of B cells into plasma cells and production of local specific antibodies (6).

The final phase of HP is marked by the development of pulmonary fibrosis and angiogenesis. These changes are mediated by a variety of different cell types, including myofibroblasts that are found in the extracellular matrix and deposit collagen and proteoglycans. TGF-β, produced by activated macrophages, also induces fibrosis and angiogenesis. Mast cells, of the connective tissue type, are found in the BAL fluid and interstitial tissue of both human and mouse models of HP. These mast cells produce a variety of cytokines that recruit monocytes and lymphocytes and promote fibrosis (6).

Factors Affecting Development of HP

Even with what is known about the pathophysiology of HP, it is not understood why there is such a wide range of reactions to antigens: ranging from no symptoms to asthma to HP. A combination of antigen characteristics, other environmental exposures, and specific host characteristics appear to play a role.

Although antigens from a large variety of sources have been implicated in the development of HP (Table 6.2), most share the characteristics of being approximately

Table 6.2 Examples of antigens associated with the development of HP

Antigen group	Examples	Potential sources
Animal protein	Avian proteins; cat hair; rodent urine	Pigeon, duck, turkey, chicken, parrot, lovebird, parakeet; cat; gerbil or rat urine
Insect protein	Silkworm larvae; *Sitophila granarius*	Cocoon fluff; wheat flour
Plants	Tobacco leaves; coffee or tea dust; pine saw dust	Tobacco dust; coffee bean dust or tea leaves; sawdust
Bacteria	*Faeni rectivirgula; Thermoactinomyces candidus or viridis; Mycobacterium avium complex; Bacillus cereus or Klebsiella oxytoca*	Moldy hay; mushroom compost; hot tub, cleaning agents; cool mist humidifiers
Fungi	*Alternaria* spp.; *Penicillium brevi-compactum; Cladosporium* spp.; *Aureobasidium pullulans; Epicoccum nigrum*	Moldy wood dust; moldy hay; sauna water; moldy water in heating, ventilation, or air conditioning system; moldy basement shower
Amoebae	*Acanthamoeba castellani, Naegleria gruberi*	Contaminated ventilation system
Chemicals	Toluene diisocyanate; pyrethrum; trimellitic anhydride	Varnish, casting, lacquer, polyurethane foam; insecticide; plastics industry
Medications	Fluoxetine, β-blockers, HMG-CoA reductase inhibitors, amiodarone, cyclosporine, sulfasalazine	Specific medications

Adapted from (2) (not a complete list)

1 μm in diameter and able to reach the distal airway. Some are able to activate complement directly, while others contain toxins that can both induce inflammation as well as modify the host's immune response (2). Other environmental conditions and exposures also appear to play a role in the development of HP. Different climates, particularly wet climates, can be associated with a higher risk of HP. Exposures to Mycoplasma, Chlamydia, and viruses have been hypothesized to play a role in the development of HP (4). Finally, cigarette smoking actually seems to be protective against the development of HP, but it does not stop the progression of HP if it is already present. Multiple hypotheses have been developed to explain this, most centering on the downregulation of alveolar macrophage response to inhaled particles in smokers (2).

Finally, a variety of genetic and molecular differences appear to influence an individual's susceptibility to HP. Increased frequency of the TNFA2 allele, an allele associated with higher production of TNF-α, has been documented in patients with Farmer's lung than in controls (7). In pigeon breeders, increased frequency of HLA-DRB1*1305, HLA-DQB1*0501, and TNF-α (308) promoter has been found in patients with disease than in those without disease (8). With further study, additional genetic and molecular differences may be found that add to the understanding of why certain individuals develop HP.

Work-Up

There is no one definitive test to establish HP; therefore, the diagnosis must be made clinically by combining patient symptoms, history of antigen exposure, and supporting diagnostic tests (Table 6.3). Guidelines for the diagnosis of HP were

Table 6.3 Diagnostic tests

Test	Most common findings in HP
Inflammatory markers	CRP, ESR, WBC – elevated in acute attacks
Rheumatologic markers	ANA, RF – positive in some subacute or chronic cases
Serum immunoglobulins	Elevation of IgG and occasionally other isotypes, but not IgE
Arterial blood gas	Hypoxemia and respiratory alkalosis in acute attacks
Serum precipitans	+IgG, IgA, or IgM precipitans if correct antigen and technique are used
Chest radiograph	Acute – bilateral interstitial infiltrates Subacute – reticulonodular pattern Chronic – fibrosis and honeycombing
High-resolution CT	Acute – ground glass opacities, micronodules Subacute – linear shadows, small nodules Chronic – interstitial fibrosis (upper and mid-lung zones)
Pulmonary function test	Restrictive pattern with decreased D_{LCO}
BAL fluid analysis	CD8+ lymphocytosis
Biopsy	Peribronchial pneumonitis with interstitial infiltrates of lymphocytes and plasma cells

proposed in 1997. These suggest that HP can be diagnosed if the patient meets four major and two minor criteria and other diseases have been ruled out. The major criteria include symptoms compatible with HP; evidence of exposure to appropriate antigen by history or lab testing; CXR or high-resolution CT scan findings consistent with HP; lymphocytosis of BAL fluid*; pulmonary histologic changes consistent with HP*; and reproduction of symptoms and lab abnormalities with exposure to the suspected environment (* = if performed). Minor criteria include bibasilar rales; decreased D_{LCO}; and arterial hypoxemia, at rest or with exertion (9). Unfortunately, these guidelines have been found to be more useful for the diagnosis of acute HP, as subacute and chronic forms may not meet all of these criteria.

Laboratory Evaluation

In the acute form of HP, nonspecific markers of inflammation such as ESR, CRP, and leukocyte count can be elevated. The leukocytosis is typically neutrophil predominant, but eosinophilia as high as 20% has been reported (3). These elevations are less likely to be found in the subacute and chronic forms. Serologic findings that can occur in later stages of HP include a positive rheumatoid factor and ANA. Elevation of serum IgG levels has been commonly described, and elevations in all other isotypes, except IgE, have also been documented.

Serum precipitan testing can be performed to confirm the presence of antibody to specific antigen. Most commonly, the precipitating antibodies are IgG, but IgA and IgM have also been reported. Unfortunately, commercial screening tests for serum precipitating antibodies are of limited usefulness, as they typically test for a small number of antigens that are usually associated with occupational HP. Thus, they are often not valuable for diagnosing HP induced by a home exposure (10). In cases where HP is suspected and commercial testing is negative, it is beneficial to obtain samples from the causal environment and test for precipitating antibodies to those specific antigens. Unfortunately, serum precipitin testing is limited by its lack of specificity, as up to 50% of exposed but asymptomatic individuals may have a positive test (3). In addition, a negative test does not necessarily rule out HP, as the correct antigen and technique must be used (10).

Radiographic Evaluation

Both chest radiography as well as high-resolution CT can be used in the diagnosis of HP. A variety of abnormalities have been described for both, as findings vary depending on the condition of the patient. Chest radiography, in acute HP, most commonly shows bilateral interstitial infiltrates; hilar lymphadenopathy may be seen in approximately 50% of these patients (10).Chest radiography may also be normal, especially if taken between episodes. In subacute HP, nonspecific reticulonodular

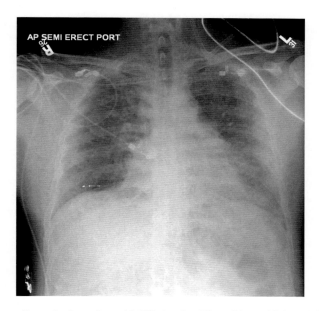

Fig. 6.2 Chest radiograph of a patient with HP, showing bilateral interstitial opacities, and alveolar opacity in the retrocardiac region, consistent with diffuse interstitial pneumonitis

patterns are more likely to be found (4). In chronic HP, chest radiography may reveal diffuse fibrosis and honeycombing (4) (Fig. 6.2). In general, high-resolution CT is more sensitive for the evaluation of HP. In the acute phase, patchy ground-glass opacities, bilateral centrilobular micronodules, and evidence of air trapping can be found (3, 4). In subacute HP, linear shadows and small nodules develop giving the reticulonodular appearance on chest radiography (3). Finally, chronic HP is characterized by interstitial fibrosis of the upper and mid-lung zones, helping to differentiate it from UIP. Pleural effusions and lymphadenopathy are rare, except for acute hilar lymphadenopathy as indicated earlier (3).

Pulmonary Function Testing

PFTs are also helpful in the assessment of HP. Classically, a restrictive pattern with decreased diffusion capacity is seen. The restrictive pattern is indicated by a decreased FEV1 and FVC, with preservation of the FEV1/FVC ratio. Early in the disease, FVC may actually be normal unless taken during an acute attack. However, with progression of disease, the restrictive findings progress and become fixed (2, 3). In addition, mixed obstructive/restrictive patterns have also been observed, particularly in the subacute form, which can lead to misdiagnosis of asthma or chronic obstructive pulmonary disease (10). Patients with HP also have abnormal diffusion capacity, indicated by a decreased D_{LCO}. This tends to be a more sensitive indicator of HP, especially early in the disease, and a better predictor of desaturation with exercise (10).

Invasive Testing

More invasive diagnostic procedures may be warranted in the work-up of HP if the diagnosis is unclear, the patient fails to respond to antigen avoidance, or other treatable diseases are suspected (4). Bronchoscopy with BAL and/or transbronchial biopsy is usually the first step if more invasive testing is pursued. BAL and biopsy can help exclude infections, malignancy, and other clinical entities such as sarcoidosis and alveolar hemorrhage (3, 10). If the information obtained from BAL and transbronchial biopsy is not sufficient to diagnose HP, VATS can be performed. VATS provides much larger tissue samples that are sometimes needed to rule out other diseases such as vasculitic processes (10). In general, VATS is safe, but should probably be avoided in patients with an FVC < 40% predicted or a supplemental oxygen requirement (4). VATS has essentially replaced open lung biopsy, as open biopsy has equivalent diagnostic accuracy but is associated with more complications (4).

BAL Fluid Analysis and Histology

Findings from the earlier invasive procedures can be valuable in the diagnosis of HP. BAL fluid analysis will typically reveal a CD8+ lymphocytosis, with a CD4+/CD8+ ratio of less than 1 (2). This is in contrast to sarcoidosis, which typically has a CD4+ lymphocytosis. However, like the clinical presentation and other diagnostic tests, the findings of BAL fluid analysis can vary with time. For instance, neutrophils tend to predominate if the sample is taken after an acute antigen exposure. Also, as the disease progresses to more chronic forms, the CD4+/CD8+ ratio increases. It is hypothesized that CD8+ lymphocytes may actually be protective against the development of fibrosis, whereas CD4+ lymphocytes may promote pulmonary fibrosis (4).

Histologic findings from lung biopsy can also vary depending on the stage of disease and the intensity and type of antigen exposure. Historically, a classic triad of "bronchiolitis or bronchiolitis obliterans, patchy NSIP, and scattered nonnecrotizing granulomas" has been described for HP (10). Although these findings can often be found, the triad is not consistently present, and a variety of other histologic findings have also been described. These findings include, but are not limited to, unresolved pneumonia with intra-alveolar exudates, foamy macrophages, pleural fibrosis, patchy interstitial fibrosis, and intra-alveolar edema. The most consistent biopsy finding in HP is a patchy peribronchial pneumonitis with interstitial infiltrates consisting of lymphocytes and plasma cells. In addition, although the inflammatory cells most commonly found in HP are lymphocytes, plasma cells, and connective tissue-type macrophages, neutrophilic and eosinophilic infiltrates have also been described. Finally, biopsy in chronic HP may reveal a predominantly fibrotic picture, including interstitial fibrosis, cystic changes, and pulmonary hypertensive vascular changes with the upper lung fields most severely affected. Unfortunately, if chronic fibrotic changes are found, it may be difficult or even impossible to differentiate HP from other forms of pulmonary fibrosis (10).

Environmental Investigation

It is exceedingly important to identify the causal antigen. Although historically a disease related to high industrial, agricultural, or hobbyist exposures, the incidence of HP in these environments has been reduced by the use of protective equipment and improved techniques. HP induced by home exposure has become more common, and identifying the causal antigen in this environment can be more challenging. To identify the inciting antigen, a careful history with directed interview questions should be used with consideration of a home inspection. Attention should be paid to details such as plumbing problems, humidifiers, hot tubs, saunas, birds and other animal exposures, roof leaks, and forced air heating and cooling system abnormalities. If home inspection is done, environmental sampling can be performed, which, depending on the technique, may both identify organisms as well as determine baseline levels of antigen (10).

Challenge Methods

A variety of challenge techniques are available to the clinician, including direct antigen inhalation, natural challenge, and in vitro challenge. A direct antigen inhalation is performed to a specific antigen in a controlled setting. Objective measurements, such as temperature, auscultation, spirometry, and WBC, are taken before the challenge. These are monitored hourly until a response is seen or an 8-h maximum time period has passed. Chest radiographs are also taken before and after the challenge. A positive response is indicated by changes on auscultation, a rise in WBC of >2,500 per mm, a decrease in FVC of 20% or greater, a temperate increase above 37.2°C, or infiltrates on chest radiograph. Direct antigen inhalation can be a dangerous test, particularly since appropriate concentrations of antigen are estimated and not based on strong scientific data, so certain criteria should be met before a patient is challenged: they should not have symptoms or be taking systemic steroids; skin prick test should be negative to the antigen in order to avoid a life-threatening allergic reaction; ideally, FVC and/or D_{LCO} should not be <50% predicted (10).

Natural or environmental challenges can be performed in a variety of different ways with different time frames, depending on the clinical presentation and circumstances of the patient. Most commonly, after a period of removal from the suspected environment, the patient is reintroduced to the environment and monitored closely. The patient's symptoms as well as objective measurements such as ESR, CRP, WBC, spirometry, and chest radiographs are followed. The advantages of this technique are that it is less expensive, has less chance of a serious reaction, does not require identifying the specific antigen, establishes the causative environment, and assesses the success of remediation. The disadvantages are that it does not identify the specific causal antigen and can be difficult to perform in patients with subacute or chronic HP (10).

Finally, challenges can also be performed in vitro by assessing lymphocyte proliferation to specific antigens. Lymphocytes gathered from BAL fluid and peripheral blood have been studied. Like serum precipitans, this technique can identify individuals who are sensitized to a specific antigen, but it cannot differentiate between asymptomatic and symptomatic individuals.

Management, Treatment, and Prognosis

The mainstay of treatment for HP is early detection and complete avoidance of the inciting antigen. Once the antigen has been identified, steps must be taken to remove the antigen from the patient's environment. This includes repairing all defects that led to antigen exposure and replacing all other affected materials. After remediation is complete, the environment should be thoroughly cleaned. When avoidance is not possible, other control measures may be used to help reduce the amount of antigen exposure. These measures may include installation of electrostatic dust filters in central air-conditioning systems and HEPA filters in select rooms. For intermittent exposures, positive pressure or dust respirators may be used. Unfortunately, none of these measures will provide completely adequate protection (10).

Systemic corticosteroid therapy has been found to help treat the acute inflammatory components of HP. Prednisone is typically used in doses of approximately 0.5 mg/kg/day for 2–4 weeks, but sometimes, higher doses or longer courses are needed (4). While prednisone can help with the symptoms in acute and subacute HP, it has not been found to alter the progression to fibrosis or end-stage lung disease, and so its use should not be considered an alternative to avoidance measures.

Most patients will improve in 1–6 months after removal from the inciting antigen. Unfortunately, there are patients who will continue to progress in their disease despite appropriate interventions. Chronic HP with fibrosis is an irreversible slowly progressive disease linked with respiratory failure, cor pulmonale, infections, and premature death (4). The emphasis of management in these patients shifts to treatment of these complications (10). The progressive nature of HP in the later stages highlights the importance of early recognition and antigen avoidance.

Questions

1. Chronic HP may include the following symptoms except:

   (a) Progressive dyspnea
   (b) Weight loss
   (c) Fevers
   (d) Nonproductive cough

2. Which components of the immune system play a role in the development of HP?

   (a) TH1 cells
   (b) TH2 cells
   (c) IgE
   (d) Eosinophils

3. What environmental factors seem to favor the development of HP?

   (a) Smoking
   (b) Dry climates
   (c) Viral infection
   (d) Antibody deficiency

4. What are among the *most common* findings on PFT in a patient with HP?

   (a) Normal FVC
   (b) Low FEV1/FVC
   (c) Increased FEV1
   (d) Low D_{LCO}

5. Which of the following has *not* been associated with HP?

   (a) Elevated CRP
   (b) Elevated IgE
   (c) Positive rheumatoid factor
   (d) Interstitial infiltrates on chest radiograph

Answers: 1. (c), 2. (a), 3. (c), 4. (d), 5. (b)

References

1. Solaymani-Dodaran, M., West, J., Smith, C., Hubbard, R. (2007) Extrinsic allergic alveolitis: incidence and mortality in the general population. *QJ Med* **100**, 233–237.
2. Fink, J.N., Zacharisen, M.C. (2003) Hypersensitivity pneumonitis. In: Adkinson NF, Yunginger JW, Busse WW, Bochner BS, Holgate ST, Simons FE,eds. *Middleton's Allergy: Principles and Practice*, 6th ed. Philadelphia, PA: Mosby, 1373–1390.
3. Gibbs, J., Craig, T.J. (2008) Hypersensitivity pneumonitis. In Mahmoudi M, ed. *Allergy and Asthma: Practical Diagnosis and Management*, 1st ed. New York: Mc-Graw Hill, 177–189.

4. Madison, J.M. (2008) Hypersensitivity pneumonitis: clinical perspectives. *Arch Path Lab Med* **132**, 195–198.
5. Woda, B.A. (2008) Hypersensitivity pneumonitis: an immunopathology review. *Arch Path Lab Med* **132**, 204–205.
6. Patel, A.M., Ryu, J.H., Reed, C.E. (2001) Hypersensitivity pneumonitis: current concepts and future questions. *J All Clin Immunol* **108**, 661–670.
7. Schaaf, B.M., Seitzer, U., Pravica, V., Aries, S.P., Zabel, P. (2001) Tumor necrosis factor-α-308 promoter gene polymorphism and increased tumor necrosis factor serum bioactivity in famer's lung patients. *Am J Respir Crit Care Med* **163**, 379–382.
8. Camarena, A., Juarez, A., Mejia, M., Estrada, A., Carrillo, G., Falfan, R., Zuniga, J., Navarro, C., Granados, J., Selman, M. (2001) Major histocompatibility complex and tumor necrosis factor-α polymorphisms in pigeon breeder's disease. *Am J Respir Crit Care Med* **163**, 1528–1533.
9. Schuyler, M., Cormier, Y. (1997) The diagnosis of hypersensitivity pneumonitis. *Chest* **111**, 534–536.
10. Jacobs, R.L., Andrews, C.P., Coalson, J.J. (2005) Hypersensitivity pneumonitis: beyond classic occupational disease – changing concepts of diagnosis and management. *Ann All Asthma Immunol* **95**, 115–128.

Chapter 7
Atopic Dermatitis

Satoshi Yoshida

Abstract Atopy can be defined as a familial hypersensitivity of skin and mucous membranes against environmental substances, associated with increased immunogloblin E (IgE) production and/or altered unspecific reactivity in different organ systems, for example, skin in the case of atopic dermatitis (AD) and lung in the case of asthma. It is a chronic, highly pruritic, inflammatory skin disease frequently seen in patients with a history of respiratory allergy and allergic rhinitis. The prevalence of AD in children has been steadily increasing since 1920s, and it now affects more than 10% of children at some point during their childhood. The term atopic dermatitis was first introduced in 1933 in recognition of the close association between AD and respiratory allergy. However, there has been considerable debate over whether AD is primarily an allergen-induced disease or simply an inflammatory skin disorder found in association with respiratory allergy. Recent studies, however, suggest that the mechanisms underlying asthma and AD have greater similarities than differences. AD is a common, potentially debilitating condition that can compromise qualityof life. Its most frequent symptom is pruritus. Attempts to relieve the itch by scratching simply worsen the rash, creating a vicious circle. Treatment should be directed at limiting itching, repairing the skin, and decreasing inflammation when necessary. Lubricants, antihistamines, and topical corticosteroids are the mainstays of therapy. When required, oral corticosteroids can be used. If pruritus does not respond to treatment, other diagnoses, such as bacterial overgrowth or viral infections, should be considered. Treatment options are available for refractory atopic dermatitis, but these measures should be reserved for use in unique situations and typically require consultation with a dermatologist or an allergist. Allergic reactions play a role in some patients but not necessarily in all. In many patients different factors such as a disturbance of skin function, infection, and mental and/or physical stresses are potentially more relevant. Immunologic disturbances are reflected in the elevated IgE production and T-cell dysregulation observed in AD. Unspecific altered reactivity is reflected in increased releasability of chemical

S. Yoshida (✉)
Yoshida Clinic and Health Care System, Tokyo, Japan
e-mail: syoshida-fjt@umin.ac.jp

M. Mahmoudi (ed.), *Challenging Cases in Allergy and Immunology*,
DOI: 10.1007/978-1-60327-443-2_7,

mediator-secreting cells and in bronchial, nasal, and skin hyperreactivity. Each disease that forms the atopic triad has important immunologic parallels. However, they involve a different regional sphere of immunologic influence, for example, the skin-associated lymphoid tissue in AD as opposed to bronchial-associated lymphoid tissue in asthma.

Keywords Kaposi varicelliform eruption • Posterior subcapsular cataract • Thrombocytopenia

Case 1

A 32-year-old man was brought to the emergency department after sudden onset of severe right shoulder pain, high fever, chills, and confusion. In the year before admission he began to have itching skin lesions on his extremities fulfilling the criteria for atopic dermatitis. He had required regular hydrocortisone 1% cream to control his symptoms. Typically he was using a 30-g tube every 3–4 weeks on his arms, neck, and face when needed. The patient appeared confused with a systolic blood pressure of 88 mmHg, nuchal rigidity, and few petechial lesions on her trunk and extremities. No smptoms related to respiratory and urinary tract infections were reported. The patient was intubated and admitted to the intensive care unit; intravenous ceftriaxone and acyclovir were initiated.

Data

The complete blood cell count revealed the following: hemoglobin, 14.2 g/dL; hematocrit, 43%;; total white blood cells count, 9,800 per mm³ with 86%; neutrophils, 12.2%; lymphocytes, and 0.6%; eosinophils; platelets, 388,000 per mm³ with normal serum chemical analysis results; and erythrocyte sedimentation rate, 10 mm. Fluorescent antinuclear antibody and anti-DNA test results were negative. The total lgE level was 968.0 IU/mL (normal value < 170; SRL laboratories, Tokyo, Japan). Transesophageal echocardiography revealed large sessile vegetation on the posterior leaflet of the mitral valve. Cerebrospinal fluid and blood cultures yielded methicillin-sensitive *Staphylococcus aureus*.

1. With the presented data, what is your diagnosis?

   (a) Anaphyraxy shock.
   (b) Invasive *Staphylococcus aureus* infections
   (c) Kaposi varicelliform eruption
   (d) Postherpetic encephalitis

Answer: (b)

2. What is your diagnosis and why?

The most appropriate diagnosis is (b). The final diagnosis of our patient's condition includes acute encepharitis and endocarditis due to *Staphylococcuss aureus.*

Discussion

The skin has been shown to be the portal of entry of *S. aureus* to the bloodstream, and *S. aureus* carriers are at higher risk for invasive *S. aureus* infections once the skin is breached. In contrast with healthy subjects, in whom the skin is colonized with *S. aureus* in less than 5%, *S. aureus* can be isolated from skin lesions of most patients with atopic dermatitis (1). Moreover, when this organism is present on intact skin, its density is usually low, whereas the density of *S. aureus* on acute exudative atopic dermatitis skin lesions can reach 107 colony-forming units per cm^2. Once attached to the skin, *S. aureus* secretes exotoxins with superantigenic properties that worsen atopic dermatitis. A deficiency in the expression of endogenous antimicrobial peptides in the skin of patients with atopic dermatitis, causing localized immunodeficiency, may account for the susceptibility of these patients to skin invasion with *S. aureus.* Therefore, atopic skin provides a favorable environment for the colonization, proliferation, and invasion of *S. aureus* (2). A possible causal relationship between atopic dermatitis and invasive *S. aureus* infection is likely because in most of the reviewed cases atopic dermatitis was present in a severe form, thus facilitating a breach of the natural cutaneous barrier and increasing the risk for *S. aureus* penetration and spread. Furthermore, the median age of patients with bacteremia was 22 years, which was much lower than that reported in other series of *S. aureus* bacteremia or endocarditis (3). Extrapolating the risk for developing invasive *S. aureus* disease from other conditions in which *S. aureus* carriage is common, atopic dermatitis is an underestimated risk factor for invasive *S. aureus* infection. In patients with known atopic dermatitis who present with acute febrile illness without an apparent source or with localized pain, the diagnosis of invasive *S. aureus* infection should be sought (4).

After 4 weeks of antibiotic treatment, the patient successfully underwent mechanical mitral valve replacement and completely recovered.

Case 2

A 9-year-old boy suffering from moderate atopic dermatitis since the age of 2 years received topical 0.005% of Cutivate Ointment of the face, neck, trunk, and limbs, twice a day for a mild eczema of the cheeks, for 3 years. He presented to the pediatric ophthalmology clinic complaining of gradual onset of blurred vision in both eyes. On examination, his vision was 6/36 in the right eye and 6/9 in the left eye, with no improvement with pinhole.

Data

Laboratory investigations showed a total white blood cell count at 20,000 ml with 90% neutrophils. C-reactive protein was normal. Blood, urine, and pustule cultures were negative. The total lgE level was 1,326 IU/mL (normal value < 170); specific lgE for dust mite was 47/3.9 IU/mL in RAST system (SRL laboratories, Tokyo, Japan).

Imaging Studies

On slit-lamp examination, he was noted to have bilateral posterior subcapsular cataract, which was worse in the left eye (Fig. 7.1). He was tested for spectacles with which his vision improved to 6/6 in the right eye and 6/9 in the left.

1. With the presented data what is your diagnosis?

   (a) Keratohelcosis
   (b) Pigment dispersion syndrome
   (c) Iridocyclitis
   (d) Posterior subcapsular cataract

Answer: (d)

2. What is your diagnosis and how do you treat this patient?

   There is no ulcerative formation in cornea. Pigment dispersion syndrome and pigmentary glaucoma are characterized by disruption of the iris pigment epithelium and deposition of the dispersed pigment granules throughout the anterior segment. The classic diagnostic triad consists of corneal pigmentation (Krukenberg spindle;

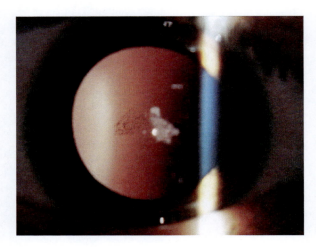

Fig. 7.1 A 9-year-old boy with posterior subcapsular cataract

slit-like, radial, mid-peripheral iris transillumination defects; and dense trabecular pigmentation). The iris insertion is typically posterior and the peripheral iris tends to have a concave configuration. The basic abnormality in this hereditary disorder remains unknown. Iridocyclitis is usually caused by direct exposure of the eyes to chemicals, particularly, lachrymators but can also be caused by ocular viral infection such as herpes zoster (i.e., herpetic iridocyclitis).

Discussion

Corticosteroids are known to cause posterior subcapsular cataract by most routes of administration. After diabetes, myopia, and glaucoma, steroid use is the fourth leading risk factor for secondary cataract and accounts for 4.7% of all cataract extractions (5). Care needs to be taken when prescribing corticosteroids, particularly in children who have a lower susceptibility to side effects. Corticosteroids are frequently required to adequately treat AD, to limit pruritus and prevent complications such as keratitis that can lead to permanent visual loss. Exacerbations of AD need to be treated aggressively. Many patients and parents have negative perceptions regarding the use of steroids, which may lead to inadequate treatment of the skin disease and increased eye rubbing. The increasing use of alternative specific immunosuppressants that lack the side effect profile of corticosteroids may reduce the incidence of cataracts in these patients.

The cataracts in these patients may have been due to the underlying disease, the treatment, or a combination of both. Cataracts secondary to AD are rare in children. In a series of 59 children, there was just one case of cataract (5). Why cataracts develop in patients with AD is not known; however, habitual tapping and rubbing of the face, a common problem in pruritic conditions, may play a role. Indeed, the presence of facial skin lesions in AD correlates with progression of the cataract. An alternative hypothesis suggests that the cataract is secondary to compromise of the blood-aqueous barrier. Patients with AD have been found to have higher levels of protein flare in the aqueous humor than controls. Posterior subcapsular cataracts may also be caused by corticosteroids used in the treatment of AD. Subsequent studies have shown that corticosteroid-induced cataracts may develop following even small doses of steroids, particularly in children. Posterior subcapsular cataract may occur at a faster rate and lower dosage in children. In addition to systemic steroids, cataracts have also been associated with ocular topical steroids, inhaled steroids, and topical steroid creams (6). When steroids are applied topically to the skin, the degree of systemic absorption depends on factors such as drug potency, the duration of application, and whether the skin is thin or damaged. Even low-potency steroid creams applied to the eyelids may result in increased intraocular pressure and cataract (7).

The mechanism of corticosteroid-induced cataract is not known but may be due to osmotic imbalance, oxidative damage, or disrupted lens growth factors. The osmotic theory suggests that corticosteroids interfere with the ionic composition of the lens. The oxidative theory proposes that corticosteroids inhibit the normal mechanisms that protect the lens from oxidative stress. Another theory of cataract formation proposes that steroids influence lens-related growth factors. Normal lens growth is mediated by growth factors such as fibroblast growth factor-2 present in the aqueous and vitreous humour. Corticosteroids may influence lens epithelial cell behavior by interfering with the normal production of growth factors. This effect may result in undifferentiated anterior epithelial cells migrating and accumulating at the posterior pole forming a posterior subcapsular cataract.

Cataract extraction in children with atopic cataract can produce excellent visual results; however, it is important to consider the presence of a coexisting retinal detachment. Retinal detachment has been reported in 8% of patients with AD and in one series, 25% of eyes with atopic cataract had retinal breaks or detachment noted preoperatively (8). A rapidly progressing cataract may mask the presence of a shallow retinal detachment, and an unrecognised retinal detachment can cause a mild cataract to progress faster. B-scan ultrasonography is a useful investigation to evaluate the anatomy of the retina in these eyes. Retinal detachment may also be associated with panuveitis or hypotony (9).

Questions

I. A 12-year-old girl presents with a 3-month history of severe persistent itching and skin lesions throughout most of her body. Physical examination revealed numerous 15–20-mm papulonodular lesions over all the extremities and trunk with some confluence (Fig. 7.2). Crusting and lichenification also were observed. No lesions were present on the face.

1. What is your diagnosis and why?

   (a) Psoriasis vulgaris
   (b) Pemphigus vulgaris
   (c) Severe atopic dermatitis
   (d) Lichen planus

Answer: (c)

Atopic dermatitis is a form of endogenous dermatitis resulting in pruritic inflammation of the epidermis and dermis, which commonly occurs in infants and children but can be found in adults. Atopic dermatitis affects more than 10% of children, and the majority of patients are affected during the first 5 years of life (10).

Psoriasis is an inflammatory epidermal proliferative disorder of the skin, which is usually not intensely pruritic. The most common lesions are papules and nodules like those shown in the photograph, but in psoriasis they are sharply demarcated and covered by silvery white scale. The lesions most commonly involve areas of the body that experience repeated minor trauma, such as elbows, knees, scalp, feet, and hands. Associated findings may include fingernail pitting or thickening (50% of cases) and arthritis (up to 10% of cases).

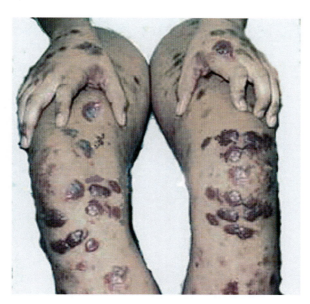

Fig. 7.2 Sever atopic dermatitis in a 12-year-old girl

Pemphigus vulgaris is an autoimmune bullous disease of the skin that usually occurs in adults and is rare in children. There is no pruritus. The lesions are flaccid vesicles or bullae that are initially localized in oral mucosa and later spread randomly to other parts of the body. This can be a serious and potentially fatal disorder.

Lichen planus is characterized by flat-topped, polygonal, violaceous papules, which are much smaller than the confluent papulonodular lesions seen in severe atopic dermatitis. The pruritus is variable. Lichen planus is uncommon in children. The common sites include wrists, shins, mucous membrane, lumbar area, and genitalia. Atopic dermatitis is frequently accompanied by a personal or family history of asthma, allergic rhinitis, or allergic skin involvement. The onset of the skin lesions is usually subacute or chronic. In infants, the extensor surface of the extremities, face, and trunk are involved, whereas children and adults have predilection for the flexural areas of the extremities, neck, and upper trunk. Patients with atopic dermatitis often have diffusely dry skin. Pruritic papules with vesicles are typical initially; these may become scaly and crusty later. Chronic lesions may have thickened lichenified skin with fibrotic papules and nodules as are seen in this case. The distribution of the lesions may become more diffuse in the chronic condition. Secondary infection is common, especially with *Staphylococcus aureus* (11). Atopic dermatitis may be confused with a number of the eczematous dermatitides including contact dermatitis, seborrheic dermatitis, and psoriasis. In dark-skinned patients, it is often difficult to differentiate the lesions from the other conditions as outlined earlier because of the lack of contrast between the lesions and uninvolved skin. In blacks, a subtype of atopic dermatitis occurs frequently where each papule involves a separate hair follicle, and is termed follicular eczema. The diagnosis of

Fig. 7.3 Blotchy purple discoloration in a 24-year-old woman

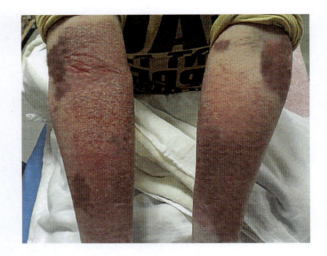

atopic dermatitis is based primarily on clinical presentation and history. No laboratory tests are available to definitively establish a diagnosis of atopic dermatitis, although patients may have elevated levels of IgE and peripheral blood eosinophilia. The histopathologic changes seen in biopsy specimens of atopic dermatitis are unspecific. Common triggers of atopic dermatitis include dry skin, infection, physical or emotional stress, sweating, and skin irritants. These irritants can include soaps, detergents, cosmetics, wool and acrylic clothing, linens, and perfumes. Symptomatic treatment consists of the use of moisturizers to prevent the itching caused by dry skin. Avoidance of any of the irritants or triggers is the cornerstone of therapy. Mild or no soap should be used when bathing. Hot baths or frequent bathing may cause drier skin and should be avoided. Oral antihistamines can help control itching. Use of H_2 blockers in cases of severe pruritus may be helpful. Topical steroid ointments or creams in addition to cool wet dressings are useful in acute flares of the disease as well as in maintenance of healing in the chronic phase. Topical or oral antibiotics should be considered when there is suspicion of secondary infection, because this may be a cause of persistent pruritus.

II. A 24-year-old woman presents with a blotchy purple discoloration affecting her hands and forearms (Fig. 7.3). She says that the marks have become increasingly noticeable over the last 5 years and are caused by minor injuries. She also has skin fragility. Apart from longstanding atopic dermatitis, she denies any other medical problems.

2. Which related medication may also cause "senile" purpura?

   (a) Carbamide cream
   (b) Antibiotic ointment
   (c) Cosmetics
   (d) Ultrapotent topical steroids

Answer: (d)

3. What investigations would you arrange?

(a) Thrombocytopenia
(b) Skin biopsy
(c) Skin sensitization against clothes
(d) Blood eosinophil count

Answer: (a)

She has been applying potent or ultrapotent topical steroids for months or years (in this case, betamethasone valerate). Signs of steroid atrophy may include skin transparency, striae, telangiectasia, skin fragility, and jagged scars. Senile or "solar" purpura arises because red cells leak into the dermis after rubbing a persistent pruritic dermatosis (in her case, atopic dermatitis). It is especially likely on sun-exposed sites, already thinned by ultraviolet radiation.

Systemic and high-dose inhaled corticosteroids may also result in cutaneous atrophy and purpura, characteristic signs of Cushing's syndrome. However, no investigations are necessary if the clinical diagnosis is obvious. If there is doubt, consider thrombocytopenia or other hematological reasons for bleeding, as these may be disastrous. If possible, discontinue topical steroids. Do this slowly to reduce the chance of rebound flare of dermatitis. Gradually select less potent products and apply less frequency, using emollients to calm itching. Ask a dermatologist for advice. Protect affected areas from the sun with clothing and sunscreens. Try not to scratch or otherwise injure the skin. It is not known if any other measures help but tretinoin, calcipotriol, and oral or topical vitamin C have been recommended.

III. A 38-year-old man with a history of atopic dermatitis is mildly unwell. The painful eruption shown in Fig. 7.4 has developed over the last 3 days.

4. What is this condition called?

(a) Impetigo
(b) Eczema herpeticum
(c) Molluscum contagiosum
(d) Verruca vulgaris

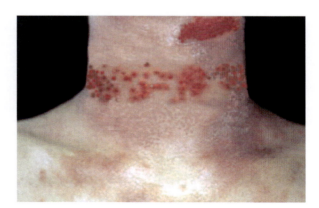

Fig. 7.4 Eczema herpeticum in a 38-year-old male

5. What is it caused by?

   (a) Herpes simplex infection
   (b) Neoplastic proliferation
   (c) Senile alloeosis
   (d) Allergic reaction

6. What medication would you use for his condition?

   (a) Antibiotics
   (b) Corticosteroid
   (c) Cauterization
   (d) Aciclovir

Answer: 4. (b), 5. (a), 6. (d)

This is eczema herpeticum (Kaposi varicelliform eruption) (12). There are characteristic clusters of umbilicated vesicles on the child's neck. Eczema herpeticum is due to primary herpes simplex infection in a patient with atopic dermatitis, or rarely, Darier's disease or other conditions in which epidermal integrity is compromised. Eczema herpeticum can also complicate facial resurfacing by chemical peel or laser. In atopics, it can arise within the dermatitis or on normal-appearing skin (13). The diagnosis can be confirmed by viral culture of blister fluid, obtained by deroofing a lesion and scraping it gently with a scalpel blade. More rapid confirmation can be obtained by immunofluorescent staining. As eczema herpeticum can become extensive and severe, the patient should be promptly prescribed aciclovir. The dose depends on severity and ranges from 200 to 800 mg five times daily for 5 days. Oral valaciclovir and famciclovir are also suitable, but not currently available in New Zealand. Intravenous aciclovir is recommended for particularly severe cases. Topical care with cold compresses using saline, weak vinegar solution, or potassium permanganate followed by emollient application can reduce discomfort and speed healing. Any involvement in and around the eye should be evaluated by an ophthalmologist. The patient should be considered contagious until the crusts fall off, which can take several weeks. Active atopic dermatitis can be treated concurrently with topical steroid and emollients according to severity. Secondary bacterial infection necessitates oral antistaphylococcal antibiotics.

References

1. Noble WC, Valkenburg HA, Wolters CH. Carriage of *Staphylococcus aureus* in random samples of a normal population. J Hyg (Lond) **65**:567–573, 1967.
2. Leyden JJ, Marples RR, Kligman AM. *Staphylococcus aureus* in the lesions of atopic dermatitis. Br J Dermatol **90**:525–530, 1974.
3. Ong PY, Ohtake T, Brandt C, et al. Endogenous antimicrobial peptides and skin infections in atopic dermatitis. N Engl J Med **347**:1151–1160, 2000.
4. Chang FY, MacDonald BB, Peacock JE Jr, et al. A prospective multicenter study of *Staphylococcus aureus* bacteremia: Incidence of endocarditis, risk factors for mortality, and clinical impact of methicillin resistance. Medicine **82**:322–332, 2003.

5. Black RL, Oglesby RB, von Sallman L, Bunim JJ. Posterior subcapsular cataracts induced by corticosteroids in patients with rheumatoid arthritis. JAMA **174**:166–171, 1960.
6. Cumming RG, Mitchell P, Leeder SR. Use of inhaled corticosteroids and the risk of cataracts. N Engl J Med **337**:8–14, 1997.
7. Garrott HM, Walland MJ. Glaucoma from topical corticosteroids to the eyelids. Clin Exp Ophthalmol **32**(2):224–226, 2004.
8. Hayashi H, Igarashi C, Hayashi K. Frequency of ciliary body or retinal breaks and retinal detachment in eyes with atopic cataract. Br J Ophthalmol **86**:898–901, 2002.
9. Lim WK, Chee SP. Retinal detachment in atopic dermatitis can masquerade as acute panuveitis with rapidly progressive cataract. Retina **24**:953–956, 2004.
10. Leung DY, Hanifin JM, Charlesworth EN, Li JT, Bernstein IL, Berger WE, et al. Disease management of atopic dermatitis: A practice parameter. Ann Allergy Asthma Immunol **79**:197–211, 1997.
11. Abeck D, Mempel M. *Staphylococcus aureus* colonization in atopic dermatitis and its therapeutic implications. Br J Dermatol **139** (Suppl 53):13–16, 1998.
12. Jarratt M. Viral infections of the skin. Herpes simplex, herpes zoster, warts, and molluscum contagiosum. Pediatr Clin North Am **25**(2):339–355, 1978.
13. Treadwell PA. Eczema and infection. Pediatr Infect Dis J **27**(6):551–552, 2008.

Chapter 8
Food Allergy

Oscar L. Frick

Abstract IgE-mediated food allergies are part of a spectrum of adverse reactions to foods including immune and nonimmune mechanisms. Anaphylaxis is the most serious and life-threatening manifestation of food allergy. Asthma, rhinitis, atopic dermatitis, and urticaria/angioedema also result from IgE-mediated reactions to foods. Not only ingestion of an allergenic food, but inhalation of food allergens may cause reactions. There are many unrecognized cross-reacting food allergens.

Keywords Food allergy • Anaphylaxis • Peanut allergy

Introduction

Adverse reactions to foods involve both immune and nonimmune mechanisms. Nonimmune reactions may be from toxins such as histamine in scombroid poisoning from spoiling fish or bacteria such as Shigella and Salmonella. There are idiosyncracies such as increased sensitivity to histamine in tomatoes and cocoa. Immune reactions are involved in Crohn's disease and ulcerative colitis, which may involve delayed or cellular immunity. IgE-mediated immediate food allergies are discussed later. There are mixed immune reactions such as eosinophilic esophagitis and celiac disease, with the latter involving IgA antibodies (1).

Allergic reactions mediated by IgE antibodies (food allergy) have increased in the past two decades. These can result in severe life-threatening anaphylaxis to lesser reactions of urticaria, angioedema, asthma, rhinitis, or oral allergy syndrome. Not only ingestion of the allergenic food but inhalation of food allergens in a sensitive individual may cause anaphylaxis. Unrecognized cross-reactivities among food allergens also can cause problems. Following are some case illustrations of such clinical situations.

O.L. Frick
University of California, San Francisco, CA, USA
e-mail: oscar_1_frick@yahoo.com

M. Mahmoudi (ed.), *Challenging Cases in Allergy and Immunology*,
DOI: 10.1007/978-1-60327-443-2_8,
© Humana Press, a part of Springer Science +Business Media, LLC 2009

Case 1

TF was a 15-year-old Filipino-American boy whom we had followed since he was a toddler with severe asthma, rhinitis, and atopic dermatitis. As an infant he had vomiting and diarrhea that lasted 6 months despite several formula and dietary changes. His asthma was under moderately good control but he had emergency room visits about every 3 months. He was taking on alternate days prednisone 10 mg/day, albuteral prn, and Claritin 10 mg/day. His atopic dermatitis was persistent affecting his arms, legs, and neck for which he was using triamcinolone 0.1% ointment twice daily. He often had a runny nose and sneezing.

One Friday, he was playing basketball with his friends and had no trouble in running, but only an occasional cough. He needed to go to the toilet and ran through the kitchen to the bathroom. After about 10 min, his friends came to the door and asked if TF was coming back to play. His mother, who was cooking dinner, realized that he was still in the bathroom. As she opened the bathroom door, she saw TF lying on the floor not breathing and blue. She called 911 and tried CPR. The EMTs arrived within 5 min and took over, but they realized that he had expired. At the ER he was pronounced deceased.

What Do You Think Happened? What Questions Would You Ask of His Mother?

What was she cooking at that time? Was he allergic to anything that she was cooking or preparing in the kitchen? Had he had any asthma symptoms that day and did he take his medications?

What If Any Work-Up Would You Have Done?

He had prick skin tests done repeatedly – last ones 1 year ago that showed him to be allergic to house dust mites, grass pollens, cedar cypress and oak tree pollens, egg, soy, salmon, cod, shrimp, walnuts, and cashews.

The family was Roman Catholic and had fish every Friday except TF who was allergic to fish. Mother was cooking fish at the time TF ran through the kitchen.

What Is Your Differential Diagnosis?

1. Severe fatal anaphylaxis from fish inhalation in this severe asthmatic boy who required alternate day oral prednisone to control his asthma
2. Severe sudden asthmatic attack

How Would You Establish the Final Diagnosis?

A markedly elevated serum beta tryptase level ($T_{1/2}$ = 90 min) indicates that the death was due to systemic anaphylaxis. Alpha and beta tryptase occur only in mast cells (2). Alpha tryptase is released slowly from normal human mast cells and is markedly elevated in systemic mastocytosis. Beta tryptase is stored in mast cell granules and is explosively released in systemic anaphylaxis. Elevated beta tryptase levels persist even postmortem for many hours and even up to days after a fatal anaphylactic reaction.

Discussion

Although TF never ate fish to which he was allergic, his mother served fish every Friday to the rest of the Catholic family. When she was cooking fish at the time when TF ran through the kitchen to the bathroom, there was enough fish protein vapor in the air that was sufficient to trigger the fatal anaphylactic reaction in TF. Severe asthmatic patients, especially those under incomplete therapeutic control, such as TF are prime candidates for fatal anaphylaxis.

Case 2

BJ was an infant whose mother had allergic rhinitis since childhood and father had childhood asthma, which is clear now. BJ was nursed for 6 months, switched to cow's milk formula, and started on cereal and fruit at 3 months. He did well with no colic or rashes. At 9 months, he was given two bites of a peanut butter cookie when he began crying, spit up, and a rash developed around his mouth that spread to his chest. He responded to Benadryl with rash gone in 3 h. His pediatrician gave his mother an Epi-Pen Jr and instructions for use.

When BJ was 15-months old, he and his mother boarded an airplane for a flight from San Francisco to San Diego (90-min flight). Once airborne for 45 min, BJ grew fussy, crying, then he developed hives over face and limbs, had difficult breathing, and became limp and cyanotic.

What Was Happening to BJ and What Was Causing His Symptoms?

It appears that he was having an anaphylactic reaction. The hostess was serving packages of peanuts to the other passengers. The mother realized that there was a peanut odor as passengers were opening their peanut packages and that sufficient aerosolized peanut protein was in the air that caused BJ'symptoms.

What Did His Mother Do?

She injected BJ in his thigh with Epi-Pen Jr. and slipped a Claritin Redi-tab under his tongue. She called the hostess for help. The hostess informed the pilot and he advised the Los Angeles Airport that he was coming in for an Emergency landing. However, they were still 15 min away. Immediately following the Epi-Pen Jr injection, BJs breathing and color improved and he began crying. He continued to improve over the next 10 min, so the pilot decided to fly on to San Diego some 30 min more.

By the time, they reached San Diego, BJ's breathing was normal and his hives were fading. This was one of the first cases reported that aerosolized peanut protein in an enclosed air space like an airplane cabin was sufficient to cause anaphylaxis in a peanut-sensitive patient. As a result, FAA recommended that peanuts on airplanes be substituted with other snacks.

Case 3

JK was a 39-year-old man who had an urticarial rash after eating shrimp. He strictly avoided shrimp and asked in restaurants about shrimp in menu dishes. Two years later, he ate in a San Francisco restaurant. After the salad course, he noted a tingling on his tongue and lips; he became flushed and hot and his lower lip became swollen. He realized that there might have been shrimp in the salad, so he injected his thigh with his Epi-Pen and took Benadryl 25 mg. His reaction did not grow worse except that his upper lip became swollen, but the reaction gradually subsided. He had asked the waiter about shrimp before he ordered and was reassured that there was no shrimp by the waiter. He returned to the restaurant 1 week later and asked the manager and chef about shrimp in the salad. This restaurant often uses a few small bay shrimp in salads, but not in his salad. However, he learned that the salad bowls were only rinsed after a salad with shrimp and the next "shrimp-free" salad. Apparently, there was sufficient shrimp protein residue in the bowl to have caused his reaction.

Two weeks later, he took some visiting friends to Fisherman's Wharf where they were going to have dinner. Upon walking past the cooking crab pots on the Wharf, he began itching and hives developed, then he began coughing and had difficulty in breathing. He was very apprehensive, and his friends noted that his voice became hoarse before he fainted onto the sidewalk.

What Happened to JK?

He was experiencing an anaphylactic reaction, probably to something in the air because he had eaten nothing in the past 4 h. Because there was a strong odor of crab in the air from the cooking crab pots, it is likely that he was reacting to crab.

What Was Done Then?

His friends called 911. One friend found his Epi-Pen in his jacket pocket and injected it into his thigh through his trouser leg.

He also started CPR. EMT arrived in 5 min and he was taken to ER.

By that time, he was breathing easier and conscious, but with marked angioedema and urticaria. He was admitted to hospital for overnight observation to make sure that he did not have a late recurrent reaction as the epinephrine wore off. He was discharged next day after an uneventful night.

Discussion

There is a strong cross-reactivity between the tropomyosin muscle protein allergens in all shellfish – shrimp, crab, lobster, and crayfish (3).

His moderate reaction to shrimp 2 weeks before his walk past the cooking crab pots increased his sensitivity to smaller doses of allergen, e.g., aerosolized crab.

He was admitted for overnight observation because there can be late-phase anaphylactic reactions many hours after an initial reaction. The effect of injected epinephrine may last only minutes to a few hours. This is why Epinephrine injectable kits usually have two doses of epinephrine. An immediate anaphylactic reaction involves muscular constriction and massive leakage of intravascular fluid into tissues causing edema, which can cause vascular collapse (shock), tracheal and bronchial constriction, asphyxia, and death. A late-phase reaction hours later is an eosinophilic inflammation of airways and tissues that responds to corticosteroids, antihistaminics, and antileukotrienes.

Case 4

YP was a 26-year-old woman who was with four coworkers who had lunch at a Pizza restaurant. She had asthma since childhood. She had had several episodes of hives after eating walnuts and pecans, so she always asked or checked the menus in the restaurant about the presence of nuts in the dishes she ordered. She perused the menu and found a mushroom, tomato pizza with pesto that she ordered. She grew up in an Italian neighborhood and had often had pizza and no problem with pizza with pesto containing pine nuts. The other women shared two chocolate sundaes with nut toppings, but YP refused any dessert.

After lunch, the girls walked two blocks to their cars. Her friend was with her to drive back to the office. It was a cool day, but she felt quite warm and her face flushed. She had a slight cough that she thought was an asthma flare, so she took two puffs of her albuterol.

What Was Happening to YP?

Was she having an asthma attack?
Was she starting to have an anaphylactic reaction?
What should she have done at this point?

Given herself an Epi-Pen injection in her thigh and taken an antihistamine.

There is a much richer vascular supply in the thigh muscle than in the arm subcutaneously that leads to more rapid uptake of epinephrine into the vascular system and dissemination through the body (4). Epinephrine constricts the capillaries that have dilated and caused vascular leakage due to histamine and platelet-activating factor (PAF) released from mast cells and basophils during an anaphylactic reaction.

Subsequent Course and Discussion

In her car, after driving several blocks, her cough worsened and she began itching – her friend noticed a rash on her face. The cough worsened and she began wheezing, so she took another puff of albuterol while driving. Her lips began to swell, so her friend pulled the car over to roadside. YP then injected herself with her Epi-Pen in her upper arm, but within minutes she passed out. Her friend called 911 on her cell phone. EMTs arrived within 5 min. She was unconscious, cyanotic, barely breathing, and had no blood pressure. In the ambulance, she stopped breathing; EMT did CPR after two more epinephrine injections – she had coded. At the ER, further emergency care brought her around and she recovered after 2 days in hospital.

Checking back at the restaurant the next week, her friend discovered that the pesto was walnut-based. YP thought it had pine nuts that are usually in pesto.

Pine nuts are related to cashew and pistachio that sometimes do not cross-react with walnuts, pecans, and filberts. However, in tree-nut sensitive patients, it is prudent to avoid all tree nuts and peanuts. Although peanuts are legumes, they are often processed in the same equipment as tree nuts in baked goods and candies. The seed proteins (2S-albumin, vicillins, etc.) (5) in tree nuts and peanuts are similar and if one can be sensitized to *one* such protein, it is possible to become independently sensitized to another.

Case 5

RB was a 7-year-old boy with moderate asthma, allergic rhinitis, and dermatitis that started when he was a toddler. His eczema was still a major problem, but better over the recent years. His asthma was controlled with inhaled corticosteroids, but attacks needing ER visits occurred twice a year.

His allergic sensitivities by prick skin tests were due to dust mites, dog and cat, grass pollen, egg, and wheat. On physical exam, he had mild lichenified eczema on his ante-cubital and popliteal fossae. His nasal turbinates were swollen. His lungs had mild expiratory rhonchi but no wheezing. He was on a strict egg- and wheat-free diet, using rice crackers for cereal. We repeatedly asked his mother about any wheat or egg sources. She insisted that she was strictly avoiding all wheat and egg products at home and at school. She avoided having wheat bread in the home. She had for years had mattress and pillow encasings, and she followed strict house dust control; there were no pets.

What Further History or Diagnostic Tests Would You Do?

Were his teacher, family relatives, and friends aware of his pet and egg and wheat allergies? Did he visit other homes with pets or did he sleep over in others' houses? Is there mold in the house, especially in his bedroom? Does he fit in the normal growth curve for his age? Were there new allergens to which he became sensitive since his last skin tests? Would a new set of prick skin tests help? Would radioallergosorbent test (RAST)s help? Would a home visit be useful?

Course and Discussion

Prick skin tests were repeated and RAST tests were done, but the same allergens were confirmed and no new allergens were observed. In frustration, we decided to make a home visit to see if there was a hidden pet and to check status of encasings and bedroom. On the house inspection, we noted that the only room in the house that was wall-papered was the dining room and that the paper was dry and peeling. We posited that perhaps the dried wheat wallpaper paste became airborne and might be contributing to RB's continued allergic problems. We suggested that the dining room wallpaper be removed, cleaned, and painted. After that was accomplished, RB's asthma and eczema improved markedly with no more ER visits. We surmised that the wheat paste powder had aerosolized and caused continued allergic symptoms in RB.

Sometimes a home visit can provide most useful diagnostic information. Several allergy clinics and practices have trained personnel to make such home visits to look for hidden allergens. We had one instance in which a child had strong cat skin test but the family insisted that there was no cat in his environment. We had a cat-sensitive resident who accompanied us on a house visit. Upon entering the house, he began sneezing indicating that there was a cat present. The family then sheepishly admitted that they had put the cat in a closet.

Case 6

AQ was a 42-year-old nurse who developed a rash and subsequent urticaria and angioedema from the latex gloves used in the OR. She had to change her nursing duties to supervisory work where she could no longer encounter latex. She did well from allergic symptoms for 10 years.

One day she ate a plum following which she developed some mouth tingling and then urticaria. This was controlled with hydroxyzine within a few hours.

If She Had Come to You for Medical Advice What Would You Have Done?

Prick skin tests for plum and other fruits and latex? Would you have used commercial extracts or prick-to-prick tests with the fruits? Would you have done RASTs? Would you have given her an Epi-Pen?

Course and Discussion

One week later, she ate a peach and again similar symptoms occurred with increasing hives. She ran to her garage to drive to the ER, but she collapsed in her yard. Her nurse housemate came home shortly thereafter and found AQ unconscious in the driveway – cyanotic and barely breathing. She rushed her to the hospital ER where resuscitation efforts were successful and AQ recovered with some residual anoxic brain damage.

The lipid transfer protein (LTP) allergen in the skin of the Rosacea family of pitted fruits (peach, plum, apricots, almond, and cherry) is also found in latex; this was the case with AQ (6). Other more closely related fruits to latex are banana, kiwi, and figs. Figure 8.1 shows relative degrees of cross-reactivity among allergenic foods (7).

Conclusion

We have presented several cases of IgE-mediated food allergies that resulted in anaphylaxis from ingested or inhaled food allergens.

Cross-reactions among food allergen families can also be a problem.

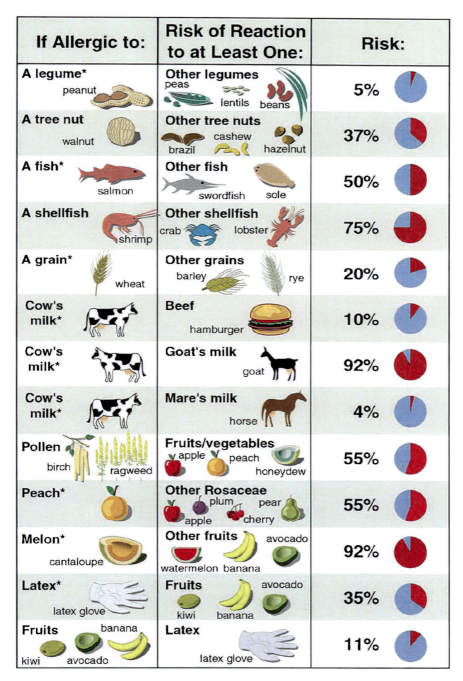

Fig. 8.1 Relative degrees of cross-reactivity among allergeinc foods, from Sicherer SH, J Allergy and Clin Immunol, 2001, 108: 881–890, Elsevier, with permission

Questions

1. A 6-year-old boy who had an anaphylactic reaction to peanut at age 3 had a cookie containing peanut butter in the school lunchroom. He began having an itchy mouth and rash on his cheeks and then he began coughing. What would you do first as cafeteria monitor?

   (a) Call 911.
   (b) Give him a Benadryl capsule.
   (c) Help to give him his Epi-Pen injection in his thigh.
   (d) Call his mother and doctor.

2. If a patient has had an anaphylactic reaction to peanut because it is a legume, one should advise the patient to:

   (a) Avoid all beans, peas, lentils, and soya
   (b) Allow soya, but avoid all other legumes
   (c) Allow all legumes in diet, except peanut
   (d) Allow all legumes in diet, except peanut, but take note of any mild reaction to other legumes

3. A 27-year-old man had an anaphylactic life-threatening reaction to a shrimp scampi dish, he need *not*

   (a) Be afraid to eat crab, lobster, and crayfish
   (b) Avoid areas where crab or shrimp are being cooked
   (c) Carry an Epi-Pen
   (d) Ask in the restaurant if there has been shrimp prepared in his salad bowl

4. A 3-year-old boy with atopic dermatitis rash on his arms, legs, and face should avoid

   (a) All foods that give a positive prick skin test reaction
   (b) All foods that give a positive in vitro or RAST reaction
   (c) Dust mites if prick skin tests to mites is positive – mattress and pillow encasings
   (d) Exposure to blooming tree and grass pollens in spring and summer

5. A 17-year-old young woman has had hives for the past 2 years at 2–3 times per week.

   (a) She is likely to be allergic to a food.
   (b) She is reacting to stresses of her college quizzes.
   (c) It is most likely to resolve in time without ever pinning down a cause.
   (d) She is likely allergic to her birth control pills.

Answers: 1. (c), 2. (d), 3. (a), 4. (c), 5. (c)

References

1. Sampson HA. Adverse reactions to foods. In *Middleton's Allergy. Principles and Practice*, 6th Ed, NF Adkinson, JW Yunginger, WW Busse, BS Bochner, ST Holgate, FER Simons (eds.). St Louis, Mosby 2003, pp. 1619–1634.
2. Schwartz LB, Metcalfe DD, Miller JS .Tryptase levels as an indicator of mast cell activation in systemic anaphylaxis and mastocytosis. N Engl J Med. 1987, 316:1622–1626.
3. Reese G, Ayuso R, Lehrer SB. Tropomyosin, an invertebrate pan-allergen. Int Arch Allergy Immunol. 1999, 119:247–258.
4. Simons FER, Roberts JR .Epinephrine absorption in children with a history of anaphylaxis. J Allergy Clin Immunol. 1998, 101:33–37.
5. Teuber SS, Dandikar AM . Cloning and sequencing of a gene encoding a vicillin-like proto-protein, Jug r 2, from English walnut kernel (*Juglans regia*): a major food allergen. J Allergy Clin Immunol. 1999, 104:1311–1320.
6. Fernandez-Rivas M, Gonzales-Mancebo E, Rodriguez-Perez R . Clinically relevant peach allergy is related to peach lipid transfer protein, Pru p3, in a Spanish population. J Allergy Clin Immunol. 2003, 112:789–795.
7. Sicherer SH. Clinical implications of cross-reactive food allergens. J Allergy Clin Immunol. 2001, 108:881–890.

Chapter 9
Drug Allergy

Anna Kovalszki and James L. Baldwin

Abstract Drug allergy and sensitivity is one of the most challenging presentations that the practicing allergist encounters. Because of the extensively complex nature of these cases and the multiply mediated forms of drug allergy, we will present two illustrative and challenging cases with two very different mechanisms.

Keywords Drug allergy • Carmine allergy • Aspirin-exacerbated respiratory disease

Case 1

A 47-year-old woman with moderate persistent asthma and allergic rhinitis with bronchitis was prescribed azithromycin, which she had tolerated numerous times previously. She ingested 500 mg at 1 P.M., and by 2:30 P.M., she had developed facial urticaria and periorbital angioedema. She took 50 mg of Benadryl and presented to the ER with marked left periorbial angioedema and wheezing. Her vital signs were HR 108, RR24, BP 132/92, and SAO2 97%. She was administered 0.3-mg IM epinephrine and was started on prednisone. She left in improved respiratory condition without wheezing, although the angioedema took several hours to clear. She was instructed to see an allergist regarding her presumptive azithromycin reaction.

Her past medical history was significant for hypertension controlled with hydrochlorothiazide, gastroesophageal reflux controlled with rabeprazole, and moderate persistent asthma treated with fluticasone/salmeterol discus 250/50 and albuterol PRN. She had been taking each of these medications for over 3 years.

A. Kovalszki (✉) and J. Baldwin
Allergy and Clinical Immunology Division, Department of Medicine,
University of Michigan, Ann Arbor, MI, USA
e-mail: vidadi@umich.edu

M. Mahmoudi (ed.), *Challenging Cases in Allergy and Immunology*,
DOI: 10.1007/978-1-60327-443-2_9,
© Humana Press, a part of Springer Science+Business Media, LLC 2009

Data

No laboratory data taken.

Imaging Studies

None initially.

Impression/Working Diagnosis

Primary doctor referred her to us for newly acquired azithromycin allergy.

Differential Diagnosis

Acute urticaria due to any number of factors (foods, insect stings, viral-induced urticaria, true drug allergy/sensitivity, excipient allergy/sensitivity, acute urticaria of idiopathic nature, contact urticaria).

Work-Up

Work-up in allergy consisted of taking an in-depth history and physical exam, followed by immediate hypersensitivity skin testing.

In-Depth Allergy History

She has seasonal and perennial allergic rhinoconjunctivitis and moderate persistent asthma, with previous skin testing positive to trees, grasses, weeds, cats, and dogs. She has been to the emergency room three times for asthma in her life. She usually takes a prednisone taper 2–3 times yearly for asthma exacerbations. She also experienced tongue itching and irritation with kiwi and pineapple.

In addition, she has had a number of adverse symptoms that she has attributed to different foods. About 1 h after ingesting raspberry flavored Whips® yogurt, red tortellini soup, and applying certain eye shadows and blushes, she has had a combination of symptoms consisting of some or all of the following: hives on her face, skin flushing, periorbital edema, and shortness of breath.

She had also developed hives following ingestion of sulfa antibiotics in the distant past.

Physical exam showed no current hives or rashes and her lungs were clear.

Skin Prick Testing

We performed skin prick to carmine, as this product is used to dye items red and it was present in all of her products, including the ingested generic azithromycin (Teva Pharmaceuticals). The results are as follows:

Appropriate negative saline control

Histamine: 4 + (11/48 mm)
Carmine: 4 + (11/42 mm) reaction to carmine
Teva Pharmaceutical coating: 4 + (9/24 mm)
Teva Pharmaceutical azithromycin tablet stripped of the colored coating: 1 + (5/8 mm)
Greer Dust Mite Mix, cochineal insect extract, Pfizer Zithromax® tablet, and Pfizer
    Zithromax® coating: All negative

Please see Figs. 9.1 and 9.2 for skin prick results.

Further work-up included oral challenge with brand name Pfizer Zithromax®, without any adverse effect. She has avoided carmine-containing foods, drugs, and cosmetics and has had no recurrence of her previously unexplained carmine reactions.

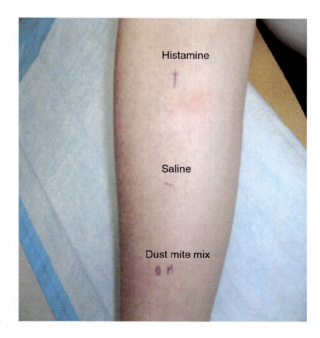

Fig. 9.1 Skin prick test:
Negative and positive controls

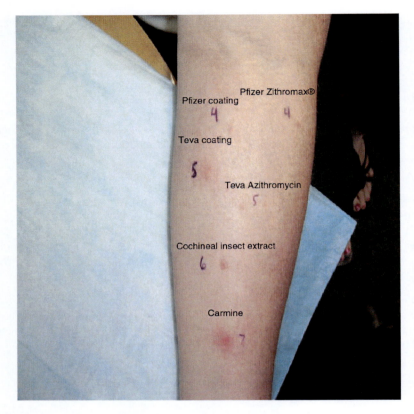

Fig. 9.2 Skin prick test: Demonstration of carmine and Teva Pharmaceutical coating allergy

Final Diagnosis

Carmine (excipient) allergy with no evidence of allergy to azithromycin itself.

Discussion

Carmine is a biogenic colorant derived from the cochineal insect. Carmine allergy has been described in carmine dye workers with occupational asthma, as well as in patients with type I hypersensitivity reactions to foods, drugs, and cosmetics colored various shades of pink, red, and purple with carmine dye (1–4). Prevalence of the disorder is not known, however, it is thought to be uncommon. In one study, factory workers were evaluated for prevalence of sensitization to carmine and occupational asthma at a natural dye processing factory where two workers had previously been given a diagnosis of carmine-induced occupational asthma. Among the 24 remaining employees, 41.6% were sensitized and 8.3% had occupational asthma as a result of carmine sensitization (1). Presentation of ingested carmine is that of immediate type hypersensitivity symptoms including hives, angioedema, bronchospasm, hypotension, and sometimes vomiting following ingestion of a product containing carmine. Additionally, localized immediate itching and swelling following application of cosmetics containing carmine also occurs.

The pathophysiology of this reaction is that of IgE-mediated allergy to carmine. Several investigators have suggested a retained insect protein as the etiologic allergen; however, no consensus exists as to the character or identity of this protein (2). Skin prick testing with carmine, along with the carmine-containing food, drug, or cosmetic in question generally confirms carmine allergy. Conversely, a carmine-specific IgE RAST has recently become available, although correlation with skin testing is unknown. Because of its exempt from certification status, carmine need not be listed by name on foods to which it has been added and can go under any of the following designations: color added, artificial color, carmine, cochineal extract, natural red 4, and E120. This makes avoidance of ingestion often problematic. The Food and Drug Administration has recommended that this allergen be listed by name on labels of foods to which it has been added, but no legislation has yet enforced this recommendation.

This case is illustrative of an excipient allergy and not a true drug allergy. Excipients are inactive substances added to a drug to confer suitable consistency or form to the drug - in this case a colorant. Another example of an excipient allergy is paraben allergy. The parabens are preservative excipients that can result in hypersensitivity reactions (types I and IV) and masquerade as a true drug allergy. The dangers of missing excipient allergy are continued reactions to the excipient, the misdiagnosis of true drug allergy, and inappropriate avoidance of medication that may be needed in the future. It was only through a careful in-depth history that this patient was properly diagnosed and treated.

Questions

1. A 10-year-old child with severe atopic dermatitis presents to her allergist's office with worsening dermatitis. The patient was placed on mometasone furoate for the first time 3 weeks prior to presentation, due to worsening atopic dermatitis. Skin exam is positive for worsening erythema and dermatitis, but no yellow scaling or pustules. What possible adverse reaction should the allergist consider? (5)

   (a) Vehicle allergy to propylene glycol
   (b) Staphylococcal superinfection
   (c) The patient is eating wheat, previously tolerated and skin prick test negative
   (d) Noncompliance with moisturization regimen

Answer: (a) Mometasone contains propylene glycol, a known excipient allergen found in some steroid creams. The clinical description of the rash is not consistent with a superinfection; the only new medication prescribed was mometasone furoate, and the patient does not have a wheat allergy. Noncompliance with moisturization should not result in worsening dermatitis, but rather in worsening dryness and scaling.

2. A 23-year-old college student presents to his dermatologist with a severely itchy dermatitis, mainly erythematous and somewhat confluent, that began after vacationing in Arizona. The student was conscientious and applied sunscreen daily during his trip. Allergic work-up is most likely to reveal which one of the following:

   (a) Solar urticaria
   (b) Positive patch testing to paraben
   (c) Erythropoietic protoporphyria
   (d) Skin prick test positivity to Bermuda grass

Answer: (b) The patient has a rash after applying sunscreen. In the allergy world, excipients in sunscreens such as parabens can cause contact dermatitis. He does not have urticaria based on the description. Erythropoietic protoporphyria has systemic complaints of abdominal pain after sun exposure and blistering as part of the clinical picture. Bermuda grass sensitivity may cause some local hives on his feet, but would not cause a persistent rash.

3. A 35-year-old man presents with a hospital-acquired pneumonia. The isolated organism is only sensitive to cefuroxime. This patient has a history of hives following penicillin (PCN) administration in his twenties. What diagnostic test is most useful in this setting, prior to treatment versus desensitization? (6)

   (a) Skin prick test to PCN major and minor determinants, and if negative, administer cefuroxime.
   (b) Skin prick test to nonirritating concentration of cefuroxime, and if negative, administer cefuroxime
   (c) Administer test dose of cefuroxime, and if no reactions occur, then full dose
   (d) Desensitize to cefuroxime

Answer: (a) The patient has a history of possible type 1 sensitivity to PCN. Even though the cross reactivity with cephalosporins is low, in a recent New England Journal article by Gruchalla et al., it is recommended that in patients with history of pencillin allergy, PCN testing be done prior to administration of cephalosporins (6). There is no validated method for evaluating the patient with cephalosporin directly, and he may not need desensitization if his prick to PCN is negative. Although administering test dose of cefuroxime would likely be done by many allergists, as there is no PCN currently available for testing, the best scientifically appropriate answer is testing to PCN first.

4. A 45-year-old woman with HIV/AIDS needs to be on trimethoprim sulfam-ethoxazole (Bactrim®), for *pneumocystis carinii* (PCP) prophylaxis. She has a history of maculopapular rash 1 week after taking Bactrim. What is our recommendation?

   (a) Avoid Bactrim®, consider aerosolized pentamidine
   (b) Start Bactrim® and treat any rashes with Benadryl
   (c) Outpatient oral desensitization to Bactrim®
   (d) Inpatient IV desensitization to Bactrim®

Answer: (c) In multiple studies, for patients who have rash caused by Bactrim®, and concurrent HIV, it is recommended that patients be desensitized over days at home to Bactrim®. Aerosolized pentamidine is not as effective as Bactrim® for PCP prophylaxis. Starting Bactrim® at full dose could result in serious rash and is not recommended without desensitization.

5. A 67-year-old man with history of rash with sulfapyridine presents with severe heart failure. The drug of choice is furosemide, another sulfa-containing product. What option does the cardiologist have? (7)

   (a) Ask the allergy department to perform skin prick testing to furosemide prior to administration.
   (b) Avoid furosemide and administer ethacrynic acid instead.
   (c) Administer furosemide with impunity.
   (d) Administer test dose of furosemide and watch for reactions.

Answer: (c) In a New England Journal Article, Strom et al. found that there is no significant cross-reactivity between sulfa antibiotic allergies and other sulfa medications, such as diuretics. Therefore, the cardiologist can administer furosemide.

Case 2

A 13-year-old Montana boy with asthma and a history of nasal polyposis developed a headache while visiting his grandparents in Michigan. He was given Excedrin Migraine® and over the next 3 h, he experienced severe shortness of breath, rhinorrhea, and wheezing unresponsive to his albuterol inhaler. He was taken to the emergency room and was noted to be in severe respiratory distress and unable to speak. Exam revealed squeaky air sounds with very shallow and tachypnic breathing with a respiratory rate of 40, poor air movement, tachycardia, severe retractions, and an oxygen saturation of 76% on room air. He was immediately intubated. He was treated with albuterol and ipratropium nebulized aerosol, corticosteroids, and antibiotics and was extubated 2 days later. We were called to evaluate him for possible aspirin (ASA) allergy.

Data

His blood gas at time of intubation: pH 7.17/PCO2 67/PO2 126/-HCO3 23.

Chest X-ray with hyperinflation and RML/RLL atelectasis, LUL atelectasis versus infiltrates.

CT Scan

CT scan was obtained prior to sinus surgery. Extensive sinus disease is present throughout the paranasal sinuses consistent with mucosal thickening, fluid, and/or polyps. Maxillary ostia are obscured.

Imaging Studies

Figure 9.3 illustrates his chest X-ray findings. Figure 9.4 is a cross section of his CT scan showing opacification of and possibly nasal polyps in his paranasal sinuses.

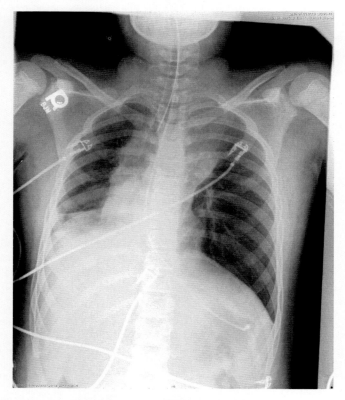

Fig. 9.3 Chest X-ray: Demonstration of hyperinflation and RML/RLL atelectasis, LUL atelectasis versus infiltrates

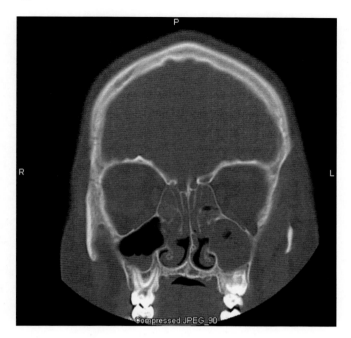

Fig. 9.4 CT scan of sinuses: Demonstration of right maxillary sinus air-fluid level, left maxillary sinus opacification, and extensive bilateral nasal turbinate hypertrophy

Impression/Working Diagnosis

Status asthmaticus secondary to pneumonia or Excedrin Migraine® in a patient with ASA-exacerbated respiratory disease

Differential Diagnosis

Drug reaction, underlying cystic fibrosis, asthma flare due to infection, drug, or allergy, pneumonia, anaphylaxis

Work-Up

We saw the patient and elicited a history of multiple sinus surgeries for recurrent and severe sinusitis as well as a history of anosmia and nasal polyposis. He had had ibuprofen one time with total body pruritus but no hives, rash, or shortness of breath. He also had never had ASA in the past. Excedrin Migraine contains caffeine, tylenol, and ASA. He has had the other two ingredients without difficulty in the past.

He was being treated for numerous allergies by serial dilution Rinkel method by his otolaryngologist in Montana (8). He had not had his shot for 3 weeks, although he had not seen much benefit after 2 years of therapy. This is not surprising, as Rinkel method is not effective than traditional immunotherapy, as demonstrated by Roger Hirsch and others (8). Records from his otolaryngologist doctor reported allergy to dandelion, poplar, ragweed, timothy grass, cottonwood, and mugwort. He had multiple food allergies listed, but he was able to eat all items mentioned including eggs, wheat, peanuts, and soybean.

His asthma had been very severe and he was using his albuterol inhaler even when relatively well controlled on montelukast and fluticasone/salmeterol 500/50 inhaled twice daily. He frequently needed oral corticosteroid for exacerbations. He had many sinus infections as well as severe rhinitis causing snoring and daytime somnolence.

He had sweat chloride and genetics checked for cystic fibrosis that were normal.

After stabilization and weaning from mechanical ventilation he returned to Montana and began seeing an allergist for his allergic rhinitis and asthma. He followed up in Michigan 3 months later for ASA challenge and potential desensitization and therapy to attempt to improve both his rhinitis/polyposis/sinusitis and possibly asthma.

On arrival we elected to challenge him to ibuprofen rather than ASA, as the former is the more accepted nonsteroidal anti-inflammatory medication (NSAID) in the pediatric population and based on the mechanism of ASA-exacerbated respiratory disease would be as effective as ASA treatment.

On our physical exam, there was a small polyp in his left nostril, but his airways sounded normal and stable, with an FEV1 of 2.08 (75% predicted), FVC 2.77 (87% predicted), FEV1/FVC ratio 75%, and FEF 25–75 1.63 (52% predicted). Baseline PEFRS were recorded the previous week with <20% variability.

He underwent Motrin® dye-free syrup challenge. His provoking dose was 80 mg and he underwent standard desensitization protocol, waiting 3 h between administrations and beginning at a lower than recommended dose, with the following doses (all in mg): 10, 20, 40, 80, 80, 80, 120, 120, 120, 160, 160, 200, 200. He had multiple reactions at the doses of 80, 120, 160, and 200 mg. Over 8 days, he was desensitized to 200 mg of Motrin® in an outpatient setting. He was instructed to take 200-mg Motrin two times daily indefinitely following desensitization.

In a follow-up phone conversation from Montana, we found him to be in good spirits and health. He has established care with a local allergist and is on classic immunotherapy. He is taking his Motrin 200 mg bid and has not needed his rescue albuterol inhaler for months. His rhinosinusitis and anosmia have also significantly improved.

Final Diagnosis

ASA-exacerbated respiratory disease

Discussion

ASA-exacerbated respiratory disease (AERD) affects 10–20% of adult asthmatics. These patients also have polypoid rhinosinusitis and respiratory reactions characterized by wheezing, rhinitis, and lacrimation within 3 h of ingestion of any NSAID that inhibits COX-1 (9). COX-2 inhibitors do not exacerbate AERD. Rarely doses of >1 g of acetaminophen will also exacerbate AERD as this dose weakly inhibits COX-1.

The pathophysiology of the disorder does not involve an immune-mediated mechanism of allergy, either through IgE or delayed T-cell mediated type reaction, but rather involves the eicosanoid pathway. Patients with AERD exhibit elevated level of cysteinyl leukotrienes and prostaglandins. Prostaglandins are produced through the COX-1 enzyme from arachidonic acid. Cysteinyl leukotrienes are made through the 5-lipoxygenase (5-LO) pathway from the same substrate. Following ingestion of an NSAID, PGE2 decreases because of COX-1 blockage, and there is a consequent increase in leukotriene production through the 5-LO pathway, which is responsible for the typical symptoms of the AERD reaction. Following desensitization and continued therapy, however, the levels of leukotrienes produced fall to normal, likely accounting for the clinical improvement seen in desensitized and treated AERD patients (9).

Work-up includes oral ASA/NSAID challenge, though some alternatives exist. Nasal and inhaled lysine-ASA preparations available in other countries are not approved here, but have been used in other countries for challenge. Nasal ketorolac challenges have been reported to be effective in diagnosis of respiratory disease and have even been used for desensitization with good results (10).

Treatment for the prevention of recurrence of polyposis and also severity of asthma includes desensitization to ASA/NSAID and continued daily therapy indefinitely. Several protocols for desensitization have been proposed. The latest practice paper from the Aspirin Desensitization Joint Task Force in 2007 suggests starting at 20.25 mg followed by 40.5, 81, 162.5, and 325 mg and giving another increased dose if no reactions occur every 90 min. FEV-1 and exam were performed prior to each dose. A 15% or more decrease in FEV-1 suggests a lower respiratory tract reaction. The 90-min interval can be spaced out to 3 h based on individual patient characteristics. Provoking doses need to be repeated prior to escalation (11).

This case is particularly challenging because of our patient's age. In general, this is a disease of adulthood, so much so that the diagnosis was questionable until confirmed with NSAID challenge. The AERD literature in children is sparse. The most comprehensive case presentation is that of five children who had well-documented ASA-induced asthma in a Journal of Pediatrics article from 1973 (12). Beyond the dearth of data, it is also uncommon to desensitize these patients at this age. Because of our firm diagnosis and parents' wishes, we elected to proceed with this treatment. As a result, he has improved significantly. He is not requiring rescue albuterol; his polypoid rhinosinusitis has stabilized and his sense of smell has returned.

Questions

1. What mediator exists in overabundance in AERD?

   (a) Complement C4
   (b) Leukotriene C4
   (c) Histamine
   (d) Tryptase

Answer: (b) Leukotrience C4 is elevated in patients with AERD as part of the cascade that is abnormal. Complement is part of the complement cascade and is sometimes elevated as an acute phase reactant in patients who are infected. Histamine and tryptase are elevated during anaphylaxis.

2. Which of these medications does not exacerbate patients with AERD?

   (a) Ibuprofen
   (b) Acetominophen
   (c) Ketorolac
   (d) Celecoxib

Answer: (d) COX-2 inhibitors do not inhibit COX-1 and therefore do not exacerbate AERD. Tylenol in high doses, >1 g, can have partial COX-1 blocking activity. Ketorolac and Ibuprofen are NSAIDs and block COX-1.

3. Many diseases cause nasal polyps. What entity does not cause polypoid rhinos inusitis?

   (a) Cystic fibrosis
   (b) Wegener's granulomatosis
   (c) Allergic rhinitis
   (d) Churg-Strauss syndrome

Answer: (b) All of the possibilities have been known to cause polyps except for Wegener's granulomatosis, which causes granulomas as implied by its name.

4. What level of FEV1 drop is considered to be a threshold value for continuance of desensitization?

   (a) 5%
   (b) 10%
   (c) 15%
   (d) 20%

Answer: (c) At 15% or more FEV1 drop, a dose needs to be repeated before escalation of dosing during an ASA challenge in an AERD patient.

5. A 50-year-old man with a history of gout presents with a rash 2 weeks after being placed on high-dose allopurinol therapy. The rash is maculopapular, somewhat dusky and confluent, with areas of wet sloughing. He also complains of sore throat and eye irritation. Physical examination is notable for oral ulcerations and

conjunctival injection. Skin biopsy of a blistering lesion is most likely to show (13) which one of the following:

(a) Subepidermal vacuole formation with full thickness epidermal necrosis
(b) Dissolution of stratum granulosum
(c) Epidermal hyperplasia and subepidermal lymphocytic infiltrate
(d) Vasculitis with occlusion of dermal blood vessels

Answer: (a) The clinical scenario is consistent with toxic epidermal necrolysis (TEN). In TEN, there is full thickness epidermal necrosis and subepidermal vacuole formation, hence sloughing of the skin. Dissolution of stratum granulosum is seen in staphylococcal scalded skin syndrome. Epidermal hyperplasia and subepidermal lymphocytic and/or eosinophilic infiltrate are seen in drug eruptions. Vasculitis is seen on pathology in vasculitis affecting the skin.

Acknowledgement We thank Dr. Matthew Greenhawt in his contribution to clinical care for one of our patients.

References

1. Tabar-Purroy, A. I., Alvarez-Puebla, M. J., Acero-Sainz, S., Garcia-Figueroa, B. E., Echechipia-Madoz, S., Olaguibel-Rivera, J. M., Quirce-Gancedo, S. (2003) Carmine (E-120)-induced occupational asthma revisited. *J Allergy Clin Immunol* **111**, 415–419.
2. Chung, K., Baker, J. R., Jr., Baldwin, J. L., Chou, A. (2001) Identification of carmine allergens among three carmine allergy patients. *Allergy* **56**, 73–77
3. DiCello, M. C., Myc, A., Baker, J. R., Jr., Baldwin, J. L. (1999) Anaphylaxis after ingestion of carmine colored foods: two case reports and a review of the literature. *Allergy and Asthma Proc* **20**, 377–382.
4. Wuthrich, B., Kagi, M. K., Stucker W. (1997) Anaphylactic reactions to ingested carmine (E120). *Allergy* **52**, 1133–1137.
5. Coloe, J., Zirwas, M. J. (2008) Allergens in corticosteroid vehicles. *Dermatitis* **19**, 38–42.
6. Gruchalla, R. S., Pirmohamed, M. (2006) Antibiotic Allergy. *N Engl J Med* **354**, 601–609.
7. Strom, B. L., Schinnar, R., Apter, A. J., Margolis, D. J., Lautenbach, E., Hennessy, S., Bilker, W. B., Pettitt, D. (2003) Absence of cross-reactivity between sulfonamide antibiotics and sulfonamide nonantibiotics. *N Engl J Med* **349**, 1628–1635.
8. Hirsch, R. S., Kalbfleisch, J. H., Cohen, S. H. (1982) Comparison of Rinkel injection therapy with standard immunotherapy. *J Allergy Clin Immunol* **70**, 183–190.
9. Stevenson, D. D., Szczeklik, A. (2006) Clinical and pathologic perspectives on aspirin sensitivity and asthma. *J Allergy Clin Immunol* **118**, 773–786.
10. Lee, R. U., Woessner, K. M., Simon, R. A., Stevenson, D. D. (2008) Intranasal Ketorolac for desensitization in patients with aspirin exacerbated respiratory disease. *J Allergy Clin Immunol* **121**, S73 (abstract).
11. Macy, E., Bernstein, J. A., Castells, M. C., Gawchik, S. M., Lee, T. H., Settipane, R. A., Simon, R. A., Wald, J., Woessner, K. M. (2007) Aspirin challenge and desensitization for aspirin-exacerbated respiratory disease: a practice paper. *Ann Allergy Asthma Immunol* **98**, 172–174.
12. Yunginger, J. W., O'Connell, E. J., Logan, G. B. (1973) Aspirin-induced asthma in children. *J Pediatr* **82**, 218–221.
13. Rapini, R. P. (2005) Reactive erythemas. Practical Dermatopathology, Philadelphia, PA: Elsevier, 61–70

Chapter 10
Anaphylaxis

Kris G. McGrath

Abstract Anaphylaxis is the most severe presentation of immediate-type hypersensitivity. It occurs rapidly and is often dramatic and unanticipated. Most episodes are not fatal; however, death may occur suddenly through airway obstruction or irreversible vascular collapse. There are at least 40 different signs and symptoms that may occur during the course of anaphylaxis. Cases related to the presentation and the management of anaphylaxis are discussed later.

Keywords Anaphylaxis • Exercise-induced anaphylaxis • Food-dependent exercise-induced anaphylaxis • Idiopathic anaphylaxis • Tryptase

Case 1

John is a 34-year-old male, who was found collapsed on the floor of a pharmacy at 9:30 P.M. The paramedics were called to the scene. John was intermittently aroused with confusion and mumbling of speech, and his face was red with swelling of the right eyelid.

Examination. His vital signs revealed a BP of 60 palpable, P 130, RR 24; T 98.7°F, O_2 sat. 88% room air. Skin: Generalized erythematous raised lesions, edema of right eyelid, redness from upper chest to face. HEENT: nonobstructing soft palate, uvular and oral pharyngeal edema. Lung auscultation: poor air movement, expiratory wheeze. Heart: regular rate and rhythm, no murmur. Extremities: mild distal cyanosis; no clubbing or edema. Abdomen: soft, nontender, no rebound/guarding/masses/organomegaly, normal bowel sounds. Neurological: arousable, mumbling speech.

K.G. McGrath (✉)
Division of Allergy Immunology, Department of Medicine, Northwestern University Feinberg School of Medicine, Chicago, IL, USA
e-mail: k-mcgrath@northwestern.edu

M. Mahmoudi (ed.), *Challenging Cases in Allergy and Immunology,*
DOI: 10.1007/978-1-60327-443-2_10,
© Humana Press, a part of Springer Science+Business Media, LLC 2009

John was left in the recumbent position with his lower extremities raised. Aqueous epinephrine 1:1,000 dilution, 0.3 mL, was administered IM in the upper lateral thigh and a large-bore IV infusion of normal saline was initiated. Oxygen 100% by nonrebreather mask was administered.

He was transported to a nearby university teaching hospital emergency department. He was alert, complaining of generalized itching, shortness of breath, and "a lump in my throat." Improvements in his initial examination included normal vital signs, generalized skin erythema, scattered urticaria, no cyanosis, and lung auscultation with faint end expiratory wheeze. Lab reports were obtained at 10:30 P.M.

Past medical history. Seasonal allergic rhinitis and intermittent asthma.

History of present illness. John recalls developing itchy red spots on his chest and back, spreading all over his body, and swelling of his right eye lid at 9 P.M. He became short of breath and felt a sensation in his throat, "like a lump." He recalled abdominal cramping and feeling "lightheaded."

Allergy history. No known previous drug/food allergy.

Medications. Albuterol inhaler two puffs q 4 h prn. Not on ACE or β-adrenergic antagonist drugs. No illicit/herbs/natural remedies. Stings/bites: None. Illness: Asthma controlled. Food/activity: Eating began at 5:30 P.M. and concluded at 8:30 P.M. The evening began with appetizers of shrimp and smoked salmon. The salad contained walnuts. The main course followed with beef tenderloin and green beans. Dessert was hazelnut cheesecake. He left the restaurant at 9 P.M. and at 9:15 P.M. went to the pharmacy for diphenhydramine for intense itching of his skin, followed by the aforementioned events. He did not exercise after eating.

Laboratory results. Normal CBC, electrolytes, blood glucose, BUN, creatinine, liver enzymes, and C4. The chest X-Ray was normal with sinus tachycardia on ECG. Serum tryptase 8.0 µg/L (nl 1.9–13.5 µg/L).

Hospital Course. With resolution of his complaints and physical findings, John was observed for 3 h and during the signing of his discharge instructions he complained of feeling *lightheaded* and developed urticaria, facial angioedema, stridor, shortness of breath, and hypotension. Reinstitution of anaphylaxis therapy ensued including recumbent positioning, IM aqueous epinephrine, two large-bore IV saline infusions, intubation, and O_2-supported mechanical ventilation. He was admitted to the medical intensive care unit.

1. With the presented information, what is your working diagnosis?

    (a) Idiopathic anaphylaxis
    (b) Food-induced anaphylaxis with a biphasic response
    (c) Exercise-induced anaphylaxis
    (d) Food-dependent exercise-induced anaphylaxis
    (e) Insect sting/bite anaphylaxis
    (f) Drug-induced anaphylaxis

2. With the presented information what is your *"differential diagnosis"* if not anaphylaxis?

    (a) Shock from other causes: Cardiogenic, endotoxic, hypoglycemic

    (b) Restaurant syndromes: MSG, sulfites, fish poisoning (scrombroidosis/sauri
        nosis)
    (c) Excessive production of histamine: systemic mastocytosis, urticaria pigmen-
        tosa, basophilic leukemia
    (d) Hereditary or acquired angioedema
    (e) Idiopathic urticaria/angioedema in an asthmatic with acute bronchospasm

Case Discussion

John had anaphylaxis with a biphasic response from food. The suspect foods ingested within 4 h of the event in sequence were shrimp, salmon, walnut, beef, green bean, and hazelnut. The nearest food to the onset was hazelnut. Upon discharge from the hospital John was educated on the necessity of avoidance of the foods he ingested within 4 h of the onset of symptoms. He was prescribed an emergency kit including two doses of self-injectable epinephrine, prednisone 40 mg q A.M., and Ceterizine 10 mg qd for 4 days. An allergy referral was given to be seen within 3–4 weeks.

Allergy consultation included a complete allergy history with confirmation of adherence and response to therapy, review of the medical records, and an examination. Prick skin testing was done only to suspect foods relative to the anaphylactic event. These included shrimp, salmon, green bean, walnut, hazelnut, histamine, and diluent control. Hazelnut resulted in a 4-mm wheal and a 30-mm flare within 10 min; all others were negative. As a precaution prick skin testing to the other tree nuts and peanut were applied, with negative results. As an action plan, John was instructed on hazelnut avoidance and to always be prepared for accidental or hidden exposure to hazelnut. He will have readily available a triple therapy kit consisting of two doses of self-injectable epinephrine, 50-mg prednisone, and 10-mg Cetirizine and seek immediate emergency care. John was informed about national organizations that provide important information and educational materials, such as the Food Allergy and Anaphylaxis Network, www.foodallergy.org, the American Academy of Allergy, Asthma, and Immunology, www.aaaai.org, and the American College of Allergy, Asthma and Immunology, www.acaai.org. A medic alert card or jewelry identification was advised (MedicAlert®, Turlock, Ca, www.medicalert.co.us) as well as a folding wallet card from the American Academy of Allergy, Asthma and Immunology anaphylaxis educational materials (www.aaaai.org).

In anaphylaxis risk assessment, John had a comorbidity of atopy and asthma increasing his risk of anaphylaxis from ingested antigens. He did not have underlying cardiac disease and was not on drugs that may interfere with anaphylaxis treatment: β-adrenergic antagonist, angiotensin-converting enzyme inhibitor, MAO, inhibitor, or tricyclic antidepressant. Clinical manifestations were those most commonly seen in anaphylaxis: cutaneous >90%, respiratory 55–60%, cardiovascular 30–35%, gastrointestinal 25–30%, and miscellaneous 5.8%. By diagnostic criteria (see Table 10.2 later) he fulfilled criteria 1 with an acute onset of an illness (minutes to several hours) with involvement of the skin, mucosal tissue, or both. In addition, John had at least one of the following: respiratory compromise or reduced blood pressure.

John's treatment was prompt and appropriate with no delay in epinephrine administration. Unfortunately, John had a biphasic response of anaphylaxis. Were there early clues in his medical history, type of trigger, timing of presentation, and physical exam in alerting the ED to observe longer? Yes, there were. The biphasic reaction occurs in up to 20% anaphylaxis, usually within 8 h of the initial presentation. The oral route is a predisposing factor with risk factors of initial hypotension, laryngeal edema, and a delay of more than 30 min between ingestion of allergen and appearance of first-event symptoms.

Food anaphylaxis is the most common cause of anaphylaxis in the community leading to emergency department visits, with 150 deaths annually in the USA. Anaphylaxis has a slower onset from food ingestion as from injected allergens, but can occur within seconds to a few hours after ingestion. Fatality, however, may occur within 25–35 min. The food trigger may not always be obvious, such as hidden, trace, or malicious. This necessitates examining ingredient lists and labels. A lack of serum tryptase elevation occurs in the majority of cases. This is likely due to basophil as opposed to mast cell mediation, and slower onset. A better serum marker for food-induced anaphylaxis may be platelet-activating factor (PAF) level or PAF-acetylhydrolase activity. Targeted from history IgE-specific skin testing should be performed 3–4 weeks after the episode, allowing mediator reformation. Circumstances may not allow skin testing, substituting with serum ImmunoCap testing (Phadia AB, Uppsala, Sweden).

John's asthma was intermittent and controlled and did not contribute to this event or impede treatment.

Case 2

Mary is a 26-year-old female who awakened at 7 A.M. with swelling of her right hand. This persisted throughout the day with development of left hand and upper lip swelling. At 10 P.M. she began to itch all over and noted red raised skin lesions all over her body. Her father brought her to the emergency department (ED). Within 30 min upon arrival she complained of throat tightness, difficulty in speaking, and difficulty in breathing. She was given 0.3-mL 1:1,000 dilution aqueous epinephrine IM, 125-mg methyl prednisolone IV, 50-mg diphenhydramine IV, and 20-mg famotidine IV. Intubation was required with O_2-supported mechanical ventilation.

Past medical history. Cholecystectomy in 2006.

Medications. None.

Allergy history. Drugs: No previous drug/food allergy. No prescription/OTC medications, illicits/herbs/natural remedies, ACE or β-adrenergic antagonist drugs.

Stings/bites. None; Illness: None; Food/activity: No food ingestion or exercise in previous 9 h.

Examination. Patient sedated on mechanical ventilation. Vital signs: BP 105/54, P 120, RR 24; T 98.9°F. Skin: Generalized urticaria, edema of upper lip. HEENT: tongue edema against endotracheal tube. Lung auscultation: CTAB. Heart: regular rate and rhythm, no murmur. Extremities: no cyanosis, clubbing, or edema. Abdomen: soft, nontender, no rebound/guarding/masses/organomegaly, normal bowel sounds. Neurological: sedated.

Laboratory results. Normal CBC, electrolytes, blood glucose, BUN, creatinine, liver enzymes, C3, C4, C1q. CXR normal. ECG sinus tachycardia. Serum tryptase 26 µg/L (nl 1.9–13.5 µg/L).

Hospital course. Hypotension and respiratory failure persisted over the next 6 h requiring IV pressors, two large-bore IVs of normal saline and continued O_2-supported mechanical ventilation. Sixty milligrams of methyl prednisolone and 50 mg of diphenhydramine were administered q 6-h IV. Over the next 6 h urticaria/angioedema resolved, pressors were weaned, and patient extubation occurred without adverse sequela.

1. With the presented information, what is your working diagnosis?

   (a) Idiopathic anaphylaxis with protracted course
   (b) Food-induced anaphylaxis
   (c) Drug-induced anaphylaxis
   (d) Mastocytosis
   (e) Hereditary angioedema
   (f) Acquired angioedema

2. With the presented information what is your *differential diagnosis* if not anaphylaxis?

   (a) Shock from other causes: Cardiogenic, endotoxic, hypoglycemic
   (b) Restaurant syndrome: MSG, sulfites, fish poisoning (scrombroidosis/saurinosis)
   (c) Excessive production of histamine: systemic mastocytosis, urticaria pigmentosa, ruptured hydatid cyst, basophilic leukemia
   (d) Flushing: carcinoid, medullary thyroid carcinoma, VIP-secreting tumor, alcohol, autonomic epilepsy

Case Discussion

Mary has idiopathic anaphylaxis (IA) with a protracted course. Her serum tryptase was elevated, which is not elevated in any other condition, except in mastocytosis. Idiopathic anaphylaxis is responsible for one-third of anaphylaxis presentations and has no external allergen trigger. It is a diagnosis of exclusion after eliminating other causes, such as anaphylaxis from food, drug, exercise, food + exercise, diagnostic agents, and insect stings/bites, and illnesses such as mastocytosis and C1 esterase inhibitor deficiency/dysfunction. The symptoms of IA are identical to known causes of anaphylaxis, and classification of IA is relative to clinical manifestations and frequency. The acute management of IA is the same as with other types of anaphylaxis with the difference occurring with outpatient management. This depends upon the IA classification. She will have readily available a triple therapy kit consisting of two doses of self-injectable epinephrine, 50-mg prednisone, and 10-mg Cetirizine and seek immediate emergency care. As in case 1, Mary was informed about the same supportive organizatons and to see an allergist.

Disease Discussion

Anaphylaxis is the most severe form of allergy and is called "the killer allergy," and defined as, "a serious allergic reaction that is rapid in onset and may cause death."

Often unanticipated, this event occurs suddenly with rapid progression. Death may occur suddenly through airway obstruction or irreversible vascular collapse. Most episodes of anaphylaxis are not fatal. Anaphylaxis requires prompt recognition and therapeutic intervention. Once treatment is initiated, the patient must be educated, provided with an action plan, and observed for protracted and biphasic anaphylaxis. Anaphylaxis is caused by sudden and progressive release of biological active mediators from mast cells and peripheral blood basophils (1–3).

The World Allergy Organization's and Simon's nomenclature eliminates the term anaphylactoid and classifies anaphylactic events as immunologic and nonimmunologic (2, 4). The most common is the immediate hypersensitivity response (IgE-dependent). This occurs from IgE fixing to FcεRI receptors on surface membranes of tissue mast cells and blood basophils. Receptor-bound IgE molecules aggregate upon allergen reexposure resulting in cellular activation and mediator response. Immunologically induced anaphylaxis can also occur through immune complex of IgG and IgM, platelets, T-cells, leukotriene formation, and activation of complement, contact, and coagulation systems. Nonimmunologic anaphylaxis (IgE-independent) occurs from factors acting directly on mast cells. These include radio contrast media (RCM), opioids, vancomycin, radiation, exercise, cold water or air exposure, and ethanol. Idiopathic anaphylaxis occurs spontaneously and is not caused by an unknown allergen; autoimmunity is likely involved. Munchausen's anaphylaxis is a purposeful self-induction of true anaphylaxis; fictitious anaphylaxis is often fabricated within history and lacks objective findings. All forms present the same, requiring rigorous allergy history-taking, diagnostic and therapeutic intervention, and the acquisition of biomarkers (4). Refer to Table 10.1 for types/causes/mechanisms of anaphylaxis.

Anaphylaxis incidence is underestimated and underrecognized. Mild episodes, though potentially fatal, may resolve spontaneously without evaluation. The incidence is rising, especially from food in the USA, Australia, and the United Kingdom (UK). The lifetime prevalence of anaphylaxis from all triggers has an estimated lifetime prevalence of 0.05–2%, and average annual incidence of 21 per 100,000 person-years. The estimated case fatality rate is 0.65%. Prescriptions for self-injectable epinephrine were estimated at 1% of the population of Manitoba, Canada. Anaphylaxis hospital admissions in the UK rose 700% from 1991 to 2004 (5–8).

Table 10.1 Some causes and mechanisms of anaphylaxis in humans

Immunologic IgE-mediated	Immunologic non-IgE-mediated
Drugs: β-Lactam antibiotics, sulfonamides, tetracyclines, cisplatinum, carboplatinum, thiopental	Blood products (blood, plasma, cells), IVIG: IgG anti-IgA antibody, IgE isotype, immune complex, complement activation by serum protein/immune aggregates, i.e., IVIG (nonimmune complex) cellular element anaphylaxis-cytotoxic (IgG, IgM)
Biological: Vaccines, enzymes, OKT3 monoclonal antibody, cetuximab, omalizumab, horse antilymphocyte globulin, Botox, herbals, bee products	
Foods: Peanut, tree nuts, cow's milk, hen's egg, soy, wheat, fish, shellfish, grains, and seeds	
Blood products: Nonatopic receives IgE to food or drug; atopic receives allergen or drug rom donor	
Food additives: Carmine	
Insect stings/bites, other bites: Venoms: Hymenoptera, fire ants, jellyfish, scorpions, snakes. Insect saliva: Mosquitoes, deer fly, pigeon ticks, triatomid bugs, green ants	
Inhalants: Grass pollen, peanut, horse, cat and hamster dander	
Seminal Fluid: Seminal proteins, transfer of partner's ingested food or drug	
Natural rubber latex: Gloves, condoms	
Immunotherapy extracts: Pollens, dust mite, mold, animal, venoms	

Nonimmune mediated: Direct release of mediators from mast cells and basophils
    Drugs: Acetylsalicylic acid, COX 1 and COX 2 nonsteroidal anti-inflamatory agents, opiates, ethanol
    Diagnostic Agents: Radiocontrast media, flouresceine, sulfobromophthalein
    Physical: Exercise, cold (air, water), heat, UV radiation

Combination of mechanisms: Immune-IgE, complement activation, immune complex, immune aggregates, cytotoxic and nonimmune direct mast cell mediator release, contact system

Drugs: Vancomycin, protamine sulfate, succinylcholine, thiopental, d-Tubocurarine, pancuronium, atracurium, vecuronium (direct mast cell release and/or IgE-mediated)

Colloid plasma expanders: Dextran (direct mast cell release and complement mediated-immune aggregates, hydroxyethyl starch)

Contact system: Dialysis exposure: AN69 membrane, bradykinin-mediated

Miscellaneous: Food-dependent exercise-induced (FDEIA), FDEIA + aspirin/NSAID

Autoimmune: Idiopathic

Forty different signs and symptoms may occur. Clinical manifestations within organ systems occur with the following frequency: skin >90%, respiratory 55–60%, cardiovascular 30–35%, gastrointestinal 25–30%, and miscellaneous 5.8%. At the onset the patient may have a sense of oppression or impending doom along with nasal, ocular, and palatal pruritus as well as sneezing and diaphoresis (1–3).

Symptoms usually begin within 5–60 min after exposure to the inciting agent. Delay in onset of several hours is less common. Anaphylaxis from an ingested antigen can occur immediately, but usually occurs within 2 h and can be delayed for several hours. The initial manifestation of anaphylaxis may be sudden loss of consciousness; death may occur in minutes. Sudden fatality has also been attributed to postural change during anaphylaxis, sitting or standing, as opposed to remaining recumbent with raised lower extremities. Deaths occurring days to weeks after anaphylaxis are often due to organ damage occurring early in the course of anaphylaxis. In general, the later the onset of anaphylaxis, the less severe. Early onset anaphylaxis may resolve spontaneously or with treatment to be followed by another "biphasic" episode. Protracted anaphylaxis lasts 5–48 h despite therapy, with an estimated rate of 23–28% or less (4).

The diagnosis of anaphylaxis is clinical; however, laboratory findings assist in confirmation. A CBC may show an elevated hematocrit secondary to hemoconcentration. Blood chemistries may reveal elevated creatinine phosphokinase, troponin, aspartate aminotransferase, or lactate dehydrogenase if there is myocardial damage. Elevation of serum/urine histamine and serum tryptase can occur, and complement abnormalities have been observed. Plasma histamine is elevated within 5–10 min of mast cell activation and returns to baseline within 30–60 min. Urinary histamine metabolites, including methyl histamine, may be found for up to 24 h. Mast cell-derived tryptase achieves a peak level at 1 h and remains elevated for up to 6 h following anaphylaxis. This necessitates collecting serum tryptase levels within 3 h. It is not elevated in other causes of death; however, it is elevated in individuals with mastocytosis. A normal serum tryptase does not exclude anaphylaxis. Food-induced anaphylaxis is seldom associated with elevation of serum tryptase, possibly due to basophil predominance over mast cells. Future availability of measuring other mast cell and basophil activation markers will be useful as a part of an "anaphylaxis panel." The ImmunoCap test (Phadia AB, Uppsala, Sweden) may be used on postmortem serum to measure specific IgE to antigens such as Hymenoptera or suspected foods (4).

A chest radiograph may show hyperinflation, atelectasis, or pulmonary edema. ECG changes other than sinus tachycardia or infarction include T-wave flattening/inversion, bundle branch blocks, supraventricular arrhythmias, and intraventricular conduction defects. Myocardial infarct/damage may occur in up to 80% of fatal cases (4).

Diagnostic criteria of anaphylaxis have been established and are shown in Table 10.2. Any one of the three criteria are expected to capture greater than 95% of the cases (9). Table 10.3 includes the differential diagnosis of anaphylaxis.

A recent antigen or substance exposure and clinical suspicion are the most important diagnostic tools. Obtain the circumstances surrounding the event. Begin with the time of the initial complaints, the sequence of complaints, and physical findings observed by the patient. Confirm these findings by witnesses and photographs. Review the medical records and note objective findings. Work backward regarding the timing of exposure and acquire past history of anaphylaxis. IgE antibody can be demonstrated in vivo by skin prick testing or in vitro by the ImmunoCap (Phadia AB, Uppsala, Sweden). Absent IgE may justify an oral graded food challenge. For agents that alter arachidonic acid metabolism such as ASA/NSAIDS and other suspected non-IgE mediated agents, carefully graded oral challenge can be done with clinical observation and measurement of pulmonary function, nasal patency, and vital signs, following informed consent and necessity of agent (3).

Table 10.2 Clinical criteria for diagnosing anaphylaxis

Acute onset of an illness (minutes to several hours) with involvement of the skin, mucosal tissues, or both (e.g., generalized hives, pruritus, or flushing, swollen lips, tongue, uvula *and at least one of the following*

  Respiratory compromise (e.g., dyspnea, wheeze-bronchospasm, stridor, reduced PEF, hypoxemia)
  Reduced BP or associated symptoms of end-organ dysfunction (e.g., hypotonia [collapse], syncope, incontinence)

Two or more of the following that occur rapidly after exposure to a *likely allergen for that patient* (minutes to several hours):

  Involvement of the skin-mucosal tissue (e.g., generalized hives, itch-flush, swollen lips, tongue, uvula)
  Respiratory compromise (e.g., dyspnea, wheeze-bronchospasm, stridor, reduced PEF, hypoxemia)
  Reduced BP or associated symptoms (e.g., hypotonia [collapse], syncope, incontinence)
  Persistent gastrointestinal symptoms (e.g., crampy abdominal pain, vomiting)

Reduced BP after exposure to *known allergen for that patient* (minutes to several hours):

  Infants and children: Low systolic BP (age-specific) or greater than 30% decrease in systolic BP[a]
  Adults: Systolic BP of less than 90 mmHg or greater than 30% decrease from that person's baseline

From J Allergy Clin Immunol 2006;117:393, with permission

PEF Peak expiratory flow, *BP* blood pressure

[a]Low systolic blood pressure for children is defined as less than 70 mmHg from 1 month to 1 year, less than 70 mmHg + [2 × age] from 1 to 10 years, and less than 90 mmHg from 11 to 17 years

Table 10.3 Differential diagnosis of anaphylaxis

Other forms of shock: Hemorrhagic, cardiogenic, endotoxic, hypoglycemic
Cardiac arrhythmia, myocardial infarction
Aspiration of foreign body
Severe cold urticaria
Redman syndrome from vancomycin
Pulmonary embolism
Seizure disorder
Vasovagal (vasodepressor) reaction
Hyperventilation
Idiopathic urticaria in an asthmatic with acute bronchospasm
Factitious allergy, panic attacks, vocal cord dysfunction, globus, Munchausen stridor, undifferentiaded somatoform anaphylaxis
Restaurant syndromes: MSG, sulfites, fish poisoning (scrombroidosis, saurinosis)
Flushing: Postprandial, carcinoid, postmenopausal, chlorpropramide, alcohol, medullary thyroid carcinoma, autonomic epilepsy, VIP-secreting tumor
Excessive production of histamine: Systemic mastocytosis, urticaria pigmentosa, basophilic leukemia, ruptured hydatid cyst, tretinoin treatment of acute promyelocytic leukemia
Hereditary and acquired angioedema
Capillary leak syndrome

Factors that increase the severity of anaphylaxis or interfere with treatment are listed in Table 10.4 (4).

The treatment of anaphylaxis should include the established principles for emergency resuscitation and is presented in Table 10.5 (4, 10).

Table 10.4 Factors that influence the severity or interfere with treatment of anaphylaxis

Asthma; not controlled, especially if FEV1 ≤ 70% predicted. COPD
Underlying ischemic cardiac disease, older individual, with rapid infusion of allergen
Mastocytosis
Vision or hearing impairment, CNS diseases
Drugs: Prescription, nonprescription, recreational, ethanol
Concomitant therapy with the following:
    β-adrenergic antagonists
    Monoamine oxidase inhibitors
    Tricyclic antidepressants
    Angiotensin-converting enzyme inhibitors
    Angiotensin II receptor blockers
Delay or inadequate dose of epinephrine administration
Psychiatric disease

Table 10.5 Treatment, education, and prevention of anaphylaxis

Immediate: Aqueous epinephrine 1:1,000 dilution, 0.3–0.5 mL (0.01 mg/kg in children: maximum 0.3 mg) IM-thigh. May repeat every 5–10 min if necessary. IV epinephrine only in dire situations when severe hypotension or cardiac collapse is unresponsive to IM doses using 5–10-μg IV bolus (0.2 μg/kg) for hypotension and 0.1–0.5-mg IV for cardiovascular collapse with toxicity monitoring; children: 0.01 mg/kg (0.1 mL/kg of a 1:10,000 solution). Consider continuous low-dose epinephrine IV infusion at 4–10 μg/min.

If sting: Tourniquet proximal to site releasing every 1–2 min every 10 min, injecting one-half dose aqueous epinephrine into site (0.1–0.2 mg)

Record blood pressure, pulse, and O2 saturation

Depending on severity, degree of response, and the individual patient:

Benadryl 25–50 mg adults, 1 mg/kg up to 50 mg children IV slowly; Ranitidine 50 mg adults, 12.5–50 mg children (1 mg/kg) IV over 5–10 min

Nasal oxygen or high-flow oxygen through nonrebreather mask or endotracheal tube

Methylprednisolone 1–2 mg/kg/day IV or Hydrocortisone 5 mg/kg (200 mg max) q 4–6 h or Prednisone 0.5 mg/kg/day PO (exact doses of corticosteroids not established)

Be prepared for intubation

For severe bronchospasm:

Inhaled β2-agonist: Nebulized; albuterol 2.5–5 mg/3 mL saline or levalbuterol 0.63–1.25 mg, unit dose. When not responsive, IV aminophyline 5 mg/kg over 30 min

For systolic blood pressure: <90 mmHg, age ≥ 10; <70 mmHg + (2× age in years), children age >1–10; <70 mmHg, infants 1–12 months; <60 mmHg, term neonates (0–28 days)

Two IV lines wide open

Vasopressors IV: Norepinephrine, metaraminol. Aortic balloon counterpulsation for myocardial dysfunction

For patients taking β-adrenergic antagonists:

Glucagon 1–5 mg IV slowly, then titrate at 5–15 μg/min infusion, emesis precaution

Atropine if bradycardia; 0.3–0.5 mg IM or IV every 10 min, maximum of 2 mg

Observation for protracted or biphasic anaphylaxis in emergency department observation unit, hospital admission, or intensive care unit. Observation period individualized on patient's severity, reliability, and access to care

Obtain serum tryptase within 3 h of onset; mark time of blood draw. If available, plasma histamine within the first hour, 24-h urinary methyl histamine, PAF and PAF-acetylhydrolase. Save frozen plasma/serum sample.

Discharge with preparedness/action plan: Avoid trigger if known; triple therapy kit: two epinephrine self-injectors, 30–50-mg prednisone, 10-mg Cetirizine, EIA and FDEIA exercise with companion, FDEIA no food within 6 h of exercise. Anaphylaxis action plan form (www.aaaai.org), medical identification (www.medicalert.co.us), referral to allergy specialist

Questions

1. What is the most common cause of anaphylaxis in the community leading to increasing visits to emergency departments?

   (a) Food
   (b) Drug
   (c) Stinging insects
   (d) Food-dependent, exercise-induced
   (e) Idiopathic

2. What is the leading cause of anaphylaxis in the hospital setting?

   (a) Radiocontrast media
   (b) Vancomycin
   (c) Aspirin and NSAIDs
   (d) During anesthesia and surgery
   (e) β-Lactam antibiotics

3. In the order of frequency, what is the most frequent manifestation of anaphylaxis?

   (a) Cardiovascular: lightheaded, faint, hypotension, myocardial infarction
   (b) Respiratory: "lump in my throat," stridor, wheezing, dyspnea
   (c) Cutaneous: itching, flushing, urticaria, angioedema
   (d) Gastrointestinal: abdominal cramping, nausea, emesis, diarrhea
   (e) Neurological: confusion, dizziness, syncope, seizure, loss of consciousness

4. What is unique about food-induced anaphylaxis?

   (a) May be mimicked by "restaurant syndromes" from MSG, sulfites, and spoiled fish (scombroidosis, saurinosis).
   (b) May occur within seconds, but generally has a slower onset than injected allergens.
   (c) Food-induced anaphylaxis is seldom associated with an elevated serum tryptase due to basophil involvement over mast cells.
   (d) Serum PAF or PAF-acetylhydrolase activity may be a better biomarker of food-induced anaphylaxis.
   (e) All of the above.

5. Characteristic of biphasic anaphylaxis is as follows:

   (a) Occurs in up to 20% of anaphylaxis.
   (b) It is most common for the second episode to occur within 8 h of the first.
   (c) The initial trigger may be immunologic, nonimmunologic, or idiopathic.
   (d) The oral route appears more of a predisposing factor.
   (e) Death can occur.
   (f) All of the above.

6. What class of drugs could the patient be taking that inhibits the endogenous compensatory mechanism of shock in anaphylaxis?

(a) β-Adrenergic antagonists
(b) Angiotensin-converting enzyme inhibitors
(c) Tricyclic antidepressants
(d) Monoamine oxidase inhibitors

7. What is the most common cause of anaphylaxis in the operating room?

(a) Latex
(b) Induction/hypnotic agents
(c) Muscle relaxants
(d) Blood products
(e) Antibiotics

8. What is not true about food-dependent exercise-induced anaphylaxis?

(a) Aspirin is an exacerbating factor.
(b) The triggering food may be ingested safely without exercise.
(c) In Japan wheat is the most common cause.
(d) Eight percent of patients have symptoms within 2 hours of eating rather than exercising.
(e) The suspect food skin test is negative in most patients.

9. Idiopathic anaphylaxis is likely caused by:

(a) An unknown food
(b) An unknown drug
(c) Recreational drug
(d) An underlying disease
(e) An autoimmune-type process

10. The most common cause of death from anaphylaxis is from:

(a) A delay in administering epinephrine
(b) Fear of administration of epinephrine in a patient with cardiac disease
(c) A delay in administration of an H1 and H2 antihistamine
(d) A delay in administration of a corticosteroid

Answer Key: 1-a, 2-e, 3-c, 4-e, 5-e, 6-b, 7-c, 8-e, 9-e, 10-a

References

1. Simons FER. Anaphylaxis, killer allergy: Long-term management in the community. J Allergy Clin Immunol 2006;**117**:367–377.
2. Simons FER. Anaphylaxis. J Allergy Clin Immunol 2008;**121**(2):S402–S407.
3. Johansson SGO, Bieber T, Dahl R, et al. Revised nomenclature for allergy for global use: Report of the Nomenclature Review Committee of the World Allergy Organization, October 2003. J Allergy Clin Immunol 2004;**113**:832–836.

4. McGrath KG. Anaphylaxis. In: Grammer LC, Greenberger PA, eds. Patterson's Allergic Diseases, Seventh Edition. Philadelphia, PA: Lippincott Williams & Wilkins 2009:205–226.
5. Poulos LM, Waters AM, Correll PK, et al. Trends in hospitalizations for anaphylaxis, angioedema, and urticaria in Australia, 1993–1994 to 2004–2005. J Allergy Clin Immunol 2007;**120**(4):878–884.
6. Lin RY, Cannon AG, Teitel AD. Pattern of hospitalizations for angioedema in New York between 1990 and 2003. Ann Allergy Asthma Immunol 2005;**95**:159–166.
7. Gupta R, Sheikh A, Strachan DP, et al. Time trends in allergic disorders in the UK. Thorax 2007;**62**:91–96.
8. Lieberman P, Camargo CA Jr, Bohlke K, et al. Epidemiology of anaphylaxis: Findings of the American College of Allergy, Asthma and Immunology Epidemiology of Anaphylaxis Working Group. Ann Allergy Asthma Immunol 2006;**97**:596–602.
9. Sampson HA, Munoz-Furlong A, Campbell RL, et al. Second symposium on the definition and management of anaphylaxis: Summary report-second national institute of allergy and infectious disease/food allergy and anaphlaxis network symposium. J Allergy Clin Immunol 2006;**117**:391–397.
10. Joint Task Force on Practice Parameters, American Academy of Allergy Asthma and Immunology, Joint Council of Allergy Asthma and Immunology. The diagnosis and management of anaphylaxis: An updated practice parameter. J Allergy Immunol 2005;**115** (Suppl):S483–S523.

Chapter 11
Eosinophilia and Eosinophilic Disorder

Massoud Mahmoudi

Abstract Eosinophilic disorders are a spectrum of diseases characterized by peripheral eosinophilia and eosinophilic infiltration in various organs. The manifestation of each disease varies by the affected organ. Here, we present two challenging cases in eosinophilic pneumonia and eosinophilic esophagitis.

Keywords Eosinophilia • Eosinophilic pneumonia • Eosinophilic esophagitis

Case 1

Our patient is a 45-year-old Asian/Caucasian male who was referred to us in 2003 for evaluation of allergy and asthma. He reported a history of intermittent "itchy lungs" since 1990s. His symptoms included dry cough triggered by certain weather conditions and occasionally in springs. There was no history of shortness of breath, wheezing, or nasal symptoms. His only medication included vitamins and supplements.

His past medical history consisted of hypertension and tonsillectomy. Drug allergy: Penicillin with unknown reaction. Family history: Mother died of breast cancer and father had hypertension.

Social and environmental history. He was married and worked as a musician. He was born in East coast and after traveling and living in Europe, Saudi Arabia, and southwest USA, he moved to northern California at age 14. He admitted to four packs per year history of smoking and consumption of a case of beer per week for 15 years. He also had a history of recreational drugs in the past but no intravenous drugs. He had lived in his present home off and on since 1982. The house was equipped with central heating and air conditioning units. He used a nonfeather pillow and a comforter. The living room and his bedroom were of hardwood. He had two indoor cats.

M. Mahmoudi (✉)
University of California San Francisco, San Francisco, CA, USA
e-mail: allergycure@sbcglobal.net

M. Mahmoudi (ed.), *Challenging Cases in Allergy and Immunology*,
DOI: 10.1007/978-1-60327-443-2_11,
© Humana Press, a part of Springer Science+Business Media, LLC 2009

Review of systems. Except dry skin, right hearing loss and neck and shoulder pain were unremarkable.

Physical examination. He appeared as a pleasant tall male, well nourished, and in no acute distress. Vitals: BP: 132/108 mmHg, pulse: 96 beats per minute (regular). HEENT: The examination revealed hyperemic eyes, blocked ear canals with cerumen, and edematous nostrils, otherwise within normal limits. Heart had regular rhythm with no murmur. Auscultation of chest revealed rough breath sounds in the right upper lung (posteriorly). Extremities: The fingernail of his first right digit had the appearance of a mycotic infection. The remaining of the examination was within normal limits.

Diagnostic testing. Prick skin testing to aeroallergens was done and no significant reaction was identified. Spirometry pre- and postbronchodialator revealed normal measurements except reduced lower airways (forced expiratory flow rate at 25–75% was 69% of predicted). After postbronchodilator, peak expiratory flow rate (PEF) increased by 10%; otherwise, there were no significant changes with other parameters.

Impression. Cough with unknown etiology, likely due to irritation, smoking, and exposure to the club environment.

Plan. He was advised to take montelukast 10-mg tablet once a daily and follow-up visit in 2 weeks.

His health history from 2003 to 2007 included several visits to our office, some with 8–11 months intervals. During this period, his primary physician started him on a blood pressure medication. He continued on montelukast for a while and then stopped it. He also tried beclomethasone inhaler with no help. He continued with cough and sinus problems. Our effort to convince him to have a chest X-ray and CT scan of the sinuses was unsuccessful. He also developed rash due to possible adverse reaction to a beta-blocker medication for his hypertension. In 2005, his dermatologist diagnosed him with lichen planus and started on accutane for several months and then retnoids and prednisone.

In January 2005, he had CBC and differentials and they were within normal limits. In April 2005, his CBC measurements included white blood cell of 16.1 (3.8–10.8) thousands per μl, lymphocytes 15% (20–45%), and eosinophil 25% (0–6%), the absolute eosinophil of 4,000 (0.015–0.500) $\times 10^{-3}$/mm^3, erythrocyte sedimentation rate (ESR) 47 (0–15) mm/h, serum iron 10 (40–190), and fructoseamine 181 (205–265) μmol/l. These abnormal numbers coincided with sickness post colon hydrotherapy (recommended by his physician) and he lost 11 lbs and developed diarrhea. The other significant history included quitting alcohol in 2006.

Our last visit with him was on March 2007. We did not hear from him till September 2007 when we got a call that he was in ICU.

Reportedly, prior to admission to the hospital, he developed nonproductive cough, malaise, and worsening shortness of breath. He had recently started a 10-days course of minocycline due to skin infection. He then saw his physician and was referred to the emergency department. In the emergency room, he appeared short of breath at rest, alert, and oriented. Vitals: BP: 109/87 mmHg, pulse: 141 beats/min, and O$_2$ saturation 88% in room air. Later on his BP was

134/91 mmHg, O_2 saturation on 4 l of oxygen was 90–92%, and temperature was 98.3°F. Abnormal findings: Heart was tachycardic (monitor 124 beats/min); chest auscultation revealed fine bibasilar rales (more on the left) and a few rhonchi.

Data

Laboratory data. The abnormal lab results are presented in Table 11.1. The EKG revealed sinus tachycardia. The two views of chest X-ray depict bilateral diffuse interstitial infiltrates, bilateral areas of consolidations, and bilateral minor pulmonary effusions.

With Presented Data, What Is Your Working Diagnosis?

This 45-year-old male presented with cough of several days duration, dyspnea, and hypoxemia. His initial chest X-ray revealed bilateral infiltrate, consolidation, and minor pleural effusion. Presented data and the exam lead us to diagnosis of *bilateral pneumonia.*

Differential diagnosis. The differential diagnosis includes malignancy, sarcoidosis, pneumocystis, histoplasmosis, coccidiomycosis, and allergic bronchopulmonary aspergillosis (ABPA).

Table 11.1 Abnormal lab findings

Test	Abnormal parameters	Range
WBC 10^3 per mm^3	20.0 H	4.8–10.8
MCH pg	31.5 H	27.0–31.0
Lymphocyte (%)	7.7 L	20.5–51.1
Eosinophils (%)	17.0 H	0.0–6.0
Eosinophil absolute number 10^3 per mm^3	3.40 H	0.0–0.5
Granulocyte absolute number 10^3 per mm^3	14.4 **H**	1.4–6.5
Glucose (mg/dl)	107 H	65–100
Sodium (mmol/l)	136 L	138–146
Calcium (mg/dl)	8.2 L	8.5–10.3
Albumin (g/dl)	2.9 L	3.2–5.0
Total protein (g/dl)	5.6 L	6.0–8.0
AST (SGOT) U/l	7 L	14–50
ALT (SGPT) U/l	8 L	10–44
Urine analysis	Hazy appearance, protein, rare RBC, WBC, bacteria	Clear color, negative (proteins, RBC, WBC, bacteria)
	Decreased specific gravity	Specific gravity (1.010–25)
Arterial blood gas	Ph: 7.43, PCO_2: 36.9 mmHg, PO_2: 65% on 4-l oxygen	Ph 7.350–7.450, PCO_2 35.0–45.0, PaO_2 75–100% in room air

L lower than normal range; H higher than normal range

Work-Up

HIV testing was negative. *Echocardiagraphy.* Ejection fraction 63%, no pericardial effusion and mild aortic insufficiency. The *pulmonary angiography* was negative for emboli. *High-resolution CT scan* of the chest: The findings included (a) extensive alveolar infiltrates in upper lobes (bilaterally) and less extensive infiltrates in dependent regions of lower lobes (bilaterally), (b) bilateral pleural effusions (more on the right), (c) extensive lymphadenopathy in mediastinum and hilar regions, and (d) a 2-cm mass-like density in posteromedial region of the right lower lobe. *Bronchoalveolar lavage (BAL)* results indicated an inflammatory background, negative stain for malignancy, and pneumocystis (Fig. 11.1).

Pleural fluid cytology. Reactive mesothelial cells, inflammation, and eosinophils were reported. There was no evidence of malignancy. *Lung biopsy.* Eosinophils were noted in biopsy of the left lung. Fungal stain was negative.

What Is Your Diagnosis and Why?

Malignancy. Although the CT imaging of our patient could have been a result of metastatic lung disease, all malignancy tests (cytology) were negative.

Sarcoidosis. Although hilar adenopathy is usually seen in sarcoidosis, the remaining data do not support the diagnosis of sarcoidosis.

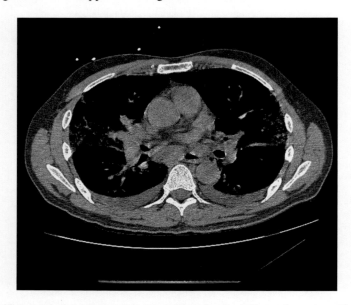

Fig. 11.1 High-resolution CT scan of the lungs. Note alveolar infiltrates in upper and lower lobes, bilateral pleural effusions, lymphadenopathy in mediastinum and hilar regions, and mass-like density in posteromedial region of the right lower lobe

Pneumocystis. Pneumocystis usually occurs in immunocompromised patients. The HIV testing and staining for pneumocystis were negative.

Histoplasmosis, coccidiomycosis. All fungal stainings were negative; also, the CT of the chest and the laboratory data do not support the diagnosis of fungal infection.

ABPA. The laboratory data (peripheral eosinophilia) and chest X-ray qualify the diagnosis of ABPA for further consideration. However, negative testing for *Aspergillus fumigatus,* the remaining data such as lung biopsy, and the acute presentation suggest a different diagnosis.

The review of clinical presentation, i.e., cough, shortness of breath, recent history of minocycline, and presented data (peripheral blood eosinophilia and presence of eosinophil agregates in the lung tissues) led us to the diagnosis of *eosinophilic pneumonia.*

Our patient had a unique presentation of eosinophilic pneumonia. He had features of various eosinophilic pneumonias. Duration of presentation was within a week and he presented with an acute episode. This presentation fits the criteria of the *acute eosinophilic pneumonia.* The symptoms were also started after several days of taking minocycline. This is a common presentation of *secondary eosinophilia* due to medication. Parasitic infections and medications may also cause an entity known as *simple eosinophilic pneumonia*; such condition, however, is usually mild and resolves without treatment. History of chronic peripheral eosinophilia (2004) and lack of atopic condition added up to the complication of his condition. Given the history of recent minocycline use and his acute presentation, however, we narrowed our diagnosis to *minocycline-induced acute eosinophilic pneumonia.*

Discussion

Eosinophilia is an abnormal accumulation of eosinophils in peripheral blood and or tissues due to various causes. Although we have identified etiology of eosinophilia in many conditions, other causes of eosinophilic diseases still remain unknown. Various anatomical structures including lung tissues are target of infiltration.

Pulmonary eosinophilia is a diverse group of eosinophilic lung diseases with peripheral blood and or lung tissue eosinophilia. There is no uniform way of classifying pulmonary eosinophilia. Perhaps the simplest way of grouping pulmonary eosinophilia is dividing the diseases into *primary* (eosinophilc lung diseases of unknown causes) and *secondary* (eosinophilic diseases of known causes). Primary eosinophilia may present as *simple, acute,* and *chronic eosinophilic pneumonia* or as *hypereosinophilic syndrome.* Secondary causes of pulmonary eosinophilia are drugs, infections, and environmental factors; Table 11.2 (1, 2).

Simple eosinophilic pneumonia (Loeffler syndrome). This form of eosinophilic pneumonia is self-limited and may develop as a result of parasitic infection, medication, smoke, or an unknown cause (idiopathic). Peripheral blood or BAL shows eosinophilia. Chest radiograph shows transient opacities. Symptoms are usually mild and treatment is usually not necessary (2, 3).

Table 11.2 Etiology of eosinophilia

Classification	Examples of causative agents
Primary (idiopathic)	
Simple eosinophilic pneumonia	Parasites
	smoke, idiopathic
Acute eosinophilic pneumonia	Idiopathic
Chronic eosinophilic pneumonia	
Hypereosinophilic syndrome	
Secondary causes	
Infections	
Bacteria	Brucella, mycobacteria
Viruses	Human T-cell lymphocytic virus, West Nile virus
Fungi	Aspergillus, Coccidia
Parasites (usually helminthes)	Round worms (Strongyloides, ascaris, toxocara, hookworm)
Malignancies	Hodgkin's and non-Hodgkin's lymphoma
Medications	
Antibiotics	Minocycline, penicillins, sulfonamide
NSAIDS	Aspirin, naproxyn, Ibuprofen
Cardiovascular	Captopril, hydrochlorothiazide, amiodarone
Environmental	Dust, smoke

Acute eosinophilic pneumonia. Patients with acute eosinophilic pneumonia usually present with 1 week or less of dyspnea, cough, and fever. Presenting symptoms may also include chest pain and myalgia. Worsening of respiratory symptoms may require intubation and ventilatory support. Diagnoses include the presence of eosinophilia in peripheral blood (not common), BAL and lung tissues biopsy (usually not necessary), and diffuse opacities, Kerley B lines, and pleural effusion in chest radiography. The affected patients do respond to corticosteroids. The relapse of this form of pneumonia is uncommon (3, 4); Table. 11.3.

Chronic eosinophilic pneumonia. Chronic eosinophilic pneumonia presents in fifth decade of life and is female dominant (male to female: 1:2). Patients with this form of pneumonia present with weeks to months of dyspnea, cough, fever, and weight loss. Respiratory failure is uncommon. Diagnosis is based on presence of eosinophilia in peripheral blood, BAL, and lung tissues as well as peripheral opacities in chest radiography. Patients respond to corticosteroids but may relapse during taper. Therefore, duration of treatment may take from months to years (5, 6) table 11.3.

Drug-induced eosinophilic pneumonia. Eosinophilic pneumonia may present secondary to use of medications. Although minocycline was a possible cause of pneumonia in our patient, a wide range of medications may cause drug-induced eosinophilic pneumonia (Table 11.2) (3, 6).The symptoms due to this type of pneumonia are usually mild (simple eosinophilic pneumonia) and may resolve after discontinuation of the offending medication. At times the affected patients present with the picture of an acute eosinophilic pneumonia and respiratory distress. Such patients need prompt attention and may need intubation to manage the respiratory distress.

Table 11.3 Classification of eosinophilic pneumonia

Characteristics	Simple pulmonary eosinophilia (Loeffler syndrome)	Acute eosinophilic pneumonia	Chronic eosinophilic pneumonia
Gender (male: female)		1:1	1:2
Mean age (year)		29	45
Duration of symptoms before presentation	1–2 weeks	Within a week	Weeks to months
Peripheral blood eosinophilia	Usually in normal range	Usually in normal range	1,000 eosinophils/mm³
BAL		Usually more than 25% eosinophils	Usually more than 25% eosinophils
Lung biopsy	Not needed	Only if BAL is negative	Only if BAL is negative
Chest radiograph findings	Transient opacities	Diffuse opacities, Kerley B-lines, pleural effusions	Peripheral opacities
Corticosteroid response	Usually not needed	Yes	Yes
Relapse	Unusual	Unusual	Usual
Prognosis	Good	Good, if treated promptly	Good but it usually relapses

BAL Bronchoalveolar lavage

Pathophysiology. Migration of eosinophils from bone marrow to target tissues is a multistep process. First, the eosinophils propagate and mature in bone marrow, then they enter circulation, and finally migrate into the target tissues. This multistep process includes participation of several cytokines, adhesion molecules, and chemoattractants. The mechanism of eosinophil recruitment to lung tissues, however, is unknown. In chronic eosinophilic pneumonia, it is proposed that an unknown stimulus triggers the initial step in recruiting Th2 cells to the lungs. This is mediated by a thymus and activation-regulated chemokine (TARC) and regulated upon activation, normal T-cell expressed and secreted (RANTES). The IL-5, produced by Th2 cells, and other cytokines, IL-6, IL-10, RANTES, and eotaxin collectively participate in accumulation of eosinophils in lung tissues (5).

Work-Up. The work-up for esoinophilic pneumonia starts with a detailed history. It is important to inquire about recent medications, infections, and travel history. The initial examination should also include pulse oximetry and arterial blood gases in case of acute presentation. The laboratory investigation should at least include a complete blood count (CBC), looking for peripheral eosinophilia, specifically, and possible sign of infections. Then other laboratory studies should include tests to exclude human immunodeficiency virus (HIV) infections, ABPA, and parasitic infections.

Imaging studies. The first imaging study is a chest X-ray. The abnormal chest X-ray should be followed by a high-resolution CT scan of the chest. The features of the chest X-ray and the CT findings may vary among different types of eosinophilic pneumonias. The chest X-ray findings may include transient, peripheral or diffuse opacities, Kerley B-lines, and pleural infusion (3). The CT findings may include peripheral consolidation, diffuse interstitial infiltrates, patchy alveolar infiltrates, ground glass infiltrates, or Kerley B-lines. At times lymphadenopathy and pleural effusion may also be present (3, 7).

Bronchoscopy. The next step is bronchoscopy and analysis of BAL. The BAL of greater than 25% eosinophils is a criterion for eosinophilic pneumonia.

Lung biopsy. It is performed when BAL is negative and to exclude other causes of lung diseases. The biopsy would show an aggregate of eosinophils.

Treatment. If possible, the underlying cause of eosinophilic pneumonia should be identified and treated. Simple eosinophilic pneumonia may resolve after discontinuation of the offending medication or treatment of the parasitic infection. It is usually a mild disease and the use of corticosteroid is not necessary. Acute eosinophilic pneumonia responds well to corticosteroid therapy. A common regiment is methyl prednisolone 125 mg every 6 h until resolution of the respiratory failure (7). Chronic eosinophilic pneumonia responds to corticosteroid as well. However, during tapering the dose, there is a chance of relapse. A starting dose of corticosteroid (prednisone) is usually 40–60 mg per day; the dose may be tapered to a maintenance in the first few weeks (3).

Summary and conclusion. Pulmonary eosinophilia is a diverse group of lung diseases with peripheral and or tissue eosinophilia. Eosinophilic pneumonia divides into simple, acute, and chronic. Although an eosinophilic pneumonia has a good prognosis, however, it should be diagnosed and treated promptly to prevent an organ damage and fatality. Corticosteroids are the mainstay of treatment for acute and chronic eosinophilic pneumonias and should be tapered cautiously in the chronic form of the disease.

Questions

1. Which one of the following is the secondary cause of eosinophilic pneumonia?

    (a) Bacterial infection
    (b) Parasitic infections with roundworms
    (c) Fungal infections
    (d) Malignancies
    (e) All of the above

2. Which of the following statements is true?

    (a) Peripheral eosinophilia is an indication of an eosinophilic disease.
    (b) Presence of eosinophiols in BAL or lung tissues is an indication of eosinophilic disease.
    (c) Presense of respiratory symptoms such as cough and shortness of breath and eosinophils in BAL or lung tissue is an indication of eosinophilic lung disease.

(d) If BAL is positive for eosinophils, lung biopsy is a logical next step in diagnosis of eosinophilic pneumonia.
(e) All patients with peripheral eosinophilia develop eosinophilic disease.

3. What is the first step in management of drug-induced eosinophilic lung disease?

(a) Decreasing the medication dose to half and watching for worsening of the
   symptoms.
(b) Stop the offending medication.
(c) Add an antiparasitic medication.
(d) Lung biopsy to confirm the diagnosis.
(e) BAL to confirm the diagnosis.

4. Which one of the following medications can cause drug-induced eosinophilic
   pneumonia?

(a) Ibuprofen
(b) Aspirin
(c) Amiodarone
(d) Captopril
(e) All of the above

5. Which one of the following is true regarding eosinophilic pneumonia?

(a) Transient opacities on a chest X-ray are characteristic of acute eosinophilic
   pneumonia.
(b) Transient opacities on a chest X-ray are characteristic of a chronic eosinophilic
   pneumonia.
(c) Transient opacities are characteristic of Loeffler syndrome.
(d) Relapse of chronic eosinophilia is unusual.
(e) Relapse of simple eosinophilia is frequent.

Answer key: 1. (e), 2. (c), 3. (b), 4. (e), 5. (c)

Case 2

P. Fulkerson and Marc Rothenberg

A 17-year-old Caucasian male presents to your office with the chief complaints of chronic dysphagia and poor weight gain for the past 7 years. The family reports that while he has been a picky eater since he was a toddler, his feeding issues were not a concern until he was 7-years old when he experienced two choking episodes involving food impaction in his esophagus. The first episode occurred when he was 7-years old when a piece of steak had to be retrieved by endoscopy from his distal esophagus, followed by a similar episode later in the same year. A third food impaction event with endoscopy required for retrieval of a piece of chicken occurred just 2 months prior to presentation. A pH probe completed after the second episode showed no prolonged episodes of esophageal acidification, but there was concern that acid reflux was underrecorded due to poor appetite during the study. An esophagogastroduodenoscopy (EGD) with biopsies revealed moderate distal esophagitis with numerous intraepithelial eosinophils and with features suggesting reflux. He was started on an antireflux medication. With treatment, the patient still complained of difficulty in swallowing and ate poorly resulting in a significant amount of weight loss. In the spring of the next year, a barium esophagogram showed normal motility and normal diameter, but EGD biopsies revealed mid-proximal to distal esophagitis and mild basal hyperplasia. At that time, prior to any steroid therapy, an esophageal brushing showed scattered nonseptate hyphal elements consistent with a Candida species. Following standard treatment for esophageal candidiasis, the patient still had poor weight gain. A gastric emptying scan later that year showed delayed emptying. The patient underwent pyloroplasty and a Nissen fundoplication at 12 years of age. After his surgeries, he refused to eat and underwent percutaneous endoscopic gastrostomy placement. He received his nutrition entirely through his gastronomy tube for over a year. Follow-up EGDs over the next 4 years showed findings that were consistent with a diagnosis of esophagitis and gastroesophageal reflux disease (GERD). With concern for an eating disorder as his weight gain continued to be poor after surgery and medical treatment, he was referred to a psychiatrist for treatment for anorexia nervosa and was prescribed an antidepressant. His mother discontinued the antidepressant and counseling after a year of therapy, as she did not believe that it made any difference in stimulating appetite or weight gain. He has also been taking Megace for the past 3 years for appetite stimulation. He has a history of an anaphylactic reaction, including chest tightness, to seafood. Although the patient has not undergone skin prick or patch testing, the family has tried food avoidance,

P. Fulkerson and M. Rothenberg (✉)
Department of Pediatrics, University of Cincinnati College of Medicine, Cincinnati, OH, USA

including peanuts, seafood, and all dairy products, but with little improvement. In addition, the patient has a history of exercise-induced asthma and allergic rhinitis that was controlled with over-the-counter medications. The family has come to you for a second opinion, as the patient has not improved with any treatment to date.

On exam, he is a thin young man, weighing 53.6 kg (5th percentile) and measuring 165.5 cm (10th percentile). In general, he was alert and in no apparent distress. His exam was essentially benign. Of note, there were bilateral allergic shiners and mild paleness of his nasal mucosa. In addition, his abdomen was soft, nontender, and nondistended with no evidence of hepatosplenomegaly, and his skin was clear with no rashes.

With the Presented Data, What Is Your Working Diagnosis?

The patient is a 17-year-old young man with a history of chronic esophagitis and allergic rhinitis. He has been treated for GERD, esophageal candidiasis, and an eating disorder with little improvement in terms of his dysphagia or his poor weight gain. Based on poor or no response to antireflux medications and surgery, he likely has allergy-related eosinophilic esophagitis (EE). Food impaction is a common initial presentation for EE.

Differential Diagnosis

A large number of conditions are associated with esophageal dysphagia and esophagitis. In addition to eosinophilic esophagitis, we should consider GERD, recurrent or cyclic vomiting perhaps associated with an eating disorder, and under-treated esophageal candidiasis. In the absence of esophagitis, congenital esophageal rings and motility disorders, such as achalasia and diffuse esophageal spasms, should be considered. The most common consideration in the differential diagnosis is GERD.

Work-Up

CBC with differential revealed an elevated eosinophil percentage and absolute eosinophil count. Serum immunoglobulins revealed an elevated IgE. In addition, his C-reactive protein was elevated to 5.44 mg/dl (Table 11.4).

Skin prick tests were performed, which showed positive responses to a number of food and environmental antigens (Table 11.5).

Patch testing was also performed to the antigens that were negative on skin prick testing and were negative by patch testing as well. An EGD was completed, which

Table 11.4 Lab results

Lab values		Normal
WBC (k/μL)	8.55	4.5–13
Hgb (g/dL)	14.3	13–16
HCT (%)	41.2	37–49
MCV level (fL)	83	78–98
Platelet (k/μL)	299	135–466
Segs (%)	60	40–62
Lymphs (%)	28	34–42
Monocytes (%)	4.8	0–10
Eosinophils (%)	7.2 H	0–5
Neutrophil absolute (k/μL)	5.13	1.8–8.0
Lymph absolute (k/μL)	2.39	1.2–5.2
Mono absolute (k/μL)	0.41	0.0–0.8
Eosinophil absolute (k/μL)	0.616 H	0.0–0.6
IgA (mg/dL)	131	68–378
IgE (IU/mL)	216 H	<114
IgG (mg/dL)	1,020	724–1611
IgM (mg/dL)	97	60–263
C3 (mg/dL)	128	71–150
C4 (mg/dL)	28.3	15–47
CRP (mg/dL)	5.44 H	<1.0
Urease	Negative	Negative

C3 complement component 3, *C4* complement component 4, *CRP* C-reactive protein *H* high

showed a mucosa in the proximal esophagus that was moderately thickened and furrowed. The middle and distal esophaguses were markedly thick and furrowed with exudate present in small, white specks. No erosions, ulcerations, erythema, or strictures were noted. Nissen fundoplication was intact. Esophageal biopsy revealed hyperplasia of basal layer, papillary elongation, and inflammatory infiltrate consisting predominantly of eosinophils with intraepithelial eosinophils >30 per high-powered field (HPF) (Fig. 11.2).

Multiple eosinophilic microabscesses, or aggregates of four or more eosinophils in a cluster, were identified in a biopsy specimen. Biopsy specimens from the stomach and duodenum were normal. Urease activity for *Helicobacter pylori* was negative.

What Is Your Diagnosis and Why?

This patient has the gross mucosal abnormalities and histopathologic features consistent with a diagnosis of eosinophilic esophagitis. Importantly, he has dense esophageal eosinophilia, including eosinophilic microabscesses, despite antireflux therapy. Also, the patient is atopic based on his history of allergic rhinitis and the presence of allergen antigen sensitization revealed by skin prick testing and elevated IgE.

Table 11.5 Skin prick test

Antigen	Skin prick (wheal/flare mm)
Diluent	0/0
Histamine	2/3
Cantaloupe	3/7
Apple	0/0
Banana	0/0
Barley	3/5
Carrot	0/0
Corn	5/20
Mustard	5/15
Sesame	5/10
Sunflower	5/7
Peanut	0/0
Tuna	5/10
Turkey	0/0
Chicken	0/0
Lamb	0/0
Beef	0/0
String bean	5/20
Pea	5/20
Squash	5/15
Tomato	3/10
Egg white	0/0
Whole egg	0/0
Mold-1	5/15
Mold-2	5/20
Ragweed	5/20
Grass	3/5
Trees-5	7/20
Trees-6	3/5
Mite mix	5/10
Cockroach	3/5
Cat	5/20

The skin prick test introduces a tiny amount of allergen into the skin. The negative control is a saline solution to which a response is not expected. The positive control solution contains histamine to which everyone is expected to react. A ruler is used to measure the diameter of the wheal and the flare is expressed in mm. A positive response has a wheal/flare ratio similar to the positive control histamine. Mold-1 allergens include alternaria, hormondendrum, helminthosporium, penicillium, and aspergillus; Mold-2 allergens include mucor, rhizopus, fusarium, and pullularia; Trees-5 allergens include oak, pecan, sycamore, and black willow; Trees-6 allergens include ash, beech, birch mix, cottonwood, elm, and black walnut

Discussion

Definition. Eosinophilic esophagitis (EE) is a clinicopathologic syndrome found throughout the world with increasing prevalence in both children and adults over the past decade with males more commonly affected than females (8). EE is

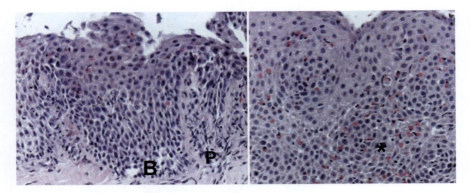

Fig. 11.2 Esophageal biopsies showing marked intraepithelial eosinophil infiltration (asterisk) associated with basal cell hyperplasia (B) and papillary lengthening (P)

characterized by esophageal and/or upper gastrointestinal (GI) tract symptoms in association with esophageal mucosal biopsy specimens containing ≥ 15 intraepithelial eosinophils per HPF in one or more biopsy specimens and a normal pH monitoring study of the distal esophagus or lack of responsiveness to high-dose proton pump inhibition. Intraepithelial eosinophil infiltration is not a specific finding for any disease entity as eosinophil infiltration of the esophageal epithelium can be found in GERD, EE, inflammatory bowel disease, and others. As such, clinical correlation is necessary for the diagnosis of EE. In addition, EE is distinguished from GERD by the magnitude of the esophageal eosinophilia, the strong association with male gender, atopy, as well as a family history of EE.

Presentation

Children most commonly present with GERD-like symptoms including heartburn and regurgitation, as well as abdominal pain and emesis. Dysphagia and food impaction are also reported with increasing prevalence with advancing age of the child. Of note, younger children with the inability to relate the feeling of dysphagia can present with feeding refusal or intolerance and failure to thrive. In adults, the most common presenting symptoms are intermittent dysphagia and food impaction. GERD-like symptoms are also common in adults. EE tends to be a chronic disease with persistent or relapsing symptoms. Esophageal strictures and small caliber esophagus, often resulting in food impaction, are the major complications of EE.

Pathophysiology

The pathogenesis of EE is incompletely understood and likely involves multiple tissues, cell types, and genes. There is a strong association between EE and allergic disease. Between 50–80% of EE patients are atopic based on presence of allergic disease (atopic dermatitis, allergic rhinitis, and/or asthma) or positive skin prick test especially to a number of different foods (9). Some EE patients also report seasonal variation in their symptoms suggesting a role for aeroallergens. In addition, treatment such as food avoidance or elemental diet can result in restoration of normal esophageal pathology, reinforcing the link between disease and an allergic etiology (8). It is believed that a local and/or systemic T helper type 2 (Th2) immune response results in eosinophil infiltration and activation in the esophagus due to overexpression of eosinophil chemoattractants and activating factors, such as eotaxin-3 (10). Like most Th2-associated diseases, environmental factors and a predisposed genetic background likely contribute to EE onset and pathogenesis (11).

Work-Up

For diagnostic work-up, a gastroesophageal endoscopy enables the best assessment of the esophageal mucosa. Endoscopy has the added benefits of permitting the detection of infection and erosions and of enabling biopsy. A number of gross mucosal abnormalities have been associated with EE, but are not pathognomonic for EE, including linear furrowing (vertical lines of the esophageal mucosa), white exudates or specks, circular rings, and esophageal strictures (proximal, middle, or distal). In the appropriate clinical context, the presence of more than one of these findings is strongly suggestive of the diagnosis of EE. Mucosal pinch biopsy specimens should be obtained from all patients in whom EE is the differential diagnosis. These biopsy specimens should be obtained regardless of the gross appearance of the mucosa, as histopathologic abnormalities are common in biopsy specimens obtained from endoscopically normal-appearing mucosa. Multiple biopsy specimens should be obtained from different esophageal locations along the length of the esophagus. To rule out other diseases, biopsy specimens should also be obtained from the stomach and duodenum. When the diagnosis of GERD versus EE is not apparent despite endoscopy and biopsy, intraesophageal pH monitoring may be of use in excluding pathologic reflux as either the primary or the concomitant cause for esophageal eosinophilia. Intraesophageal pH testing will be normal in a vast majority of patients with EE. Importantly, an upper endoscopy after 6–8 weeks of high-dose proton pump inhibitor (PPI) treatment is nearly universally required for the diagnosis of EE, as this rules out a primary role for acid-induced esophagitis. Esophageal manometry does not provide diagnostic value in patients with EE as it has been shown to be abnormal in half of adult EE patients, but normal in children (8). In patients with dysphagia, an upper GI contrast study may identify the presence of a stricture.

Because of the high rate of atopic predisposition in EE patients, a complete assessment of atopy by analysis of blood samples and skin prick testing for antigen sensitization should be completed. Peripheral blood eosinophilia may provide supportive evidence for the presence of EE but is not diagnostic. As allergy testing may predict the response to pharmacotherapy, aeroallergen-specific IgE warrants evaluation. Skin prick testing for foods and environmental allergens should be considered so that potential allergens can be identified.

Treatment

Systemic and topical corticosteroids effectively resolve the acute clinical and histologic features of EE; however, the disease generally recurs when therapy is discontinued. Currently, topical use of corticosteroids, such as fluticasone and budesonide, can be effective in inducing remission when continued for at least 6–8 weeks. The method of administration and using age-adjusted dosing is important. Patients should be instructed to administer the metered-dose inhaler (MDI) without the use of a spacer and swallow the powder without rinsing their mouth and not eating or drinking for at least 30 min after treatment. Systemic corticosteroids can be utilized in emergent cases involving dehydration and weight loss secondary to difficulty in swallowing or hospitalization for dysphagia. Although gastric acid is not thought to be the primary mediator associated with the pathogenesis of EE, acid suppression is useful as a part of fulfilling the diagnostic criteria for EE. Importantly, PPI therapy should not be considered as a primary treatment for patients with EE. In children diagnosed with EE, dietary therapy, including removal of specific antigens or utilization of elemental formula, should be considered. As this treatment plan can involve significant lifestyle modification, the patient's lifestyle and family resources needed to be considered. A registered dietician consultation is recommended to ensure maintenance of proper calories, vitamins, and micronutrients. In the future, novel biologic therapies will target the molecule receptors that influence the production, migration, and activation of eosinophil to reduce the esophageal eosinophil inflammation.

Questions

1. The most common initial presentation of EE in older children and adults is which one of the following:

   (a) Heartburn
   (b) Abdominal pain
   (c) Intermittent dsyphagia and food impaction
   (d) Emesis

2. Feature(s) that distinguish EE from GERD:

   (a) Magnitude of the esophageal eosinophilia
   (b) Strong association with male gender
   (c) Atopy
   (d) All of the above
   (e) None of the above

3. To effectively induce remission of EE, topical corticosteroids should be continued:

(a) Until acute clinical and histologic features resolve
(b) For 1–2 weeks
(c) For 6–8 weeks
(d) For 6–8 months

4. Intraepithelial eosinophil infiltration of the esophagus is pathognomonic of EE:

(a) True
(b) False

5. Diagnostic work-up for EE should include the following:

(a) Endoscopy with mucosal pinch biopsies
(b) Endoscopy after 6–8 weeks of high-dose PPI treatment
(c) Esophageal manometry
(d) All of the above
(e) (a) and (b)
(f) (a) and (c)

Answer key: 1. (c), 2. (d), 3. (c), 4. (b), 5. (e)

References

1. Feong YF, Kim K-IL, Seo IF, Lee CH, Lee KN, Kim KN, Kim FS, Kwon WF. (2007) Eosinophilic lung diseases: a clinical, radiologic, and pathologic overview. RadioGraphics 27, 617–639.
2. Katz U, Shoenfeld Y. (2007) Pulmonary eosinophilia. Clin Rev Allerg Immunol 34, 367–371.
3. Allen JN. (2004) The eosinophilic lung diseases, in Baum's Textbook of Pulmonary Diseases, 7th edition, Crapo JD et al. (eds.). Philadelphia: Lippincott Williams & Wilkins, 521–537.
4. Alberts WM. (2004) Eosinophilic interstitial lung diseases. Curr Opin Pulm Med 10, 419–424.
5. Alam M, Burki NK. (2007) Chronic eosinophilic pneumonia: a review. Southern Med J 100, 49–53.
6. Cottin V, Cordier J-F. (2005) Eosinophilic pneumonis. Allergy 60, 841–857.
7. Allen J. (2006) Acute eosinophilic pneumonia. Semin Respir Crit Care Med 27, 142–147.
8. Furuta GT, Liacouras CA, Collins MH et al. (2007) Eosinophilic esophagitis in children and adults: a systematic review and consensus recommendations for diagnosis and treatment. Gastroenterology 133(4), 1342–1363.
9. Noel RJ, Putnam PE, Rothenberg ME. (2004) Eosinophilic esophagitis. N Engl J Med 351(9), 940–941.
10. Blanchard C, Wang N, Stringer KF et al. (2006) Eotaxin-3 and a uniquely conserved gene-expression profile in eosinophilic esophagitis. J Clin Invest 116(2), 536–547.
11. Rothenberg ME. (2004) Eosinophilic gastrointestinal disorders (EGID). J Allergy Clin Immunol 113(1), 11–28.

Chapter 12
Occupational Asthma

Jonathan A. Bernstein and I. Leonard Bernstein

Abstract Occupational asthma is believed to be responsible for up to 15% of all new cases of asthma in the United States. Evaluation of patients with asthma, therefore, requires a careful and complete work history to identify or exclude potential causes or triggers for asthma. It is important for the clinician to have a strong understanding of how to evaluate and manage work-related asthma induced by both high and low molecular weight agents. The following clinical cases are designed to provide a template of how patients suspected with occupational asthma should be evaluated in order to definitively confirm this diagnosis.

Keywords Occupational asthma • Egg lysozyme • Benzalkonium chloride

Case 1

A 26-year-old man employed in an area of a plant which exclusively manufactured egg white-derived lysozyme presented with progressive shortness of breath and wheezing, which began 8 months after starting this job. The subject was rotated between different areas of the work process, which involved processing egg whites, including a drying step of hot air blowers that released a lysozyme powder into the air. When working in the final drying stage of egg lysozyme powder processing, he wore a protective mask. Six months prior to the initial evaluation, he stopped working directly near the driers as they were causing respiratory symptoms. An initial history revealed that the worker experienced chest tightness and shortness of breath during exposure to egg lysozyme powder. These symptoms improved a few hours after leaving work and periodically he missed workdays. He was never

J.A. Bernstein (✉) and I.L. Bernstein
Division of Immunology/Allergy Section, Department of Internal Medicine,
University of Cincinnati College of Medicine, 231 Albert Sabin Way M.L. #563,
Cincinnati, OH 45267-0563, USA
e-mail: Jonathan.Bernstein@uc.edu

M. Mahmoudi (ed.), *Challenging Cases in Allergy and Immunology*,
DOI: 10.1007/978-1-60327-443-2_12,
© Humana Press, a part of Springer Science+Business Media, LLC 2009

hospitalized for these symptoms. He has a 4-year pack/history of cigarette smoking but no documented prior history of allergic rhinitis, asthma, or eczema.

One day after exposure to egg lysozyme his physical exam revealed diffuse wheezing in all lung fields but was otherwise normal.

Laboratory Data

The subject received skin pricks to several seasonal and perennial aeroallergens, indicating atopy. Total serum IgE was elevated at 907 kU/L. The total peripheral eosinophil count was 75×10^6/L (normal 45–330 $\times 10^6$/L). No previous laboratory results for IgE or eosinophils were available for comparison.

Initial Impression

Probable occupational asthma secondary to egg lysozyme.

Differential Diagnosis

Conditions that should be considered in the differential diagnosis include (a) occupational asthma secondary to lysozyme from egg white or other egg proteins used in the manufacturing process and (b) aggravation of nonoccupational asthma.

Work-Up

Further skin testing to egg white, egg yolk, ovalbumin, ovomucoid ovalbumin, conalbumin, and lysozyme was conducted. Skin prick tests were done at concentrations of 50 μg/mL for each reagent. Histamine hydrochloride 10 mg/mL was used as the positive control and saline was used as the negative control. A skin test was considered positive if there was a 3 mm wheal greater than the negative saline control. Five negative control subjects (defined as exposure to egg lysozyme but no symptoms) were also skin tested to lysozyme. Prick skin tests at 50 mg/mL were positive to lysozyme, ovomucoid, ovalbumin, and conalbumin antigens and negative to whole egg yolk and egg white.

Direct Enzyme-Linked to Immunosorbent Assays

Serum obtained from the subject was divided into 1-mL aliquots and evaluated by a standard enzyme-linked immunosorbent technique for IgG- and IgE-specific antibodies using IgG and IgE alkaline phosphatase immunoconjugates (Kirkegaard and Perry Laboratories, Gathersburg, MD). The serum of a sensitized egg-processing worker with IgE to a spectrum of egg white proteins served as a positive control and negative control subjects included a pooled sera sample of exposed asymptomatic egg processing workers and a similar pooled sera sample of nonexposed asymptomatic laboratory personnel. The subject had increased specific IgE antibody to egg lysozyme and ovomucoid protein, whereas ovalbumin, conalbumin, egg white, and egg yolk yielded low IgE binding. Negative control subjects exhibited low IgE binding to the panel of egg proteins and enzymes.

Enzyme-Linked Immunosorbent Assay Inhibition

The patient's serum was diluted to a concentration of 1:10 with phosphate buffered saline and preincubated with various concentrations of proteins (cellulase, lysozyme, ovalbumin, ovomucoid, conalbumin, whole egg white, and egg yolk) for 1 h at room temperature. The preinhibited serum was then added to plates coated with lysozyme (10 µg/mL) and an enzyme-linked immunosorbent assay (ELISA) was performed, as previously described. IgE ELISA inhibition using egg white proteins as inhibitors demonstrated >50% inhibition of lysozyme-specific IgE binding by lysozyme at a concentration of 2.4 mg/mL. Egg white, egg yolk, cellulase, ovalbumin, and conal-bumin proteins did not inhibit at this concentration. Repeat IgE ELISA inhibition studies performed using the subject's serum obtained after prolonged work avoidance (1 year) were negative to the panel of egg proteins. Inhibition of lysozyme-specific IgE using ovomucoid as the inhibiting agent was observed at tenfold greater concentration (20 mg/mL). Heat inactivation of egg lysozyme did not affect its capacity to inhibit.

Physiologic Studies

Initial evaluation and pulmonary function testing revealed a baseline FEV_1 of 2.78 L/min (71% predicted), which improved after beta agonist medication to 3.27 L/min (83.7% predicted). Lung volumes were normal. Pulmonary function tests repeated 2 weeks after avoiding work revealed that the baseline FEV_1 increased to 4.02 L/min (31% improvement). A methacholine provocation test performed after a week absence from work was positive at a provocative concentration of methacholine causing a 20% drop in FEV_1 from baseline (PC_{20}) of 0.8 mg/mL, confirming the presence of bronchial hyperresponsiveness. Serial peak flow readings, recorded while the worker was at work during an 18-day period, revealed decreases during exposure to egg lysozyme powder. The subject's peak expiratory flow rate consistently decreased during lysozyme exposure and improved away from work. Specific provocation to egg lysozyme was performed after he ceased work for

2 weeks. The FEV_1 was unchanged in response to lactose powder placebo performed on a separate control test day. The FEV_1 decreased from 4.2 to 2.2 L/min 15 minutes after exposure to sifting 50 mg of egg lysozyme. Serial peak flow determinations monitored hourly for 9 h after the initial early airway response revealed no evidence of a late onset asthmatic response.

With the Presented Data, What Is Your Diagnosis?

Occupational asthma secondary to egg lysozyme.

Discussion

Allergic reactions to ingested egg proteins have been well described with allergenic food allergens (1–4). Egg allergens are also potent airborne allergens (1–4). Occupational asthma due to the inhalation of egg white aerosols have been described in bakers. Occupational asthma has also been reported to occur among egg processing workers in association with inhalation exposure to egg white aerosols and powder resulting in sensitization to multiple egg white proteins, including ovalbumin, ovomucoid, conalbumin, and lysozyme (1–4). In these workers, positive percutaneous reactivity and serum specific IgE and IgG antibodies were demonstrated to all of these egg white proteins, including egg white lysozyme (1, 5). Egg white extracted lysozyme is used in the pharmaceutical industry as an enhancer of antibiotic activity and as a preservative (1). This interesting case of occupational asthma induced by sensitization to inhaled egg lysozyme powder occurred in a pharmaceutical plant. Diagnosis was confirmed by significant shifts in the subject's peak expiratory flow rates on days at work compared to nonexposure days at home and by positive single-blinded placebo-controlled bronchoprovocation challenge tests to egg lysozyme (1). The subject exhibited immediate airway responsiveness 15 minutes after exposure without a delayed airway response. The lack of a late airway response is consistent with the subject's clinical course as delayed respiratory symptoms were not noted after avoidance measures. However, the bronchoprovocation challenge was performed several months after complete avoidance of the egg lysozyme powder, at which time a late airway response could have subsided (1, 6). Specific IgE was demonstrated in vivo by positive prick/puncture cutaneous reactivity to egg lysozyme and in vitro by serum specific IgE binding to lysozyme protein. ELISA inhibition of lysozyme-specific IgE by lysozyme, confirmed that the worker's IgE antibody response was for egg lysozyme (1, 7). Although the subject was skin test positive to several egg proteins, ovomucoid was the only other egg protein that resulted in elevated direct serum-specific IgE binding. Ovomucoid also inhibited specific IgE binding to lysozyme but at a twofold higher concentration than lysozyme. This could be explained by the subject being sensitized to ovomucoid protein during the work process, the early stages of which involved extracting lysozyme from a whole egg white. It is also possible that a shared epitope between lysozyme and ovomucoid could result in cross-reactivity.

In summary, this case is a well-documented example of occupational asthma caused by a high molecular weight enzyme that was being manufactured for use in the pharmaceutical industry. It illustrates that airborne egg proteins (enzymes) are potent inhalant allergens that can induce occupational asthma.

Questions

1. ELISA inhibition assays are important for:

   (a) Confirming whether clinical symptoms are related to specific antibody responses
   (b) To demonstrate specificity of the antibody response to the causative agent
   (c) Determine if blocking IgG antibodies are interfering with the ELISA assay
   (d) To demonstrate that a specific immune response is Th-2 mediated

Correct answer: (b)

2. All of the following are important egg proteins except:

   (a) Lysozyme
   (b) Conalbumin
   (c) Glucomannan
   (d) Ovomucoid
   (e) Ovalbumin

Correct answer: (c)

3. All of the following help establish a diagnosis of occupational asthma except:

   (a) Review of MSDS sheets
   (b) Cross-shift peak expiratory flow rate monitoring
   (c) Methacholine challenge
   (d) Skin testing to common seasonal and perennial allergens
   (e) Clinical assessment in and out of the workplace

Correct answer: (d)

4. Risk factors for high molecular weight proteins known to induce occupational asthma are:

   (a) Smoking
   (b) Female gender
   (c) Atopy
   (d) Family history of asthma
   (e) Pre-existing asthma

Correct answer: (c)

5. True statements regarding specific provocation in occupational asthma include all of the following except:

   (a) Early phase airway responses correspond to acute activation of mast cells leading to the release of bioactive mediators
   (b) The absence of an early phase response to a suspected agent excludes a diagnosis of occupational asthma
   (c) Dual, early and late, phase airway responses can be observed in up to 40% of patients with occupational asthma
   (d) Specific provocation should only be conducted by experienced personnel in a controlled environment with emergency therapy readily available

Correct answer: (b)

Case 2

A 22-year-old woman working in a factory that manufactured household cleaning products was first seen with acute onset of fever, shortness of breath, chest tightness, nonproductive cough, and arthralgias, which began 7 months after initiating employment. Physical exam revealed mild cervical lymphadenopathy, conjunctivitis, tachypnea, bibasilar rales, bilateral knee effusions, and erythematous papulovescular skin lesions.

Laboratory Data

Results of routine laboratory tests and sedimentation rate, complement levels, autoantibody screen, rheumatoid factor, and cryoglobulins were normal. Results of bacterial, fungal, and viral cultures for blood, skin, sputum, and synovial fluid were also negative. Serial chest X-ray during her hospitalization revealed bibasilar pulmonary infiltrates. Pulmonary function tests and measurements of lung volumes and diffusion capacity were normal. Skin and transbronchial biopsy specimens demonstrated nonspecific inflammatory infiltrates without vasculitic changes. Empiric treatment with IV intravenously administrated antibiotics and corticosteroids resulted in complete resolution of skin, joint, and pulmonary symptoms. However, after returning to work, she experienced recurrent wheezing and shortness of breath, which began shortly after re-exposure to the cleaning products.

Initial Impression

Hypersensitivity pneumonitis.

Differential Diagnosis

Potential causes include occupational asthma, serum sickness reaction, hypersensitivity pneumonitis, bacterial pneumonia, and pulmonary infiltrates with eosinophilia (PIE syndrome).

Her symptoms of fever and arthralgia/arthritis coupled with a cutaneous rash suggest a serum sickness reaction, but markers of immune complex disease were not demonstrated. A cell-mediated immune response similar to hypersensitivity pneumonitis is supported by bilateral lower lobe infiltrates on chest X-ray and lymphocytic infiltration observed in skin and bronchial biopsy specimens. The possibility of occupational asthma requires further evaluation.

Work-Up

Single-blind, placebo-controlled, open room challenges were performed for each of the cleaning products that she was using in the workplace on separate days to determine the specific agent responsible for her symptoms. Within 5 min after exposure to a liquid toilet bowl cleaner containing benzalkonium chloride, a diffuse erythematous, pruritic, urticarial rash appeared on her face, neck, and chest. She also experienced chest tightness and dyspnea. Pulmonary function testing revealed a 38% decrease in her forced expiratory volume in 1 s (FEV_1) after 10 min with a maximum drop of 50% after 45 min. This slowly improved to baseline over 3 h. The patient was unwilling to cooperate with monitoring for a late-phase airway response. Her FEV_1 responses remained unchanged in response to placebo, a drain declogging solution, a window cleaner, and an air freshener.

Immunologic Studies

Percutaneous challenge tests were also performed with the individual components of the liquid cleaner. Within 15 min after exposure to a 1:1 mixture of N-alkyl dimethylbenzyl and N-alkyl dimethylbenzyl ammonium chloride, the worker had a 15-cm erythematous pruritic urticarial reaction, which persisted for several days. Lung changes were not seen after challenge on repeat chest radiographs. She was unreactive to the other agents and chemical constituents tested on separate days. A control subject had negative responses to pulmonary and percutaneous challenges.

With the Presented Data, What Is Your Diagnosis?

This case represents an instance of occupational asthma induced by toilet bowl cleaner containing the quaternary amine, benzalkonium chloride (8).

Discussion

The precise mechanisms responsible for induction of bronchial sensitivity to quaternary amines are unknown. However, this case emphasizes the point of recognizing that reactive chemicals can cause bronchial reactions in the workplace (9–12).

There are 40 different primary, secondary (diethanolamines), and tertiary (triethanolamines) amine compounds that have been found in the workplace that can cause occupational asthma (9, 10). Quaternary ammonium compounds are used as preservatives in contact lens cleaning solutions, aerosolized asthma medications, and household products, such as soaps, skin ointments, disinfectants, and sanitizers (11, 12). Numerous cases of cutaneous and mucosal delayed hypersensitivity reactions to agents containing the quaternary and benzalkonium chloride (BAC) have been reported (11, 12). BAC is also associated with paradoxical bronchial constriction in patients with asthma using aerosolized ipratropium bromide and beclomethasone dipropionate (11, 12). Data from many surveillance studies for work-related asthma have consistently listed cleaning products as a major cause of asthma in the workplace (13–18). In fact, the third National Health and Nutrition Examination Survey (NHANES3) database found that the highest asthma prevalence among nonsmokers occurred in the hospital industry (15, 16). Workers most commonly reported exposure to disinfectants and cleaning agents. The European Community Respiratory Health Survey Study reported that one of the highest risks for asthma occurred in cleaners (17). A subanalysis survey designed to characterize workers exposed to high and low molecular weight agents revealed that 304 workers of the total population surveyed (n = 4,492) were involved in domestic or commercial cleaning and 84% were female (17). Also, a cross-sectional survey conducted in 4,521 individuals eliciting information regarding respiratory symptoms and cleaning history revealed that asthma was more prevalent in women who were employed in domestic cleaning work compared to women who had never worked in cleaning (18).

Cleaning agents also contain a number of irritant chemicals, such as bleach, ammonium, hydrochloric acid, and volatile organic compounds that can cause or aggravate asthma as well as irritate nonatopic, nonasthmatic individuals (14). In our case, appropriate controls were utilized for the subject's exposure test as well as comparative studies in nonexposed negative controls. These investigations also excluded other potential causative agents.

In summary, this case illustrates that low molecular weight chemicals are capable of inducing immunologic and non-immunologic occupational asthma. In fact, many low molecular weight chemicals are known to induce occupational asthma including isocyanates (used in spray painting as well as foaming and hardening processes), acid anhydrides (used in manufacturing of plastics, coatings, and resins), Chloramine T (used as a sterilizing agent in the food industry), diazonium salts (used in the photocopying process), ammonium persulfate (used in the hairdressing industry), glutaraldehyde (used to sterilize medical equipment), and colophony (used in the electronics industry). It is believed that they induce occupational asthma through

IgE mediated mechanisms and perhaps through described for reactive airways dysfunction syndrome (RADS) (irritant-induced asthma), a condition, which results in airway hyperresponsiveness without a latency period after a large or chronic exposure to a chemical agent.

Questions

1. True statements regarding benzalkonium chloride include all of the following except:

   (a) It is a commonly used preservative in medications.
   (b) It can cause bronchoconstriction in susceptible individuals.
   (c) It has been demonstrated to elicit immunologically mediated reactions.
   (d) All of the above.

Correct answer: (d)

2. All of the following statements regarding volatile organic compounds are true except:

   (a) They are respiratory irritants.
   (b) They are derived from chemical compounds only.
   (c) They should be regulated below 25 mg/m^3 to promote a "nonirritating" work or home environment.
   (d) Cleaning agents are a common cause of occupational asthma.

Correct answer: (b) (VOCs are also microbial derived)

3. Amines are commonly used in the manufacturing of all of the following products except:

   (a) Cosmetics
   (b) Paints
   (c) Detergents
   (d) Pharmaceuticals
   (e) Rubber products

Correct answer: (c) (enzymes are the major constituent in detergents)

4. The most common mechanism by which chemicals cause occupational asthma is:

   (a) Immune-complex mediated
   (b) Direct stimulation of the immune system to produce IgE antibodies
   (c) Linkage to endogenous proteins to form a new antigen capable of inducing specific IgE sensitization
   (d) Cell-mediated

Correct answer: (c) (low molecular chemicals commonly act as haptens and form conjugates with endogenous proteins that act as allergens)

5. All of the following statements are true except:

(a) Chloramine T is a sterilizing agent used in the food industry.
(b) Diazonium salts are used in the beverage industry.
(c) Ammonium persulfate is used in the hairdressing industry.
(d) Glutaraldehyde is used to sterilize medical equipment.
(e) Colophony is used in the electronics industry.

Correct answer: (b) (diazonim salts are used in the photocopying process)

Case 3

For ten years, a 29-year-old male welder was regularly exposed to chromium vapors emanating from fumes of stainless steel welding during both occupational and nonoccupational activities. The onset of his illness was ascribed to an incident at work during which he was exposed for several hours to a chromium trioxide mist accidentally discharged from an adjacent chrome electroplating plant. His initial symptoms were skin and eye irritation and slight shortness of breath. He was treated with antihistamines and corticosteroids with gradual improvement. Upon return to similar work 5 months later, he noted both chest tightness and slight shortness of breath 6 h after arriving at work. Two months later, similar symptoms appeared after arc welding stainless steel materials at home.

His past medical history included two previous episodes of mild periorbital edema and urticaria associated with ingestion of raw onion. He denied other personal or family history of rhinitis symptoms, eczema, asthma, or other allergies. He had a 5 pack/year history of smoking, but quit 5 years ago.

He was first examined 2 weeks after the last episode. Physical examination revealed normal ears, nose, and throat. His chest was clear to percussion and auscultation.

Laboratory Data

A complete blood count with differential was normal. A nasal smear was negative for eosinophils. PA and lateral chest X-rays revealed slightly enlarged calcified hilar nodes and increased bronchovascular markings in both lower lung fields but was interpreted as normal. Liver profile and urinalysis were both normal. Complete pulmonary function tests, including spirometry, total lung volumes, and single breath carbon monoxide tests were normal. A methacholine challenge test performed approximately 4 weeks after the last occupational episode was normal (provocative concentration of methacholine that causes a 20% decrease in FEV_1 from baseline (PC_{20}) 25 mg/mL).

Initial Impression

Probable occupational asthma due to hexavalent chromium exposure.

Differential Diagnosis

The recurrent symptoms of chest tightness and dyspnea are strongly suggestive of bronchial hyperresponsiveness. The negative methacholine challenge test indicates that bronchial hyperresponsiveness is no longer present, although it possibly could have subsided or disappeared after the last occupational exposure. The normal chest X-ray and single breath carbon monoxide test mitigate against the possibility of chronic hypersensitivity or chemical pneumonitis. However, such entities as bronchitis, chemical- or irritant-induced asthma, resolving COP (cryptogenic organizing pneumonia), bronchiolitis obliterans, siderosis, or a small bronchial carcinoma must still be considered.

Work-Up

Skin prick testing to common aeroallergens was done to assess his atopic status, which was negative. A high resolution CAT scan, obtained to exclude the entities discussed under the differential diagnosis, was normal without evidence of abnormal masses, interstitial changes, or bronchiectatic areas.

A single-blinded inhalation test was arranged. On day 1, the subject inhaled a sterile solution of 0.9% sodium chloride. On day 2, he received an aerosol containing 1.25 μg/mL of sodium dichromate for 5 min, and on day 3, an aerosol containing 29 μg/mL of sodium dichromate for 25 min. Stable concentrations of the chromium salts were confirmed by sampling the delivery system from a Plexiglas chamber, before, during, and after the challenge. He experienced no unusual symptoms or pulmonary function changes on or after the first two challenge days. On the third challenge day, within 10 min after the cessation of challenge, there was a 12% decrease in FEV_1 that returned to baseline values by 20 min. This was not accompanied by symptoms of dyspnea, cough, or wheezing. Six hours later, a late occurring reduction in FEV_1 (40% reduction from the initial saline control of FEV_1) occurred. At this time, physical examination revealed faintly audible wheezing. He was given a hand-held nebulizer treatment with albuterol but 15 min later, he still demonstrated a 20% reduction in FEV_1. A second hand-held nebulizer treatment was then instituted. This resulted in clinical improvement and a return of his FEV_1 to baseline values within 1 h. On the fourth challenge day, 24 h after the positive response noted on day 3, a repeat dose–response methacholine challenge test was performed. Bronchial hyperresponsiveness was demonstrated at a PC_{20} of 4 mg/mL.

Two previously unexposed volunteers were challenged with similar levels of aerosolized sodium chromate according to the same protocol and did not exhibit bronchospasm or irritant effects, despite the fact that one of these volunteers was known to have nonspecific hyperresponsiveness as assessed by a dose–response methacholine challenge test (PC_{20} = 4 mg/mL).

Immunologic Studies

Prick tests were performed with 0.1, 1, and 10 mg/mL solutions of sodium chromate or nickel sulfate 1 week after provocation testing and were all negative. Intracutaneous skin tests to chromium and nickel human serum albumin (HSA) conjugates (1:100 dilutions) revealed a large wheal (9 mm diameter) and flare (20 mm diameter) over the chromium-HSA site after 15 min. The nickel-HSA site was negative compared to saline control. An ELISA performed for chromium-HSA test was markedly positive whereas the saline control, HSA control, and nickel-HSA tests were all negative. Patch tests to 0.5% potassium chromate and 2.5% nickel sulfate solutions were negative after 48- and 96-h readings. Specificity of the ELISA tests was determined by preincubating unconjugated sodium chromate and nickel sulfate, respectively, with patient's serum 1 h before the patient's serum was added to the ELISA wells. Only preincubation with chromium sulfate caused significant inhibition (80%) of the ELISA test assay. No inhibition after preincubation with nickel sulfate was observed.

The concentrations of sodium chromate used for bronchial challenge tests were less than the recommended 50-μg/m^3 threshold limit value proposed by the American Council of Government Industrial Hygienists for noncarcinogenic hexavalent chromium compounds (19).

With the Presented Data, What Is Your Diagnosis?

The initial workplace symptoms of this patient suggested an irritative response since it occurred after exposure to an accidental discharge of chromium trioxide mist from an adjacent plant. Since he also performed welding activities at home, the initial exposure could be considered a toxic one involving chiefly the skin, eyes, and possibly the lungs. Such symptoms are not unusual in welders. However, when chest symptoms recurred after returning to work, one had to suspect that occupational exposures were causing his repetitive symptoms. Of particular significance in this case was the worker's exposure to stainless steel welding fumes, which are known to contain significant concentrations of both chromium and nickel. Such exposures could have induced any one of the conditions discussed in the differential diagnosis above, including lung cancer. Although the initial chest X-ray was interpreted as normal, the description of prominent calcified lymph nodes and increased bronchovascular markings could have been consistent with several of the entities mentioned in the differential diagnosis. Normal pulmonary function tests were reassuring by appearing to rule out either restrictive or obstructive lung disease. The methacholine challenge test was also within normal limits but bronchial hyperresponsiveness may not be demonstrable, albeit rarely, even in naturally occurring asthma. Moreover, in this particular case, it is possible that mild hyper-responsiveness occurring 1 month prior to the test might have subsided by the time the test was done. Before proceeding with further diagnostic tests, it was therefore essential that a high-resolution lung CAT scan evaluate possible structural abnormalities, which was normal. Having established this, a specific bronchial challenge test was conducted. The protocol was based on single-blinded, well-controlled exposure to known concentrations of sodium dichromate (well within the time-weighted exposure recommendations of the American Council of Governmental Industrial Hygienists for noncarcinogenic hexavalent chromium compounds) with provisions for evaluating the patient's acute and delayed responses. In addition, two unexposed control volunteers were assessed by the same challenge protocol. The patient exhibited an isolated late-phase 40% reduction of FEV_1 on the third day of challenge. Twenty-four hours later, his methacholine challenge test was markedly positive ($PD_{20} = 4$ mg/mL). Neither of the control subjects demonstrated a similar response. The possible immunologic significance of the positive specific bronchial challenge was pursued by testing the worker to HSA conjugates of sodium chromate and nickel sulfate salts. A positive intracutaneous skin test to the chromate conjugate was confirmed by an ELISA assay, the specificity of which was also verified by an inhibition test with unconjugated sodium chromate. Positive ELISA results to nickel sulfate conjugates were not observed nor did unconjugated nickel sulfate inhibit the chromate positive ELISA assay. Taken together, the diagnostic evaluation confirmed the initial impression of occupational asthma, which in this case was also characterized by IgE-mediated chromate-specific skin and in vitro tests.

Discussion

Low molecular weight agents in the workplace may either aggravate or induce asthma. Workers are exposed to these substances through aerosols, mists, and gases primarily by inhalation, although it can be demonstrated that highly potent sensitizing agents may stimulate innate and adaptive immune mechanisms initially thorough epidermal exposure. Toxic vapors of organic acids, alkalis, and dense wood smoke are more likely to be associated with irritant-induced asthma without a latent period (i.e., the RADS), while other low molecular weight chemicals (acid anhydrides, isocyanates) that have high sensitization potentials require a latency period (sensitization) and subsequent re-exposure (elicitation) (20). The essential element of the latter compounds (or their degraded metabolites) is the presence of highly reactive chemical moieties, which will readily conjugate to appropriate sites in body proteins. Included in this category are salts of transition metals such as nickel, chromium, palladium, and platinum.

In 1993, the United States National Survey estimated that over 6 million workers have potential exposure to chemical or metal asthmagens throughout the United States (21). More than one million workers worldwide are exposed to welding fumes. Respiratory illnesses commonly occur in these workers (22). Such conditions as acute or chronic bronchitis, asthma, siderosis, and possible lung cancer have been reported (23). Centrilobular nodules may be demonstrated by high-resolution computer tomography in welders who develop pneumoconiosis. Welders may be sensitized to acid anhydrides contained in painted metals and there is a report of a welder who developed RADS after a documented acute episode of metal fume fever. Welders' asthma is more likely to occur after exposure to fumes emanating from stainless steel welding rather than those from "mild steel." (24). This apparently is due to the fact that stainless steel welding fumes contain significantly higher amounts of chromium and nickel alloys than "mild steel."

Chromium is a transition metal that is widely used for electroplating processes, metal alloys, pigments, tanning of leather, cement, and production of chromate salts (22). Chromium-plated metal is nonallergic with respect to contact dermatitis, whereas chromate salt solutes are often found to be causative agents in occupational contact dermatitis. Chromium salts exist naturally in three valence forms: 2, 3, and 6. Bivalent compounds are unstable and have little commercial value. Hexavalent chromium compounds (e.g., chromium trioxide and mono-and bichromates), as compared to trivalent chromium compounds (e.g., chromium chloride), have an increased potential for allergic contact dermatitis because they are more stable, soluble, and presumably gain easier penetration of the epidermis. Although chromium salts are uncommon causes of occupational asthma, hexavalent chromium oxide fumes emitted from electric arc and oxygen welding of chromium-containing stainless steel alloys are proven causes of occupational asthma. Some of these cases have been shown to be IgE mediated. It is estimated that 400,000 workers are potentially exposed to hexavalent chromium. Workplace standards distinguish between carcinogenic and noncarcinogenic species of hexavalent chromate. The workplace environmental limit for noncarcinogenic hexavalent chromium is a time-weighted average of 0.05 mg/m^3 for up to an 8-h workday (19). The signifi-cance of concomitant exposure to nickel sulfate present in the workplace or released during stainless steel welding is yet unknown. Cross-reactions between nickel and chromium salts have been proposed but not proven (25). IgE-mediated reactions to nickel (e.g., positive immediate intracutaneous skin tests) are well documented in addition to the more common propensity of this agent to cause contact dermatitis.

The spectrum of pulmonary reactions occurring after exposure to metallic compounds includes acute and chronic obstructive symptoms, which in some cases may mimic asthma. The inhalation of fumes or dust of many metallic salts may cause chemical tracheobronchitis or pneumonitis with a general clinical picture resembling the adult respiratory disease syndrome. One of the confusing syndromes in this category is metal fume fever, which may also occur in association with super-imposed bronchial asthma. The occurrence of acute or chronic symptoms of dyspnea, cough, chest tightness, and/or wheezing should alert the clinician to a possible occupational inciting event. As with naturally occurring asthma, the physical signs may be variable. In fact, in the case of occupational asthma, there may be no evidence of wheezing if the patient has been away from work for a few days or weeks.

In the illustrative case, skin and laboratory tests revealed that IgE sensitization had occurred as a result of the initial chromium trioxide exposure. Subsequent re-exposures to small amounts of chromium in welding fumes caused clinical respiratory symptoms. The specific bronchial challenge was of interest in this case because there was an almost exclusive late onset asthmatic response. Many industrial allergens cause immediate or rapid onset responses, both in pulmonary function decrements and clinical symptoms. Some agents cause a dual type of response with manifestations of a late onset response within a time period of 6–12 h after the initial exposure (26). An isolated dual response, such as observed in this case, can also occur and is not that unusual (26).

It is important to note that either nonspecific (irritant-induced) or specific IgE-mediated asthma may occur after exposure to small molecular weight agents including chromate salts. In the current case, the mechanism of IgE-induced asthma was confirmed by positive skin and in vitro tests to HSA-conjugated chromium salts. The fact that positive skin and in vitro tests were obtained only with HSA-conjugated chromium salts and not with unconjugated chromium illustrates the fact that small mass molecules are rarely immunogenic – platinum salts being the main exception to this rule – unless conjugated to a known body protein (27). Such low molecular weight metallic compounds are, however, antigenic, as illustrated by the fact that a solution of unconjugated chromate salts inhibited the in vitro-specific IgE reaction in this patient by 80%. Such tests are not routinely available on a commercial basis but certain occupational diagnostic centers may offer guidance. If metal exposed workers have concurrent hand or generalized dermatitis, patch tests are essential to determine the presence of allergic contact dermatitis. Patch tests denote a special type of cell-mediated immunity and cannot be used to corroborate the significance of possible IgE-mediated asthma. In animal models of contact dermatitis, however, there is evidence that IgE immune responses may be a precursor of the cell-mediated response, which may develop later. As was demonstrated in this case, the temporal status of bronchial hyperresponsiveness may depend on the degree or activation of underlying allergic inflammation.

Avoidance of further exposure is the only practical treatment option in this particular situation. This patient could not return to his former occupation (and hobby) and has been asymptomatic since cessation of exposure. It should be noted that IgE-mediated instances of allergic asthma pose grave potential risks if the patient continues the exposure. There have been a number of cases of fatal anaphylaxis occurring after patients failed to follow avoidance advice.

Questions

1. Of the following, which would be the most useful diagnostic adjunct for the diagnosis of potroom asthma:

   (a) Specific in vitro IgE tests to aluminum fluoride
   (b) Positive immediate skin tests to $K_3ALF_3AlF_6$
   (c) Positive patch tests to 10% cryolite ($Na_3Al F_6$) alumina
   (d) High levels of postshift urinary fluoride
   (e) An eNO of 40 ppb

Correct answer: (e) (A high exhaled nitric oxide indicates airway inflammation, which is a central feature of asthma, whereas the other tests may indicate sensitization but do not confirm a diagnosis of asthma)

2. All of the following are true regarding chromium-induced occupational disease except?

   (a) Commonly observed in cement and leather workers
   (b) Hexavalent chromium salts are more likely to cause allergic contact dermatitis than trivalent salts
   (c) Workers can exhibit specific IgE antibodies
   (d) Unconjugated chromium salts are immunogenic

Correct answer: (d) (Platinum salts are the only transition metals known to be immunogenic when unconjugated)

3. Cement worker asthma is most often associated with:

   (a) Silicone
   (b) Cobalt
   (c) Chromium
   (d) Cadmium
   (e) Nickel

Correct answer: (c)

4. Welders may develop asthma after exposure to all of the following except:

   (a) Chromates
   (b) Toluene diisocyanate
   (c) Trimellitic anhydride
   (d) Nickel
   (e) Colophony

Correct answer: (b)

5. Which of the following hazardous air pollutants is more likely to aggravate rather than induce occupational asthma?

   (a) Maleic anhydride
   (b) Diethanolamine

(c) Chromium sulfate
(d) Hexamethylene diisocyanate
(e) Volatile organic compounds

Correct answer: (e) (VOCs are primarily irritants as discussed in Case 2; acid anhydrides and isocyanates as causes of OA are discussed in Cases 2 and 3; diethanolamine as an asthmagens is discussed in Case 2)

References

1. Bernstein JA, Kraut A, Bernstein DI, Warrington R, Bolin T, Warren CPW, Bernstein IL (1993) Occupational asthma induced by inhaled egg lysozyme. *Chest* **103**, 532–5.
2. Langeland T (1983) A clinical and immunological study of allergy to hen's egg white: I. A clinical study of egg allergy. *Clin Allergy* **13**, 381–2.
3. Smith AB, Bernstein DI, Aw TC, Gallagher JS, London M, Kopp S, et al (1987) Occupational asthma from inhaled egg protein. *Am J Ind Med* **12**, 205–18.
4. Smith AB, Bernstein DI, London MA, et al (1990) Evaluation of occupational asthma from airborne egg protein exposure in multiple settings. *Chest* **98**, 398–404.
5. Sarlo K, Clark ED, Bernstein DI (1990) ELISA for human IgE antibody to Subtilisin A (alcolase): correlation with RAST and skin test results with occupationally exposed individuals. *J Allergy Clin Immunol* **86**, 393–9.
6. Pepys J, Hutchcroft BJ (1975) Bronchoprovocation tests and etiologic diagnosis and analysis of asthma. *Am Rev Respir Dis* **112**, 829–59.
7. Bernstein DI, Smith AB, Moller DR, et al (1987) Clinical and immunologic studies among egg processing workers with occupational asthma. *J Allergy Clin Immunol* **80**, 791–7.
8. Bernstein JA, Stauder T, Bernstein DI, Bernstein IL (1994) A combined respiratory and cutaneous hypersensitivity syndrome induced by work exposure to quaternary amines. *J Allergy Clin Immunol* **94**, 257–9.
9. Hagmar L, Bellander T, Eng M, et al (1982) Piperazine-induced occupational asthma. *J Occup Med* **24**, 193–7.
10. Malo JL, Bernstein IL (1993) Other chemical substances causing occupational asthma. In: Bernstein IL, Malo JL, Yeung MC, Bernstein DI, eds. *Asthma in the Workplace*. New York, NY: Marcell Dekker, pp. 481–502.
11. Zhang YG, Wright WJ, Tam WK, et al (1990) Effect of inhaled preservatives on asthmatic subjects. II. Benzalkonium chloride. *Am Rev Respir Dis* **141**, 1405–8.
12. Sly RM (1990) Effect of inhaled preservatives on asthmatic subjects. II. Benzalkonium chloride. *Am Rev Respir Dis* **142**, 1466–7.
13. Rumchev K, Spickett J, Bulsara M, et al (2004) Association of domestic exposure to volatile organic compounds with asthma in young children. *Thorax* **59**, 746–51.
14. Pappas GP, Herbert RJ, Henderson W, et al (2000) The respiratory effects of volatile organic compounds. *Int J Occup Environ Health* **6**, 1–8.
15. Pechter E, Davis LK, Tumpowsky C, et al (2005) Work-related asthma among health care workers: surveillance data from California, Massachusetts, Michigan, and New Jersey, 1993–1997. *Am J Ind Med* **47**, 265–75.
16. Rosenman KD, Reilly MJ, Schill DP, et al (2003) Cleaning products and work-related asthma. *J Occup Environ Med* **45**, 556–63.
17. Kogevinas M, Anto JM, Sunyer J, et al (1999) Occupational asthma in Europe and other industrialised areas: a population-based study. European Community Respiratory Health Survey Study Group. *Lancet* **353**, 1750–4.
18. Zock JP, Kogevinas M, Sunyer J, et al (2002) Asthma characteristics in cleaning workers, workers in other risk jobs and office workers. *Eur Respir J* **20**, 679–85.

19. ACGIH (2002) *Threshold Limit Values for Chemical Substances and Physical Agents and Biological Exposures Indices.* Cincinnati, OH: American Conference of Governmental Industrial Hygienists.
20. Bernstein IL, Bernstein DI, Chan-Yeung M and Malo, J-L (2006). Definition and classification of Asthma in the Workplace In: Bernstein IL, Chan-Yeung M, Malo JL, Bernstein DI, eds. *Asthma in the Workplace*, 3rd ed. New York, NY: Taylor and Francis, pp. 1–8.
21. Seta JA, Young RO, Bernstein IL, Bernstein DI (1993) The United States National Exposure Survey (NOES) data base. In: Bernstein IL, Chan-Yeung M, Malo JL, Bernstein DI, eds. *Asthma in the Workplace*. New York, NY: Marcel Dekker, pp. 627–34.
22. Bernstein IL, Merget R (2006) Metals In: Bernstein IL, Chan-Yeung M, Malo JL, Bernstein DI, eds. *Asthma in the Workplace*, 3rd ed. New York, NY: Taylor and Francis, pp. 525–54.
23. Sorahan T, Harrington JM (2000) Lung cancer in Yorkshire chrome platers, 1972–97. *Occup Environ Med* **57**(6), 385–9.
24. Sobaszek A, Boulenguez C, Frimat P, et al (2000) Acute respiratory effects of exposure to stainless steel and mild steel welding fumes. *J Occup Environ Med* **42**(9), 923–31.
25. Bright P, Burge PS, O'Hickey SP, et al (1997) Occupational asthma due to chrome and nickel electroplating. *Thorax* **52**(1), 28–32.
26. Fernandez-Nieto M, Quirce S, Carnes J, et al (2006) Occupational asthma due to chromium and nickel salts. *Int Arch Occup Environ Health* **79**(6), 483–6.
27. Novey HS, Habib M, Wells ID (1983) Asthma and IgE antibodies induced by chromium and nickel salts. *J Allergy Clin Immunol* **72**, 407–41.

Chapter 13
Asthma Conundrums

Michael Schivo, Amir A. Zeki, Nicholas J. Kenyon, and Samuel Louie

Abstract Difficult-to-control asthma in adult patients is a conundrum encountered frequently in clinical practice. Recognizing the range of asthma case presentations and conundrums can improve asthma treatment plans and better patient outcomes.

Keywords Asthma • Asthma comorbidity • Refractory asthma

Objectives

Upon reading this chapter, the asthmatologist should be better able to:

1. Recognize the conundrums of difficult-to-control asthma in adult patients, including challenge in diagnosis and management of asthma and common associated comorbidities.
2. Recognize the importance of ascertaining the patient's objective and subjective response to interventions to reduce impairment and risk for exacerbations in asthma, including the use of the Asthma Control Test™ and office spirometry.
3. Discuss the differential diagnosis of difficult-to-control asthma.

Introduction

The majority of asthma patients in the United States (US) report poor control of asthma despite the general perception among physicians that most asthma is mild, intermittent, and can be easily controlled with a beta-2 agonist with or without an anti-inflammatory controller drug. Using the construct from the NIH-NAEPP guidelines, up to 77% of patients in the US have moderate to severe persistent disease (1). The REACT study

M. Schivo, A.A. Zeki, N.J. Kenyon, and S. Louie (✉)
Division of Pulmonary and Critical Care Medicine, Department of Internal Medicine, University of California, Davis Health System, 4150 V Street, PSSB Suite 3400, Sacramento, CA 95817, USA
e-mail: sylouie@ucdavis.edu

M. Mahmoudi (ed.), *Challenging Cases in Allergy and Immunology*,
DOI: 10.1007/978-1-60327-443-2_13,
© Humana Press, a part of Springer Science +Business Media, LLC 2009

found that 55% of 1,812 patients assessed through an Internet-based survey had uncontrolled asthma using the Asthma Control Test™ (ACT) to stratify cohorts. These patients with very poorly controlled disease or "continuous asthma exacerbations" often have evidence of persistent expiratory airflow obstruction (FEV1 < 60% predicted) despite high medication use and nonsmoking status.

"Refractory asthma" was adopted by the American Thoracic Society in 2000 to describe these patients (2). However, the University of California, Davis Asthma Network (UCAN™) prefers the term "difficult-to-control" asthma based on our experience that control is very often improved and achieved within 6 weeks with the correct diagnoses, asthma education, and effective therapeutic trials (3). We define "difficult-to-control" asthma in adult patients as persistent impairment, e.g., need for albuterol or an alternative short-acting bronchodilator, such as ipratropium bromide if albuterol is ineffective, for more than 2 days a week; an ACT™ scores less than 20; FEV1 less than 80% predicted; and increased risk from poorly controlled asthma despite 3 months of preferred treatments of asthma recommended by the NIH-NAEPP EPR 3 (http://www.nhlbi.nih.gov/guidelines/asthma/index.htm) and/or two or more acute asthma exacerbations requiring rescue treatment, including prednisone, in the past year.

The NIH-NAEPP EPR3 at Steps 3–6 and whenever patients experience difficulty achieving asthma control recommends referral to an asthmatologist. We recommend asking specific questions (Table 13.1) during consultation of an asthma conundrum (Table 13.2).

Table 13.1 Questions to ask in consultation	Is this allergic asthma?
	Childhood or adult-onset?
	Is his asthma controlled?
	Is compliance a problem?
	Is his technique using delivery devices a problem?
	Is patient education important in this case?
	Is a change needed in his asthma controller drugs?
	Is there another disease or comorbidity to be concerned about?
	Is a written asthma action plan needed?

Table 13.2 Conundrums in difficult-to-control asthma	Asthma–COPD overlap syndrome
	COPD
	GERD
	Rhinosinusitis
	Vocal cord dysfunction
	Allergic bronchopulmonary aspergillosis or mycosis (ABPA/ABPM)
	Chronic and subacut infection, e.g., *Mycoplasma*, RSV, *Bordatella*
	Diastolic and systolic heart dysfunction
	Bronchiolitis obliterans
	Pulmonary embolism
	Pulmonary arterial hypertension
	Tracheobroncheomalacia
	Muchausen syndrome
	Churg–Strauss syndrome

Case 1

A 35-year-old registered nurse with prednisone-dependent severe persistent asthma requiring daily prednisone is referred for difficult-to-control asthma for more than 3 years. Her chief complaint is dyspnea and the inability to exercise. She has a history of childhood asthma and gastroesophageal reflux (GERD). Her mother also has asthma. There is no history of osteoporosis or cigarette smoking and a study did not reveal sleep disordered breathing. In the past 4 weeks, she has been unable to work because of severe shortness of breath and reports waking up at night once or twice a week. Oral prednisone has improved her breathing but caused weight gain. ACT™ score is 13.

She takes her current medications daily including albuterol in a metered dose (inhaler MDI), prednisone 20 mg daily, salmeterol 50 mcg inhaled twice daily, zileuton 600 mg orally four times daily, and omeprazole 20 mg daily. She takes her medications every day. Her inhaler technique is very good. She has no written asthma action plan. The review of symptoms was negative for cough, hemoptysis, or sputum production.

Physical examination revealed a young lady weighing 170 lb, 71 in. tall with Cushingoid facies. Her sinuses were not tender to percussion and no nasal polyps or oral thrush were found. The chest was clear to auscultation and no heart murmurs were heard. No peripheral edema or skin rashes were found.

Recent spirometry and lung volumes are normal. Carbon monoxide diffusing capacity (DLco) equal to 104% was predicted (Fig. 13.1). The flow volume loop was normal in appearance. FEV1 was 4.08 L (111% of predicted), FVC was 5.16 L (115% predicted), and FEV1% was 79%. No improvement in FEV1 or FVC was found after albuterol treatment. FEF 25–75% increased from 4.03 to 5.12 L, a 27% improvement after albuterol. Chest X-ray was normal in appearance. There was no record of a RAST panel or total serum IgE level.

What Is Your Working Diagnosis?

The differential diagnosis in this patient with normal pulmonary function tests and chest X-ray includes asthma and diseases that mimic asthma. Churg–Strauss syndrome is very rare but should be included in the differential diagnosis of any patient requiring prednisone daily. Medications that can trigger cough or cause lung disease, e.g., ACE-inhibitors and amiodarone, respectively, should be sought. Chronic lung infection cannot be ruled out entirely, such as latent *Mycoplasma pneumoniae*, but *Bordatella pertussis* is unlikely given the persistence of symptoms over years. Diastolic heart dysfunction and pulmonary arterial hypertension cannot be fully excluded. COPD and allergic bronchopulmonary aspergillosis (ABPA) are unlikely.

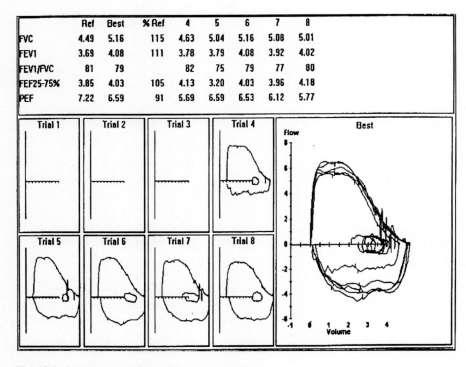

	Ref	Best	% Ref	4	5	6	7	8
FVC	4.49	5.16	115	4.63	5.04	5.16	5.08	5.01
FEV1	3.69	4.08	111	3.78	3.79	4.08	3.92	4.02
FEV1/FVC	81	79		82	75	79	77	80
FEF25-75%	3.85	4.03	105	4.13	3.20	4.03	3.96	4.18
PEF	7.22	6.59	91	5.69	6.59	6.53	6.12	5.77

Fig. 13.1 Spirometry and Flow Volume Loops *Case 1*

What Tests or Treatment Would You Recommend Next?

Review of old medical records for prior investigations and treatments is essential. Reasonable investigations depending on clinical judgment include a chest CT scan, an echocardiogram, or a 24-h pH probe testing to confirm GERD. Methacholine challenge may be considered to rule out asthma. Fiberoptic bronchoscopy would be indicated only if prior investigations are unrevealing. A serum RAST panel for seasonal and perennial aeroallergens and total IgE was ordered anticipating the need for omalizumab.

In addition, all flow volume loops from pulmonary function testing (PFT) were requested for review from the hospital laboratory during the clinic visit (Fig. 13.1).

What Is Your Final Diagnosis and Why?

1. Moderate to severe persistent asthma.
2. Vocal cord dysfunction (VCD).
3. GERD.

VCD is often overlooked when spirometry is normal which measures only expiratory flow rates. The complete flow volume loop is essential for detecting inspiratory flow obstruction. On further questioning, the patient admitted to have more difficulty taking a breath in than exhaling a breath out during her "asthma attacks." GERD, laryngopharyngeal reflux, and postnasal drip are well-known triggers.

The key to this case was to review all of the flow volume loops before ordering additional tests or changing treatment. Pulmonary laboratory technicians are instructed to print the "best effort" by the patient and Trial 6 (Fig. 13.1) was printed in the final report. Trial 6 is normal in appearance. Trial 4 illustrates most dramatically a variable extrathoracic large airway obstruction. There is also evidence of an intrathoracic large airway obstruction suggested by the flattening of the top of the expiratory limb in several of the flow volume loops. This can be classified as a fixed large airway obstruction, but this did not correlate with the patient's clinical history or physical examination. The flow volume loop pattern of a variable extrathoracic upper airway obstruction may be evident with only 25% of efforts. The diagnosis of VCD requires videographic evidence of closure of the anterior two-third of the vocal cords with a small posterior vocal cord opening ("diamond-shaped") during inspiration. Her laryngoscopy was done and confirmed a normal larynx and vocal cord closure with inspiration (paradoxical movement) and partial adduction on expiration.

Methacholine challenge can be positive in patients with VCD. A chest CT scan would be predicted to be normal and an echocardiogram would likely not be helpful given the normal physical examination. A 24-h pH probe is the definitive test for GERD but is seldom required if the patient derives dramatic benefit from treatment and elevation of the bed to 45°. The correct diagnosis in this patient averted unnecessary studies and asthma drug therapy, which would not have treated the underlying problem.

The average time to correct diagnosis in clinical reviews has been reported to be around 5 years. The majority of patients are women in their 40s and many are healthcare professionals. While rare in the general population, it is very common in difficult-to-control asthma patients in our experience at UC Davis.

Treatment of VCD requires treatment of its triggers, including postnasal drip from rhinosinusitis and/or GERD and stopping any unnecessary drug treatments, e.g., prednisone. Inhaled or oral corticosteroids have no role in treatment of VCD unless asthma is present. Triggers for VCD are often the same triggers for asthma in the same patient, e.g., exercise, breathing air pollution, and exercise in cold air. Stress and anxiety are also common, though the signs and the symptoms of VCD are not the result of conscious malingering or factitious disorder.

Speech therapy is often necessary to improve the synchrony needed in normal breathing, i.e., relaxing the larynx with synchronized thoracic and abdominal breathing. Botulinum Toxin Type A injections are rarely indicated and only in the most refractory cases. Treatment of GERD in this patient was intensified with a proton-pump inhibitor together with a H2-blocker during sleep in this patient dramatically improved asthma control over a period of 6 weeks. The patient was eventually liberated from oral corticosteroids in 9 months and is currently on a low-dose inhaled corticosteroid, a long-acting beta-2 agonist daily, and a proton-pump inhibitor to maintain well-controlled asthma and GERD. A written asthma action plan was provided with education. Zileuton was discontinued without loss of asthma control and, in retrospect, may have contributed to worsening GERD in this patient.

Case 2

A 26-year-old surgeon with prednisone-dependent severe-persistent asthma, allergic rhinosinusitis, and a latex allergy is referred for difficult-to-control asthma despite strict adherence to medications. His chief complaint is a nagging productive cough occurring 2–3 times per hour. He uses his albuterol inhaler 2–3 times per week with only temporary relief of cough and has nighttime coughing about 5 times per week. ACT™ score is 13 and his personal peak flows, normally 500 L/min have notably decreased in the past few months. He does not have a written asthma action plan.

A prior RAST panel demonstrated allergies to latex, dust mites, and a variety of tree and grass antigens. He denied any exposure to latex due at the hospital and does not smoke cigarettes. No history of hemoptysis, epistaxis, joint swelling, skin rashes, fevers, or recurrent pneumonias was found. Current medications include fluticasone/salmeterol 500/50 mcg one puff twice daily, mometasone 50 mcg nasal spray, loratadine 10 mg, and 15 mg of prednisone orally every other day. He uses nasal rinses twice daily. Cromolyn, montelukast, and zileuton were ineffective.

He is weighed 170 lb and is 69 in. tall. Vital signs are normal and he has wheezing but not in acute distress. Frontal sinuses were not tender but nasal turbinates were red and swollen. Posterior oropharynx was slightly erythematous and mucosa cobble-stone in appearance. He coughed violently during the examination. Bilateral wheezing is heard without evidence of stridor.

Office spirometry showed no evidence of a variable extrathoracic upper airway obstruction. FEV1 was 3.54 L (80% predicted), FVC was 4.61 L (87% of predicted), and the FEV1% was 76.8%. Serum IgE was >1,400 IU/mL just before prednisone was started. Complete blood count was normal without eosinophilia. Chest X-ray was normal. Serum antibodies to *Aspergillus* were negative as was an *Aspergillus* extract skin prick test.

What Is Your Working Diagnosis?

This young man with normal spirometry and chest X-ray has severe asthma and possibly an unidentified comorbid condition which could affect asthma control and cause incessant coughing. Asthma mimics to consider in this case are allergic bronchopulmonary aspergillosis/mycosis (ABPA/ABPM), Churg–Strauss syndrome, Wegener's granulomatosis, early sarcoidosis, and heart disease. GERD and recent infections, such as a viral infection (RSV, parainfluenza, rhinovirus), can exacerbate his asthma as well as *Mycoplasma* spp., *Chlamydiophila* spp., or *B. pertussis*. Several of these conditions can be excluded based on the current history and work-up. Heart disease is unlikely given the history and physical as is Churg–Strauss syndrome and Wegener's in the absence of specific diagnostic clinical and laboratory criteria though tissue biopsy would be required for confirmation. Sarcoidosis is with a normal chest X-ray but could manifest in his nasopharynx. Clinical history does not support severe GERD, but up to 50% of asthmatics have silent GERD which may worsen their asthma control (4). ABPA/ABPM is a consideration given the high IgE levels, though a negative skin prick test, negative serum precipitins to *Aspergillus*, and lack of central bronchiectasis argue against it. Lung infections caused by viruses, *Mycoplasma* spp., *Chlamydiophila* spp., and *B. pertussis* remain possible in this patient.

What Tests or Treatment Would You Recommend Next?

A high-resolution chest CT scan; serologic testing for *Mycoplasma pneumoniae*, *Chlamydiophila*, RSV, and *B. pertussis*; sputum culture; and eosinophil count are reasonable tests for the first visit. Fiberoptic bronchoscopy for intractable coughing and 24-h pH probe to evaluate for GERD were considered for later.

What Is Your Final Diagnosis and Why?

1. Severe persistent asthma, poorly controlled
2. Possible lower respiratory tract infection
3. Allergic rhinosinusitis
4. Possible GERD

In the absence of prior antibiotic treatment, the surgeon was empirically prescribed a course of azithromycin 500 mg orally for the first day followed by 250 mg orally for 4 more days. Plan was made to prescribe a proton-pump inhibitor if azithromycin was ineffective after completion. A high-resolution CT scan was not ordered because of the normal chest X-ray. Sputum culture was considered pending the serologic analysis, and a pH probe was deemed unnecessary in a patient who has not undergone a trial with a proton-pump inhibitor.

He returned 2 weeks later and reported better breathing during his course of azithromycin. His peak flows increased significantly and he coughed and wheezed much less. ACT™ score improved to 18. Serologic testing was positive for *M. pneumoniae* IgM 1.03 Units/L (>0.96 U/L unequivocally positive) as well as IgG for *B. pertussis* though IgA was equivocal. *Chlamydiophila* antibodies were negative. RSV IgG was positive though IgM was negative indicating past RSV infection. Given the persistent poor control, a proton-pump inhibitor was added which brought his asthma into the well-controlled category albeit still on prednisone.

The key to this case is recognizing that this patient's asthma control worsened significantly during the past 2 months despite strict adherence to his action plan. His productive cough and fatigue are not typical of asthma. The link between respiratory infections and severe asthma has been established in both animal models and humans (5). In one recent study, 55 stable asthmatics were found to have either *Mycoplasma* spp. or *Chlamydia* (*Chlamydiophila*) spp. infection upon evaluation, a significantly higher percentage than nonasthmatics. Another found nearly 40% of asthma cases presenting to the Emergency Department were associated with an acute atypical infection, mostly *Mycoplasma*. The association between asthma and *B. pertussis* infection is less clear but the latter is increasingly recognized as a cause of chronic cough, which can mimic asthma. Adults do not present with the typical paroxysmal cough and inspiratory whoop seen in children (6). Diagnosis can be a challenge because serologic testing for *B. pertussis* is not as specific for acute infection as nasopharyngeal cultures are: sensitivity 15–80% and specificity of 100% when *B. pertussis* is cultured.

Viruses have been implicated in asthma exacerbations, including influenza, parainfluenza, RSV, adenovirus, and rhinoviruses. Whether they directly aggravate airway hyperresponsiveness or worsen airway inflammation is not clear. There is limited therapy for viral infections, except for influenza A and B with neuraminidase inhibitors.

Case 3

A 36-year-old church pastor and former paramedic with prednisone-dependent severe persistent asthma for more than 4 years is referred for assessment and initial treatment with omalizumab which was recently approved by his health insurance. He has been on prednisone daily for a year because of unrelenting dyspnea requiring inhaled albuterol 3–4 times a day. He was diagnosed with asthma at age 12. Past history is notable for chronic rhinosinusitis, osteoporosis, and at least ten lifetime episodes of acute pneumonia, the most recent one in the past 12 months. He never smoked cigarettes and a recent 24-h pH probe testing was negative for GERD. Bronchoscopy recently revealed normal tracheobronchial anatomy and no VCD. No infection was found. He had consulted with four pulmonologists in the past year and his family practitioner for asthma exacerbations. He does not have a written asthma action plan.

In the past 4 weeks, his asthma has kept him away from work and he wakes up at night twice a week with cough and wheezing, which he treats with inhaled albuterol. He needs inhaled albuterol 3–4 times per day and feels immediately better afterward. Prednisone has improved breathing in the patient's opinion but caused unwanted weight gain. His personal best peak flow has recently ranged from 450 to 500 L/min having fallen from 700 L/min a year ago. He and his wife have kept daily records of his peak flow measurements. ACT™ is 11.

Current daily medications include albuterol MDI, prednisone 20–25 mg, fluticasone/salmeterol 500/50 mcg, montelukast 10 mg, tiotropium 18 mcg, and he irrigates his nose with saline daily. He cannot taper his prednisone without experiencing shortness of breath and a fall in his peak flow. He does not wheeze even with severe asthma attacks. His inhaler technique is very good.

Physical examination reveals a young gentleman weighing 159 lb, 64 in. tall with cushingnoid facies. Nasal passages were swollen and inflamed. No nasal polyps were found. Sinuses were nontender to percussion. Chest was clear to auscultation and no heart murmurs were heard. No peripheral edema or skin rashes were found.

Office spirometry measured the FEV1 at 3.16 L (103% of predicted), FVC 3.66 L (102% predicted), FEV1% equal to 86%. No improvement in FEV1 or FVC was found after albuterol treatment. The flow volume loops were normal. Recent chest X-ray at the time of consultation and chest CT scan done 3 months ago were both normal in appearance except for a borderline enlarged cardiac silhouette on chest X-ray. RAST panel was positive for perennial aeroallergens and total serum IgE level was recently 33.9 IU/mL on prednisone.

What Is Your Working Diagnosis?

As with our previous two cases, the differential diagnosis in this patient with normal pulmonary function tests and chest X-ray includes asthma and diseases that mimic asthma. Churg–Strauss syndrome is very rare with an incidence of 3 in 1,000,000, but it should be included in the differential diagnosis of difficult-to-control asthma patients requiring prednisone for new onset asthma or newly worsening asthma control. The history of transient pulmonary infiltrates on chest X-ray is one of the diagnostic criteria for Churg–Strauss syndrome. Our case never had documented peripheral eosinophilia or other subsequent evidence of a small and medium vessel eosinophilic vasculitis, e.g., skin rash with purpura, mononeuritis multiplex, or kidney disease with proteinuria from glomerulonephritis. All his pneumonias were treated with antibiotics with successful outcomes.

The American College of Rheumatology has established criteria for the diagnosis of Churg–Strauss syndrome. A patient should have four of the six criteria listed in Table 13.3. Treatment of Churg–Strauss syndrome is often life-long with prednisone and cyclophosphamide or azathioprine. Chronic lung infection in this patient cannot be ruled out entirely, e.g., latent *Mycoplasma pneumoniae*, but no serology was ordered by his physicians. He has been treated with several courses of azithromycin 250 mg daily for months. COPD is unlikely given his spirometry but allergic bronchopulmonary aspergillosis (ABPA) is a possibility with the history of recurrent pneumonias. The absence of bronchiectasis on chest CT makes ABPA less likely. Early interstitial lung disease with a "normal" chest X-ray has not been excluded. Pulmonary

Table 13.3 Clinical criteria for Churg–Strauss syndrome (required four of six criteria)	Asthma
	Eosinophilia (>10% on differential WBC count)
	Mononeuropathy
	Transient infiltrates on chest X-rays
	Paranasal abnormalities
	A biopsy containing a blood vessel with extravascular eosinophils

arterial hypertension is also less likely given the presented data, but the enlarged cardiac silhouette may warrant a screening echocardiogram.

What Tests or Treatment Would You Recommend Next?

Old medical records and a high-resolution chest CT scan to evaluate for early interstitial lung disease were ordered. We could consider another RAST panel for different environmental and occupational aeroallergens. A methacholine challenge test would be appropriate if asthma was in doubt. An echocardiogram to evaluate for heart dysfunction is reasonable. Bronchoscopy would be considered again, but this is only likely to reveal new information if biopsies are done.

What Is Your Final Diagnosis and Why?

1. Severe persistent asthma, very poorly controlled
2. Allergic rhinosinusitis
3. Cushing's syndrome

The patient was informed of the risks and benefits of omalizumab with the FDA medication guide, including anaphylaxis and cancer. After consent was obtained, 150 mg was administered subcutaneously without adverse reaction during a 2-h observation period. He received instruction on the proper use of an epinephrine pen for potential anaphylaxis from omalizumab (0.2% incidence). Given the long time to therapeutic effect with omalizumab, the patient entered a "clinical trial of one" with zileuton 1,200 mg twice daily in an attempt to improve his asthma control and reduce his need for oral corticosteroids. Montelukast was the only medication discontinued from his original regimen. A p-ANCA and c-ANCA were ordered in addition to serology for *B. pertussis* and the patient was asked to return in 1 month or another injection of omalizumab.

Within a week the patient reported improved peak flow measurement (390–440 L/min to over 800 L/min daily) and a reduction in his need for daily albuterol. Unexpectedly, the patient was able to reduce his prednisone dose from 25 mg daily to 4 mg daily without any loss of asthma control, albeit still very poor. He had previously been unable to drop below 10 mg of prednisone a day. He was no longer taking prednisone by the end of the second month of asthma management. His ACT™ score increased from 11 to 20 by the beginning of the fourth month of consultation. He returned to running, weight lifting, and his sermons. His asthma control did deteriorate for a week during the second month of management when zileuton was briefly unavailable through his pharmacy, and this withdrawal confirmed his therapeutic response to the 5-lipoxygenase inhibitor. His liver function tests remained normal during the first 3 months on zileuton. He remains on zileuton and omalizumab monthly in addition to fluticasone/salmeterol 500/50 mcg twice daily, tiotropium 18 mcg once daily, and inhaled albuterol as needed for asthma symptoms. His need for albuterol decreased to 5 times a week instead of 6–8 times a day.

The importance of the 5-lipoxygengenase pathway in this patient illustrates the heterogeneity in asthma syndromes. Eicosanoids and leukotrienes are potent eosinophil chemoattractants and activate neutrophils which may play a more significant role in adult-onset asthma and in cases of severe persistent asthma. 5-Lipoxygenase inhibition with zileuton and CysLT1 receptor antagonism with montelukast or zafirlukast are important alternative treatments to preferred treatment with inhaled corticosteroids and long-acting beta-2 agonists.

Omalizumab is indicated for adults and adolescents aged 12 years and older with symptomatically uncontrolled moderate to severe asthma (despite inhaled corticosteroids) who have an elevated IgE level and a positive skin test or *in vitro* reactivity to perennial aeroallergens. Omalizumab is recommended at Step 5 in the NIH-NAEPP EPR3 as add-on therapy to high-dose inhaled corticosteroids combined with long-acting beta-2 agonists before considering daily oral prednisone. Omalizumab is also recommended as add on to Step 6 treatments if asthma control is still not achieved. A clinical benefit from omalizumab in this patient may be manifest by a further decline in his need for weekly inhaled albuterol at which time an attempt to step down from the high dose of his inhaled corticosteroids to reduce adverse effects is indicated. Omalizumab has been shown to decrease the incidence of asthma exacerbations. Omalizumab injection should be given in a healthcare setting by clinicians prepared to manage anaphylaxis that can be life threatening.

Case 4

A 57-year-old preschool teacher with a history of childhood asthma, cigarette smoking (50 pack-years), and recently diagnosed COPD was referred for unremitting exertional dyspnea. She had breast cancer 2 years earlier and has since been hospitalized numerous times for severe dyspnea. No history of orthopnea, cough with sputum production, hoarseness, sinus disease, GERD, or heart disease was found. She was recently treated for acute COPD exacerbation and *Haemophilus influenzae* community-acquired pneumonia.

She uses fluticasone 220 mcg twice daily and an albuterol/ipratropium combination inhaler up to five times daily for acute dyspnea, with only modest symptomatic relief. Levalbuterol nebulizer treatment is used 2–3 times per week with similar results. Corticosteroid bursts with short-term tapers result in considerable symptomatic improvement. Remaining medications include anastrozole for her breast cancer and alendronate. She lives with birds and cats inside her home. Family history is notable for two children and her father with asthma.

She was in no acute distress with normal vitals signs and pulse oximetry. Body-mass index and physical examination were normal. No wheezing, rhonchi, or crackles were heard. Office spirometry revealed FVC at 1.73 L (69% predicted), FEV1 at 0.78 L (38% predicted), FEV/FVC ratio at 45%, and peak expiratory flow (PEF) at 1.96 L/s

Ht (in): 62.0   Wt (lb): 128   Complaint/Diag: **DYSPNEA**

Spirometry(BTPS)			PRE		POST		
		PRED	BEST	%PRED	BEST	%PRED	% CHG
FVC	Liters	2.91	2.06	71	2.69	92	30
FEV1	Liters	2.36	0.86	36	1.12	47	30
FEV1/FVC %		81	42	52	42	51	-0
FEV6	Liters		1.68		2.10		25
FEV1/FEV6%			51		53		4
PEF	L/sec	5.58	3.09	55	3.45	62	11
FEF25-75%L/sec		2.52	0.26	10	0.29	11	13
FET100% Sec			11.81		17.05		44
FIVC	Liters	2.91	1.86	64	2.47	85	33
PIF	L/sec	5.58	2.64	47	3.50	63	33
MVV	L/min	75					
Lung Volumes(BTPS)							
SVC	Liters	2.91	2.06	71			
IC	Liters	1.92	1.60	84			
ERV	Liters	0.96	0.54	57			
FRC PL	Liters	2.64	4.67	177			
RV	Liters	1.80	4.13	230			
TLC	Liters	4.73	6.20	131			
Raw	cm H20 L/sec	<3.06					
IC/TLC	%		26				
RV/TLC	%	38	67	177			
Diffusing Capacity(STPD)							
DLCO	mL/mmHg/min	22.0	11.3	52			
DL Adj	mL/mmHg/min	(Hb:)gm/dL	11.3				
DL/VA AdjmL/mHg/min/L		4.81	3.30	69			
VA	Liters	4.73	3.44	73			

Fig. 13.2 Pulmonary function test, 1-year prior to presentation

(21% predicted). Complete PFT performed 1 year prior (Fig. 13.2) shows severe obstructive airways disease, with a positive bronchodilator response, hyperinflation, air-trapping, and severely reduced DLCO. Chest X-ray, laboratory chemistries, and complete blood count with differential were all normal. Baseline peak expiratory flow rates (PEFR) are 200–250 L/min. ACT™ score was 10.

What Is Your Working Diagnosis?

Asthmatics who smoke are excluded in most asthma clinical studies and, in our experience, not often treated adequately for the COPD component of their airway disease. A reasonable working diagnosis is the *asthma–COPD overlap syndrome*. Bronchiectasis, tracheobroncheomalacia, or bronchiolitis obliterans are all improbable given the information presented. Other causes of dyspnea, such as VCD, anemia, heart disease, pulmonary embolism, recurrent lung infections, or collagen-vascular disease are also unlikely. Coexisting pulmonary arterial hypertension has not been excluded.

What Tests or Treatment Would You Recommend Next?

The patient should be evaluated for both asthma and COPD with particular attention to complications from emphysema. Smoking cessation, pulmonary rehabilitation, and a written asthma and COPD action plan are recommended. RAST panel and serum IgE level should be measured. A 6-min walk can document exercise capacity and uncover moderate to severe hypoxia, i.e., SpO2 <90% and <80%, respectively. Echocardiogram to assess pulmonary arterial pressure can evaluate for right heart dysfunction or pulmonary hypertension. Inhaled corticosteroids remain the mainstay for her asthma but their role in COPD remains controversial. Adding a long-acting beta-agonist (LABA) to her current inhaled corticosteroids, as well as a scheduled once daily long-acting muscarinic receptor blocker, e.g. tiotropium, may reduce symptoms, improve lung function and exercise capacity, and reduce exacerbation rates. Symptomatic treatment with short-acting beta 2-agonists (SABA) (albuterol or levalbuterol) and ipratropium can be used for breakthrough symptoms as needed.

What Is Your Final Diagnosis and Why?

Asthma–COPD overlap syndrome:

Questions commonly faced with asthmatic smokers include: Does this patient have COPD with abnormal bronchial hyperreactivity? Is this severe remodeled asthma that has progressed to irreversible or partially reversible obstruction? Or, is this overlapping COPD and asthma, the so-called *asthma–COPD overlap syndrome*. Finally, does making these distinctions matter?

Key differences in the inflammatory signatures and structural changes occur with respect to the epithelium, bronchial smooth muscle cells, mast cell myositis, reticular basement membrane, and presence of emphysema (7). The Dutch Hypothesis holds that asthma and BHR predispose patients to the development of COPD later in life. It states that asthma and COPD are different expressions of a single disease entity. The British Hypothesis, conversely, holds that asthma and COPD are distinct diseases that develop by unique mechanisms. Some authorities argue that obstructive lung disease is a continuum that begins in early childhood progressing into adulthood when COPD becomes the final common pathway.

The *asthma–COPD overlap syndrome* is not clearly defined. It is a syndrome in which older adults with a significant smoking history (≥10 pack-years) have both asthmatic and COPD features to their obstructive airways disease. Epidemiologic studies report an estimated prevalence of 20–25% in the US (8). Patients with overlap syndrome have poorer lung function (e.g., FEV1% <70%), hyperinflation, and more respiratory symptoms than either disease alone. They also consume more medical resources compared to asthma or COPD alone, as much as 2–6 times higher for combined disease (9).

Airway remodeling and the lung's limited repair responses in small airways may account for some of the pathological similarities that are reported in asthma and COPD (10). Severe bronchial asthma with fixed obstruction is often accompanied by an increased number of neutrophils in the airway mucosa similar to COPD. Eosinophil inflammation in COPD may play a substantial role and be associated with greater postbronchodilator reversibility. Chronic bronchitis or emphysema patients with airway eosinophilia tend to have more airway reversibility and respond more readily to corticosteroid therapy. In smokers with severe obstructive bronchitis, sputum eosinophilia predicted a beneficial response to prednisone treatment. Adult asthmatics who smoke have more neutrophils than eosinophils in their airways resembling COPD. Lastly, airway mucosal eosinophils increase in acute exacerbations of COPD, a feature normally seen in asthma (7). There is a dearth of recommendations for this conundrum but both asthma and COPD must be treated concurrently to prevent further impairment and risk for acute exacerbations from both.

Review Questions for Asthma Conundrums

1. A 34-year-old woman presents with recurrent episodes of unexplained dyspnea and wheezing. Triggers include strong soaps and perfumes, cleaning products, and emotional stress. She admits to GERD symptoms and has a hiatal hernia. Trials of beta 2-agonists, inhaled corticosteroids, and leukotriene receptor antagonists (LTRA) have provided virtually no relief. The next most appropriate step in her evaluation is:

   (a) Skin testing and a RAST panel
   (b) High-resolution chest CT
   (c) pH probe for 24-h monitoring
   (d) Direct laryngoscopy with or without a cold-air challenge
   (e) Bronchoscopy with endobronchial biopsy

2. A 21-year-old college student presents with difficult-to-control asthma. He was diagnosed with asthma during adolescence and has had multiple ER visits and one hospitalization in the past for asthma. He cites cigarette smoke, spring blooms, and cats as asthma triggers. Asthma Control Test™ score is 12. Current medications include budesonide/formoterol combination MDI and albuterol, though he thinks he may have other medications prescribed. He uses his albuterol inhaler 5–6 times per day. He is uncertain if he had RAST testing and he may have had allergy shots. The next best step in management is:

   (a) Admit the patient for intravenous steroids and continuous nebulized broncho dilators
   (b) Place the patient on oral corticosteroids for 2 weeks and see him in followup
   (c) Assess his inhaler technique, adherence to therapy, and understanding of his disease
   (d) Add a leukotriene receptor blocker and reassess him in 4 weeks
   (e) High-resolution chest CT to assess for bronchiectasis

3. A 46-year-old woman with severe persistent asthma presents for evaluation. She has been hospitalized several times in the past 3 years and has been intubated twice for status asthmaticus. Currently she takes oral and inhaled corticosteroids, inhaled long- and short-acting beta 2-agonists, theophylline, and an inhaled anticholinergic. ACT™ score is 10. The most bothersome symptoms are dyspnea

and cough productive of brownish sputum. She occasionally has fevers and scant hemoptysis. A previous IgE level was 1,500 IU/mL. The next best step in her management is:

(a) A skin-prick test for reactivity to *Aspergillus* antigens
(b) Open lung biopsy containing a blood vessel to demonstrate extravascular eosinophils
(c) A high-resolution chest CT to assess for bronchiectasis and mucous plugging
(d) (a) and (c)
(e) All of the above

4. A demented elderly man is brought into clinic by his daughter for coughing and wheezing. His daughter described the onset of his symptoms a week ago after her father fell forward while trying to stand from his wheelchair. The patient appeared well, though he did incur facial lacerations after striking a table. Chest X-ray shows right lower lobe atelectasis and an irregular calcification in the right perihilar area. Inhaled albuterol have been ineffective. On exam, there is focal wheezing over the right posterior chest. The next best step in management is:

(a) Bronchoscopy
(b) Addition of inhaled corticosteroids
(c) High-resolution chest CT
(d) Measurement of serum total IgE
(e) Addition of high-dose oral steroids

5. A 38-year-old farmer presents for evaluation of cough and dyspnea. The symptoms have occurred three times in the past year and include dyspnea, fever, cough, and chest tightness. He has received beta 2-agonists and prednisone in the past which have provided relief. Between episodes he does not take medication. His latest episode occurred a week ago and the patient was hospitalized and treated for an asthma exacerbation and pneumonia. On exam the patient is mildly tachypnic but not labored. He has fine crackles in the bilateral lower lobes, though he has no wheezing. Office spirometry shows a restrictive pattern. The next best step in management should be:

(a) High-resolution chest CT
(b) Serum precipitins for IgG and IgM
(c) Bronchoscopy
(d) A detailed history
(e) All of the above

Answers to Questions

1. Answer (d) The younger age, female gender, and association with reflux symptoms all suggest VCD. Direct visualization is necessary to confirm this. Additionally, a methacholine challenge may enhance the response. A flow-volume loop may

suggest VCD by a flattened inspiratory limb; however, a normal flow-volume loop does not rule-out VCD. As both reflux and postnasal drip can exacerbate VCD, both should be treated if suspected.

Skin testing is not necessary unless the patient gives specific allergic symptoms or demonstrates allergic rhinosinusitis. Chest imaging is also unwarranted unless allergic bronchopulmonary aspergillosis, bronchiectasis, or pulmonary vascular/rheumatologic disease is suspected. A 24-h pH probe is utilized for patients with GERD who fail conventional therapy with a proton-pump inhibitor. It is too aggressive at this stage for this patient. There is no indication of a foreign body or pulmonary parenchymal disease to warrant bronchoscopy.

2. Answer (c) Given a younger patient with a chronic disease and a complicated medication regimen, adherence is likely an issue. Greater than 50% of young patients are not adherent to their asthma regimen. Reasons include complicated medication schedules, lack of understanding of the disease, delayed onset of action of some medications, and a lowered motivation to change behaviors. These factors are coupled with inadequate action plans and education. This patient presents enough ambiguity that a detailed assessment of his technique, adherence, and understanding of his disease is necessary.

Though his ACT™ score is low, indicating poor control, nothing in the vignette indicates that the patient should be admitted. Oral steroids or a leukotriene receptor blocker may be needed, but only after an assessment of adherence can one designate a patient "refractory" to current therapy. There is no indication for imaging at this time.

3. Answer (d) This case illustrates the asthma mimic Allergic Bronchopulmonary Aspergillosis (ABPA). ABPA is present in 1–2% of severe asthmatics and is higher in patients with cystic fibrosis. The hallmarks of this disease are severe asthma, elevated sputum production (presumably from bronchiectasis), and an elevated total IgE. Other features include skin reactivity to *Aspergillus* antigen, precipitating serum antibodies to *A. fumigatus*, peripheral eosinophilia (absolute count >500/mm^3), lung infiltrates, central and upper lobe-predominant bronchiectasis, and elevated specific IgE and IgG to *A. fumigatus*. This patient has severe asthma, an elevated IgE, and sputum production. Of the choices, both a skin-prick test and a high-resolution chest CT would help make the diagnosis. CT may also show infiltrates, atelectasis, mucous impaction, and peripheral mosaic airtrapping. A complete blood count with differential would also help to demonstrate eosinophils.

An open lung biopsy may be helpful if looking for Churg–Strauss syndrome (CSS) only after an extensive workup prior to this. The severe asthma and elevated IgE do suggest CSS, but the lack of neurologic and/or skin vasculitic findings, plus the increased sputum production, argues against CSS which is extremely rare compared to ABPA

4. Answer (a) This scenario represents an adult foreign-body aspiration (FBA). Most likely the patient fell forward, chipped a tooth or his dental appliance, and

aspirated it into the right lower lobe (the most common site of aspiration). As opposed to FBA in children, adults with FBA generally do not present acutely unless symptoms are severe. Often they present with chronic cough, wheezing, refractory asthma, hemoptysis, or recurrent pneumonia. In this case, the best modality to confirm FBA is bronchoscopy. In general, flexible bronchoscopy can be safely performed to diagnose and localize the FBA, and it often can be used to remove the object (if removal can be performed safely). Rigid bronchoscopy in an operating room is preferred if the obstruction is large, comprised of fragmented material, or associated with significant inflammation. All the other choices are unnecessary as removal of the object is usually curative.

5. Answer (e) This is a good example of the clinical exam and data *not* matching that of asthma. Asthma generally presents with dyspnea and wheezing, and spirometry is either normal or shows airways obstruction. In this vignette, the patient presents with dyspnea and crackles, and spirometry shows a restrictive pattern. The clinical exam points to an interstitial lung disease and spirometry supports this. The best interstitial disease which fits here is hypersensitivity pneumonitis (HP), presumably a farm-worker's lung. Acute HP can be confused with asthma due to its rapid onset, associated dyspnea, and response to corticosteroids. But the diagnosis and management of HP is quite different than asthma. Identification of the inciting allergen (often organic material or fungal) is difficult but specific avoidance is key in disease management. Radiography can be variable, and often small nodules and ground glass opacities are seen. Serum precipitins are helpful, though they are neither sensitive nor specific. Bronchoscopy with bronchoalveolar lavage may show a lymphocytosis with a low CD4:CD8 ratio, and transbronchial biopsies may show poorly defined granulomata. Infection should be excluded. A thorough history linking the symptoms to a specific exposure is above all of them to solving this conundrum.

References

1. Fuhlbrigge AL, Adams, RJ, Guilbert, TW, et al. The burden of asthma in the United States. Level and distribution are dependent on interpretation of the National Asthma and Education and Prevention Program Guidelines. *Am J Respir Crit Care Med* 2002; **166**: 1044–1049.
2. American Thoracic Society. Proceedings of the ATS Workshop on refractory asthma. Current understanding, recommendations, and unanswered questions. *Am J Respir Crit Care Med* 2000; **162**: 2341–2351.
3. Mealey FH, Kenyon NJ, Avdalovic MV, Louie S. Difficult-to-control asthma in adults. *Am J Med* 2007; **120**: 760–763.
4. Kiljander TO and Laitinen JO. The prevalence of gastroesophageal reflux disease in adult asthmatics. *Chest* 2004; **126**(5): 1490–1494.
5. Martin RJ, Kraft M, et al. A link between chronic asthma and chronic infection. *J Allergy Clin Immunol* 2001; **107**(4): 595–601.
6. Hewlett EL and Edwards KM. Clinical practice: pertussis- not just for kids. *N Engl J Med* 2005; **352**(12): 1215–1222.
7. Jeffery, P.K. Remodeling and inflammation of bronchi in asthma and chronic obstructive pulmonary disease. *Proc Am Thorac Soc* 2004; **1**: 176–183.

8. Soriano JB, Davis KJ, Coleman B, Visick G, Mannino D, Pride NB. The Proportional Venn diagram of obstructive lung disease: Two approximations from the United States and the United Kingdom. *Chest* 2003; **124**: 474–481.
9. Shaya FT, Dongyi D, Akazawa MO, Blanchette CM, Wang J, Mapel DW, Dalal A, Scharf SM. Burden of concomitant asthma and COPD in a medicaid population. *Chest* 2008; **134**: 14–19.
10. Mauad T, Dolhnikoff M. Pathologic similarities and differences between asthma and chronic obstructive pulmonary disease. *Curr Opin Pulm Med* 2008; **14**: 31–38.

Chapter 14
Mastocytosis

Bettina Wedi

Abstract Mastocytosis is a neoplastic disease involving mast cells (MC) and their CD34+ progenitors and consists of a heterogeneous group of diseases with a clinical spectrum ranging from localized mastocytoma to generalized forms such as mast cell leukemia. In 80% of mastocytosis, the skin is involved. Cutaneous mastocytosis (CM) has to be distinguished from systemic mastocytosis. CM is divided into maculopapular CM (= urticaria pigmentosa), diffuse cutaneous mastocytosis, teleangiectasia macularis eruptive perstans, and solitary mastocytoma of skin. All forms of mastocytosis can result in systemic symptoms induced by IgE-dependent or -independent degranulation of MC mediators (e.g., induced by hymenoptera stings or histamine liberating drugs). In this chapter, two cases of cutaneous and systemic mastocytosis are discussed.

Keywords Cutaneous mastocytosis • Urticaria pigmentosa • Teleangiectasia macularis eruptive perstans • Serum tryptase

Case 1

A 48-year-old man consults the allergy department because 6 months ago he experienced a severe anaphylactic reaction including generalized urticaria, angioedema of the face, dyspnea, and hypotension with consciousness for few minutes developing 10 min after he was stung by a yellow jacket into the right arm. In addition, he reports unexplained severe anaphylactic reaction with hypotension during intubation anesthesia about 10 years ago. For the first time consulting a dermatologist with

B. Wedi
Department of Dermatology and Allergology, Hannover Medical School, Ricklinger Street 5, 30449, Hannover, Germany
e-mail: wedi.bettina@mh-hannover.de

M. Mahmoudi (ed.), *Challenging Cases in Allergy and Immunology*,
DOI: 10.1007/978-1-60327-443-2_14,
© Humana Press, a part of Springer Science+Business Media, LLC 2009

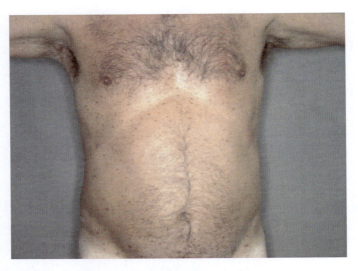

Fig. 14.1 Cutaneous maculopapular mastocytosis (urticaria pigmentosa)

this complaints he also wants to demonstrate his nevi that appear to have proliferated during the last year. He explains that after a hot bath they become more reddish and a little bit itchy.

He presents laboratory results from his practitioner with elevated specific IgE to yellow jacket but not to honey bee venom.

Physical examination shows multiple symmetrically distributed reddish-brown macules and papules of 1–7 mm in diameter with enhancement over the trunk (Fig. 14.1). Gentle rubbing of these papules produced localized pruritic wheals (Fig. 14.2). Everything else beside skin is normal. Mean blood pressure is 140/80 mmHg.

Data

Histology of lesional skin demonstrates a perivascular infiltrate with diffuse oval- to spindle-shaped mast cells in the reticular dermis (Giemsa staining). Additional single mast cells are found between the collagen fibres in the deeper dermis.

Bone marrow biopsy shows normocellular bone marrow. Toludine staining and immunhistochemistry demonstrate loosely scattered mast cells throughout the whole bone marrow, in some locations perivascular mature mast cells. Absence of Multifocal compact MC infiltrates, consisting of at least 15 cells, were absent and there was no diffuse mast cell infiltration.

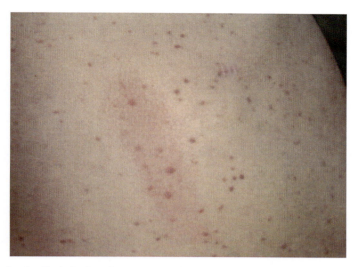

Fig. 14.2 Postive Darier's sign after gentle rubbing of lesional skin

Abdominal and lymph node ultrasounds are normal. Biopsies of the gastric, colon, and duodenal mucosa do not demonstrate increased mast cell numbers. Osteodensitometry and X-ray of bones are normal.

Laboratory results demonstrated elevated serum tryptase of 48 µg/l (normal <11.4 µg/l, CAP-FEIA, Phadia, Uppsala, Sweden). Complete blood count, coagulation parameters, and serum chemistry are normal. Total IgE is 21 kU/l (normal <100 kU/l; CAP-FEIA, Phadia, Uppsala, Sweden); specific IgE to yellow jacket venom is 14 kU/l (RAST class 3; normal <0.35 kU/l) but not detectable to honey bee venom. Titrated skin test with hymenoptera venoms demonstrates no reactivity to honey bee venom (prick up to 100 ng/ml, intradermal test 1 µg/ml) but demonstrates positivity to 100 ng/ml in the prick test with yellow jacket venom.

With the Presented Data, What Is Your Working Diagnosis?

History is consistent with immediate type allergy to yellow jacket venom which is confirmed by specific sensitization demonstrated by yellow jacket venom-specific IgE and positive titrated skin test. The physical examination demonstrated reddish-brown macules and papules including wheal development after gentle rubbing (positive Darier's sign) which is consistent with cutaneous mastocytosis, namely urticaria pigmentosa. Mast cell degranulation induced by specific IgE-mediated sensitization to yellow-jacket venom and histamine liberating drugs during intubation anesthesia are likely to have caused the described anaphylactic reactions.

Differential Diagnosis

Other dermatologic diseases resembling cutaneous mastocytosis can be distinguished by histology. Potential differentials are lentigines, syndrome of dysplastic nevi, histiocytoma, leiyomyoma, cutaneous lymphoma, langerhans cell histiocytosis, papular (hemorrhagic) exanthema, erythrodermia.

What Is Your Diagnosis and Why?

The scenario of brown-reddish maculopapular skin lesions, positive Darier's sign, elevated serum-tryptase, and increased mast cells in lesional skin biopsy is consistent with cutaneous maculopapular mastocytosis (urticaria pigmentosa). Diagnosis is delayed at the age of 48 years because the patient was nearly asymptomatic with the exception of two anaphylactic reactions, one during intubation anesthesia and the other after a yellow jacket sting. Immediate type allergy to yellow jacket venom is confirmed by the demonstration of specific IgE to yellow jacket venom in the titrated skin test and the CAP-FEIA (RAST).

Discussion

The term mastocytosis (1–3) covers a heterogeneous group of rare diseases that are characterized by increased and in part morphologically striking mast cells in one or different organs (Table 14.1). In most cases, mast cells are proliferated in the skin [cutaneous mastocytosis (CM)], in systemic mastocytosis additionally or solely internal organs, most frequently the bone marrow, lymphatic organs, gastrointestinal tract, liver, or lung are involved. In childhood, the skin is almost exclusively involved and around puberty mastocytosis disappears or improves.

The incidence of mastocytosis is estimated at seven new cases per one million of the general population per year. About two-third are children and one-third are adults. In childhood, manifestation is usually within the first 2 years of life. The onset in adults is usually between 20 and 40 years of age (1–3).

CM is divided into maculopapular CM (MPCM = urticaria pigmentosa, UP), diffuse cutaneous mastocytosis (DCM), teleangiectasia macularis eruptive perstans (TMEP), and solitary mastocytoma of skin (2). Grading of the skin symptoms is recommended (Table 14.2).

The skin lesions in UP, the most frequent CM, are red-brown macules, papules, and plaques, most commonly on the trunk, but all sites can be affected. The number of lesions varies from 10 to 1,000, but the extent of involvement is not predictive for systemic disease. Usually, the face, head, palms, and soles are spared. The Darier's sign (urtication or dermatographism, rarely blistering following rubbing of the pigmented macule; Fig. 14.2) is not always present in CM.

Table 14.1 WHO classification of mastocytosis (16)

Group	Subtype
Cutaneous mastocytosis (CM)	Urticaria pigmentosa (maculopapular cutaneous mastocytosis, MPCM)
	Teleangiectasia macularis eruptive perstans (TMEP)
	Diffuse cutaneous mastocytosis (DCM)
	Mastocytoma
Indolent systemic mastocytosis	"Smoldering" mastocytosis
	Isolated bone marrow mastocytosis
Systemic mastocytosis with associated hematologic disease	Myeloproliferative disease or myeloic leucemia
Aggresive systemic mastocytosis	Lymphadenopathic systemic mastocytosis with eosinophilia
Mast cell leukemia	Aleukemic mast cell leucemia
Mast cell sarcoma	
Extracutaneous mastocytoma	

Table 14.2 Grading of skin symptoms[a] in mastocytosis (16)

Grade	Definition
0 = No symptoms	Prophylaxis[b]
1 = Mild, infrequent	Prophylaxis, therapy if needed
2 = Mild/moderate, frequent	Daily therapy
3 = Severe, frequent	Daily and combination therapy often suboptimal
4 = Severe adverse event	Requires immediate therapy and hospitalization

[a] Pruritus, flushing, blistering, and bullae formation
Ball patients with mastocytosis are advised to avoid precipitating factors and events – for most of them, prophylactic antihistamines (H1 and H2 histamine receptor antagonists) are recommended

In adults an often overlooked, more unimpressive type of CM is TMEP which is characterized by nonpruritic erythematous macules with telangiectasias with a widespread distribution. It may be found in association either with systemic mastocytosis or with various hematological abnormalities, such as myelodysplasia, myeloproliferative disorders, acute myeloid leukemia, and lymphoproliferative disease.

In contrast, single mastocytoma and diffuse mastocytosis are more common in childhood (4). Mastocytomas, accounting for 10–15% of all pediatric CM generally occur before the age of 1 year. Typically, they present as single lesions, although cases of multiple mastocytomas in different locations are possible. Clinically, mastocytomas appear as an indurated red-brown macule, papule, plaque, or tumor up to 4 cm in diameter. Darier's sign is usually positive because solitary mastocytomas generally have the highest concentration of mast cells compared with all types of CM. Diffuse CM is a rare severe variant of CM that occurs predominantly in infants (4). The skin is infiltrated by mast cells in a generalized pattern leaving a thickened, doughy appearance that accentuates skin folds, but blistering and generalized erythroderma are also reported.

Frequent symptoms in CM include not only cutaneous flushing, blistering, pruritus, but also shortness of breath, asthma exacerbations, hypotension, and gastrointestinal symptoms, including acid reflux, peptic ulcer disease, and diarrhea. These symptoms are caused by the release of mast cell mediators, particularly histamine. In systemic mastocytosis, different symptoms are possible depending on the infiltration of the respective organs, e.g., anemia, leukopenia, pathologic fractures, hepatosplenomegalia.

It is not explained why several patients with systemic mastocytosis have no symptoms ("indolent"), whereas others have significant disease ("aggressive").

Recent studies suggest that in more than 50% of adult patients, urticaria pigmentosa is associated with systemic involvement, mainly bone marrow infiltration (1–3). However, progression to malignant disease appears to be rare. Absence of abnormalities in blood-cell counts (low erythrocyte and platelet counts, increased leukocyte counts) indicates that malignant transformation has not occurred.

Lesional biopsies of the skin show an increase of mast cells in the dermis (1–3). They are spindle-shaped, and their granules stain metachromatically with toluidine blue or Giemsa stain. Biopsies should be performed with minimal trauma and perhaps even without epinephrine to improve the number of stainable mast cells.

Serum tryptase levels are an indicator of mast cell load (5). There are two main types of mast cell tryptase, α-tryptase and β-tryptase. α-tryptase is secreted constantly from the cell and levels reflect the total tryptase baseline correlating with the mast cell number, whereas β-Tryptase is stored in mast cell granules and found to be elevated only after mast cell activation, such as anaphylaxis. The level of total serum tryptase (α and β) that is measured by the CAP-FEIA (Phadia, Uppsala, Sweden) correlates closely with the cumulative mast cell burden.

Pediatric CM unlike adult CM is believed to represent a transient dysregulation of local growth factors rather than a genetic mutation. In adults, a mutation of the activating KIT-receptor on mast cells is important (6, 7). Actually, more than ten mutations of c-kit, the gene for KIT, have been described. The most common mutation is D816V, in which asparaginase is replaced by valin at codon 816. Mutation of the KIT-receptor results in activation with subsequent accumulation and increased survival of mast cells. However, a second so far unknown hit is necessary in the pathogenesis because c-kit but not mastocytosis is observed in other hematologic disorders.

In contrast to normal mast cells, mast cells in mastocytosis express adhesion molecules such as CD2 and CD25 that can be detected by immunohistochemistry or flow cytometry.

A curative treatment of mastocytosis is not available (1–3). The c-kit receptor is resistant against the c-kit inhibitor imatinib. The systemic adult mastocytoses with hypereosinophilia and FIP1L1-PDGFRA rearrangement are the only imatinib sensitive forms.

Symptomatic treatment focuses on mast cell mediators. Most important is patient education about the disease, prophylactic treatment, and avoidance of mast cell activators. Potential triggering factors of symptoms are heat, cold, excessive UV exposure, mechanical skin irritation, exercise, stress and fear, hymenoptera venoms, histamine-rich food, alcohol, and several drugs (e.g., ASA and other NSAIDs, morphine and derivatives, amphotericin B, polymyxin B, quinine, muscle relaxants, radio contrast media, dextrans, betablocker). Emergency medications including epinephrine should be prescribed.

Severe anaphylactic reactions particularly to insect venom are more common in patients with mastocytosis (8–11). Therefore, in patients with hymenoptera venom allergy (systemic allergic reaction and demonstration of IgE-mediated sensitization), specific immunotherapy with insect venom is very important and possible in most cases (8, 12). Not rarely, cutaneous mastocytosis or indolent mastocytosis is for the first time diagnosed when serum-tryptase levels are routinely assessed after a severe hymenoptera sting reaction and found to be increased (skin lesions overlooked by the patient and nondermatologist) (13).

Basic drug treatment consists of H1 antihistamines with or without concomitant H2-antihistamines, which prevent the wheal and flares, pruritus, and flushing. H2-antihistamines can suppress gastric hypersecretion and the development of peptic ulcer. Mast cell stabilizers like topical cromolyn and ketotifen are indicated in gastrointestinal symptoms with diarrhea.

Oral and perhaps also bath 8-methoxypsoralen plus ultraviolet-A irradiation (PUVA) but particularly high-dose UVA1 are effective in reducing numbers of mast cells and levels of histamine and leukotriene in the skin. However, lesions recur within several weeks.

Mastocytosis in childhood is usually healing spontaneously. Therefore, awaiting is justified.

Questions

1. Which statement is incorrect?

   (a) Urticaria pigmentosa is the most common subtype of cutaneous mastocytosis in adults.
   (b) Bone marrow biopsy was not indicated in the above-mentioned case as usually the bone marrow is not involved in cutaneous mastocytosis.
   (c) Serum-tryptase level indicates mast cell load.
   (d) Darier's sign occurs after gentle rubbing of the reddish-brown macules/papules.
   (e) Systemic reactions to hymenoptera stings are more severe in patients with mastocytosis.

2. Which statement is correct?

   (a) Histology is able to distinguish mastocytosis from other dermatologic diseases such as papular exanthema or langerhans cell histiocytosis.
   (b) Total IgE is increased in more than 90% of patients with urticaria pigmentosa.
   (c) Elevated tryptase levels indicate severe allergic reactions to hymenoptera venoms.
   (d) Specific immunotherapy with hymenoptera venom is indicated in every patient with mastocytosis irrespective of specific sensitization.
   (e) Specific immunotherapy with hymenoptera venom is too dangerous in patients with elevated serum-tryptase levels.

3. What is incorrect?

   (a) Urticaria pigmentosa is a common subtype of cutaneous mastocytosis in adults.
   (b) TMEP is a common subtype of cutaneous mastocytosis in infants.
   (c) Solitary mastocytoma is a common subtype of cutaneous mastocytosis in children.
   (d) Diffuse mastocytosis is a common subtype of cutaneous mastocytosis in children.
   (e) If cutaneous mastocytosis manifests in early childhood prognosis, spontaneous healing is possible.

4. Which statement is correct?

   (a) Serum histamine levels are a better indicator for disease activity in UP than serum tryptase.
   (b) Diagnosis of UP can be delayed if skin lesions are not prominent and systemic symptoms are missing.
   (c) All patients with UP should receive regular treatment with systemic corticosteroids.
   (d) Imatinib treatment should be started early in childhood.
   (e) c-kit mutations are more common in childhood mastocytosis compared to adults.

5. Which statement is incorrect?

   (a) Palms and soles are predominantly affected in UP.
   (b) Normal blood-cell counts indicate that malignant transformation has not occurred.
   (c) H2-antihistamines are helpful in histamine-mediated gastric hypersecretion.
   (d) Cromolyn may be used if diarrhea is present.
   (e) It is not explained why several patients with systemic mastocytosis are asymptomatic (indolent), whereas others have significant disease.

Answers

1. (b)
2. (a)
3. (b)
4. (b)
5. (a)

Case 2

Marianne Frieri

Keywords Mast cells • Systemic mastocytosis • Histamine • Tryptase

A 25-year-old adult Caucasian female presents with fatigue, headache, cognitive dysfunction, and arthralgias. Past medical history was positive for atopic dermatitis at age 2 with positive skin tests to eggs, peanut, and dust mites. At age 15, she experienced recurrent episodes of flushing and anaphylaxis which were thought to be related to hidden peanut ingestion or insect allergy. Family history was positive for allergic rhinitis in her mother, father with coronary heart disease, and a sister with leukemia. Physical examination revealed a thin female, afebrile with a blood pressure of 125/70 mmHg, pulse of 60/min, respirations of 12/min, and weight of 100 pounds. Head and neck findings revealed no flushing, telangiectasia, but cervical lymphadenopathy. Skin revealed numerous brownish red pruritic macules with a positive Darier's sign (Fig. 14.3). Cardiopulmonary findings revealed clear lung fields and normal heart sounds. Examination of the abdomen revealed hepatosplenomegaly two finger breaths below the right costal margin and a palpable spleen tip. Extremities revealed some tenderness in her left hip and femur. Peripheral pulses and neurologic examination was intact.

Data

CT scan demonstrated hepatosplenomegaly with some retroperitoneal adenopathy. Bone radiography and scan was abnormal with sclerotic lesions in the left hip and femur (Fig. 14.5).

Laboratory evaluation revealed a complete blood count of 3,500 white blood cells ($N = 6.0–17.5$k/mm^3), 50% neutrophils ($N = 38–80\%$), 30% lymphocytes ($N = 15–49\%$) 15% monocytes ($N = 0–8\%$), and 5% eosinophils ($N = 0–8\%$). Hemoglobin was 8.0 g/dl ($N = 13.2–17.1$ g/dl) with a hematocrit of 25% ($N = 38.5–50.0\%$),

M. Frieri
Department of Medicine, Nassau University Medical Center, State University of New York, Stony Brook, New York, NY, USA
e-mail: mfrieri@numc.edu;mfrieri@nyit.edu

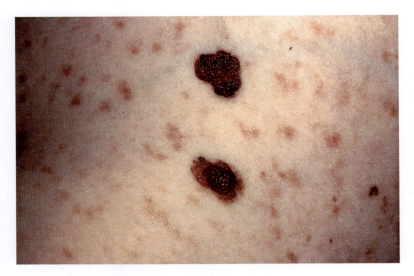

Fig. 14.3 Cutaneous lesions in systemic mastocytosis

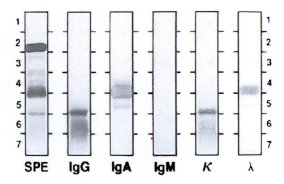

Fig. 14.4 Immunofixation pattern revealing an IgGκ and IgAλ biclonal gammopathy pattern [modified from Frieri et al. (14)]

180,000 platelets (N = 140–400k/mcL), and sedimentation rate of 50 mm/dl (N = 0–20 mm/dl). Liver function revealed an elevated alkaline phosphatase of 150 U/l (N = 40–115 U/L), serum transaminases, calcium, and urinalysis were normal. Plasma, urinary histamine, and tryptase were elevated at 105 ng/ml (N = ≤11.5 ng/ml). Quantitative immunoglobulin levels revealed elevated IgG of 2,000 mg/dl (N = 639–1,349 mg/dl), normal IgA and IgM. Serum protein electrophoresis was negative for a monoclonal gammapathy. However, in an earlier study, we had demonstrated a biclonal gammapathy (14) (Fig. 14.4). A skin and lymph node biopsy showed paratrabecular fibrosis, aggregates of fusiform mast cells mixed with lymphocytes and eosinophils. On immunostaining, tryptase was positive in mast cell aggregates.

With the Presented Data, What Is Your Working Diagnosis?

The history is consistent with flushing and recurrent anaphylactic episodes.

The physical examination revealed cutaneous brownish red pruritic macules and a positive Darier's sign consistent with cutaneous mastocytosis. However, due to the cervical lymphadenopathy, hepatosplenomegaly, and abnormal sclerotic lesions in the left hip and femur, this condition is more than urticaria pigmentosa. Further laboratory data revealed anemia, elevated sedimentation rate, liver function tests, plasma, urinary histamine, tryptase, and IgM level.

Differential Diagnosis

Other dermatologic conditions but without skin lesions are shown in Table 14.3 (15).

What Is Your Diagnosis and Why?

The cutaneous, systemic findings and abnormal hematologic, liver function and elevated histamine, tryptase levels and increased skin mast cells are consistent with systemic mastocytosis.

The patient was treated with fexofenadine, a nonsedating antihistamines, combined with, ranitidine, an H2 antagonist; epinephrine as needed for anaphylaxis; and oral cromolyn sodium or gastrocrom, which has been reported to improve gastrointestinal symptoms and bone pain (16).

Clinical course. The patent was referred to a Hematologist–Oncologist for follow up and possible cytoreductive therapy with cladribine. Other possibilities might include Imatinib if D816Vck mutation is negative, or the new tyrosine kinase inhibitor, PKC412.10 (14).

Discussion

Systemic mastocytosis is a hematologic condition due to pathological accumulations and activation of mast cells in skin, bone marrow, liver spleen, and lymph nodes (17). Most patients with mastocytosis exhibit the D816 V point mutation in

Table 14.3 Common differential diagnoses systemic mastocytosis without skin lesions (15)

Mast cell disorders	Aggressive systemic mastocytosis
	Mast cell leukemia
	Systemic mastocytosis with clonal hematologic non mast cell lineage disease
	Isolated bone marrow mastocytosis
Endocrine disorders	Adrenal tumor; Vasointestinal peptide tumor
	Gastrinoma
	Carcinoid syndrome
	Diabetes mellitus
	Medullary thyroid carcinoma
	Estrogen–testosterone deficiency
Gastrointestinal disorders	Peptic ulcer; Helicobactor pylori infection
	Ulcerative colitis
	Hepatitis
	Cholecystolithiasis
	Parasitic disease
	Gluten-sensitive enteropathy
Cardiovascular disorders	Allergic disease
	Idiopathic anaphylaxis
	Cardiac disease, aortic stenosis
	Essential hypertension
	Vasculitis
Neoplastic or oncologic disorders	Malignant lymphoma
	Myeloma
	Histiocytosis
	Bone or tumor/metastases
	Hypereosinophilic syndrome

Modified from Valent et al. (15)

the tyrosine kinase domain of the transmembrane receptor protein kit, leading to its constitutive activation in bone marrow or lesional skin tissue (17). Detection of a codon 816 c-kit mutation is included as a minor diagnostic criterion in the World Health Organization's diagnostic criteria for systemic mastocytosis and determining mutational status of the c-kit gene also has pharmacogenomic implications in patients considered for investigational mast cell cytoreductive therapies (17). The disease has been found to be associated with abnormal pre-beta lipoproteins, oligo-clonal immunoglobulins, and malignancy (18, 19). Mastocytosis could result from an innate defect in a hematopoietic stem cell triggered by growth factors that could lead to abnormal mast cell proliferation (19). Symptoms that occur in mastocytosis are related to spontaneous or triggered release of mast cell mediators or clonal expansion of the hematopoietic clone which gives rise to mast cells (20). Systemic mastocytosis can occur with or without skin lesions which may be absent in 20% of patients and in addition to histamine release, heparin can lead to massive gastrointestinal bleeding in children and can influence lymphocyte function (21). In contrast to adults, most children with urticaria pigmentosa with onset of lesions before age 2 have limited cutaneous disease and can present with severe bullous lesions (22). Almost all adult patients with urticaria pigmentosa and some children

Fig. 14.5 Abnormal sclerotic hip lesion in a patient with systemic mastocytosis [modified from Frieri et al. (18)]

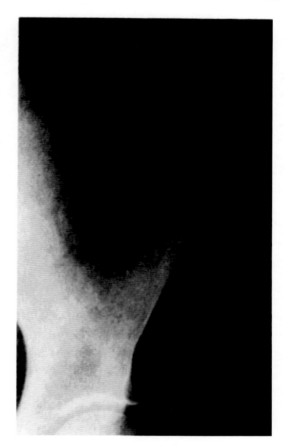

particularly with the late onset of skin lesions have pathological mast cell collections in bone marrow and internal organs (17). Lesions of urticaria pigmentosa may be absent and especially in those with advances and aggressive categories of disease (17). In these patients, when the index of suspicion for systemic disease is high, bone marrow biopsy and aspirate are recommended to check for presence of the World Health Organization diagnostic criteria for systemic mastocytosis (17).

Mastocytosis should be suspected when a child or adult presents with a pruritic cutaneous rash diagnosed as urticaria pigmentosa, exhibits an unexplained abnormality in a blood count, hepatosplenomegaly, lymphadenopathy, flushing, anaphylaxis, diffuse bone remodeling, or pathologic fractures incidentally or after diagnostic workup of bone pain (17). The skeleton is one of the most frequently involved extracutaneous organs and patterns of skeletal scintigraphy have been correlated with plasma and urinary histamine levels, which reflects the general severity of the disease process compared to radiographic or laboratory studies of bone metabolism (23) (Fig. 14.6).

Fig. 14.6 Anterior whole-body multifocal areas of increased tracer accumulation [modified from Rosenbaum et al. (23)]

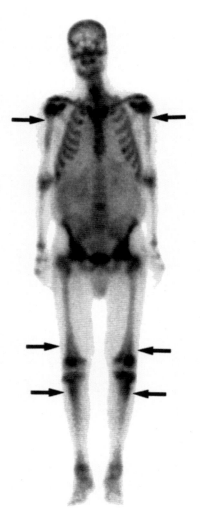

Approximately 20% of patients with systemic mastocytosis are diagnosed after a bone marrow biopsy which can reveal diagnostic mast cell collections associated with myelodysplastic syndromes, but myeloma, lymphoma, acute leukemias, and other lymphoproliferative disorders can be diagnosed (17) (Fig. 14.7).

Mast cell-mediated events have also been suggested to play a role in innate and acquired immunity including wound healing and tumor angiogenesis. The systemic infiltration by mast cells often results in protein clinical manifestations that can obscure the underlying disease. A consensus classification adopted by the World Health Organization in 2001 is widely used as a reasonable approach to the classification and therefore diagnosis of the disease (Table 14.4) (15). If at least one

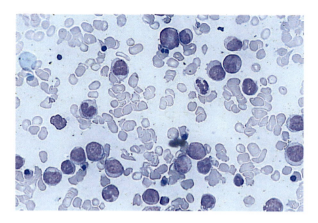

Fig. 14.7 Peripheral smear illustrating acute myelomonocytic leukemia in a patient with systemic mastocytosis [modified from Frieri et al. (14)]

major and one minor criterion or three minor criteria are fulfilled, the diagnosis of systemic mastocytosis can be established (15). These criteria include one major and four minor criteria. Demonstration of the major and one minor or three minor criteria is needed before the diagnosis of systemic mastocytosis is confirmed. Bone marrow is the preferred tissue source to evaluate the presence of the World Health Organization criteria. The major criteria (i.e., multifocal mast cell collections of 15 or more cells) is present in more than half of patients with systemic mastocytosis (17). D816V c-kit mutation is detectable in around 70% of patients with systemic mastocytosis in bone marrow mononuclear cells although enrichment of lesional mast cells by cell sorting or microdissection significantly increased detectability. According to the World Health Organization guidelines, demonstration of only one of four minor criteria is required for the diagnosis of systemic mast cell disease in the presence of the major criteria. In a patient with multifocal mast cell clusters consisting of 15 or more cells in the bone marrow biopsy (major criteria), morphological examination of the biopsy or aspirate smear for atypical spindle-shaped mast cells or a serum tryptase level greater than 20 ng/ml usually satisfies the World Health Organization diagnostic criteria (17).

Most patients with systemic mastocytosis are initially evaluated by dermatologists with cutaneous symptoms of flushing and pruritis associated with typical skin findings (15).

The mastocytosis WHO consensus classification is shown in Table 14.1. This classification is clinically useful in categorizing variants of the disease and divides systemic mast cell diseases into five categories of increasing clinical aggressiveness in addition to extracutaneous mastocytoma. Cutaneous mastocytosis or urticaria pigmentosa can be maculopapular, diffuse, or present as a mastocytoma. The first systemic category is indolent which occurs in most patients. Table 14.3 presents a

Table 14.4 Criteria for the diagnosis of systemic mastocytosis (15)

Major
Dense multifocal infiltrates of mast cells in bone marrow or other organs
Minor
Mast cells in bone marrow or other extracutaneous organs with an abnormal spindle
    morphology
Codon 816 c-kit mutation D816V in extracutaneous Organs and other activating mutations at
    codon 816
Mast cells in the bone marrow express CD2, CD25, or both
Serum tryptase >20 ng/ml, does not count in patients who have an associated hematopoietic
    clonal non- mast cell lineage disease

Modified from Valent et al. (15)

Table 14.5 Diagnostic evaluation of suspected mastocytosis-A [practical guide (15)]

Initial sign-symptom	Recommended diagnostic procedures
Pediatric urticaria pigmentosa like skin lesions tryptase	Skin biopsy (analysis of c-kit D816V) and serum
Adult Urticaria Pigmentosa – like skin lesions tryptase[a]	Bone marrow examinations, skin biopsy, and serum
	For systemic mastocytosis complete staging of the gastrointestinal tract, bone radiographs, abdominal ultrasound, complete blood count, chemistry, coagulation parameters, c-kit mutation status
Mediator-related symptoms without skin lesions	Serum tryptase[a]
	Bone marrow examination, if systemic mastocytosis
	Staging of systemic mastocytosis
	Serum tryptase[a]
	Repeat serum tryptase a few weeks later
Unexplained severe allergic or anaphylactoid reaction	Bone marrow examination, if systemic mastocytosis
	Systemic mastocytosis staging

Modified from Valent et al. (15)
[a]>20 ng/ml in most systemic cases

summary of disorders to be considered in the differential diagnosis in patients with aggressive mast cell disorders with no skin lesions. In these conditions, symptoms are often nonspecific and confused with other disorders such as endocrine, gastrointestinal, cardiac, pulmonary, allergic, infectious, immunologic, rheumatologic, and oncologic disorders.

The following practical guidelines are proposed in the evaluation of an adult patient without skin lesions but with an increased serum tryptase level (Table 14.4) (15). Patients experiencing an unexplained hypotensive (anaphylactoid) event, the tryptase measurement should be repeated a few weeks after the episode. If the serum tryptase level is still increased, a bone marrow examination should be performed (Table 14.5) (15). In all other patients without a severe hypotensive episode at the time of serum sampling, the bone marrow should always be examined to diagnose or exclude systemic mastocytosis or another myeloid tryptase positive neoplasm (15). In early childhood, the interpretation of the serum tryptase determination might be more difficult than in adults because of a different hypothetic ratio of mast cell granule volume/whole body volume and of total volume of skin mast cells/total body

Table 14.6 Cytoreductive treatment in systemic mastocytosis (15)

Variants of disease	Treatment options
Typical indolent systemic mastocytosis	No cytoreductive treatment required (exception: consider IFN-α2b for severe osteoporosis, if no histology documenting aggressive systemic mastocytosis is available)
Smoldering systemic mastocytosis	Mostly watch and wait. In select cases (e.g., progressive organomegaly) IFN-α2b ± glucocorticoids can be considered
Systemic mastocytosis-associated hematologic clonal non-MC lineage disease	Treat as if no systemic mastocytosis is present and treat systemic mastocytosis as if no associated hematologic clonal non-MC lineage disease associated hematologic clonal non-MC lineage disease was found. Consider splenectomy if hypersplenism prohibit therapy
Aggressive systemic mastocytosis	IFN-a2b ± glucocorticoids or cladribine with slow progressive therapy
	Consider splenectomy if hypersplenism prohibit therapy
Aggressive systemic mastocytosis: rapid progression; patients who do not respond to IFN-α2	Polychemotherapy (± IFN- α2b) or cladribine; bone marrow transplantation for select cases
	Consider splenectomy if hypersplenism prohibit therapy
Aggressive systemic mastocytosis: without c-kit D816V or with the FIPL1-PDGFRA fusion gene (+eosinophilia)	Consider STI571 (Imatinib) therapy as alternative treatment
Mast cell leukemia	Polychemotherapy or cladribine (± IFN-α2b)
	Consider bone marrow transplantation splenectomy if hypersplenism prohibit therapy. Consider hydroxyurea as palliation

Modified from Valent et al. (15)

volume. Thus, it is not known whether a serum tryptase level somewhat exceeding 20 ng/ml is an indicator for systemic mastocytosis in this patient population. Therefore, consideration should be given to monitoring the serum tryptase level over time and to not performing a bone marrow puncture unless other signs of a systemic hematologic disease or aggressive subtype of mastocytosis (organomegaly, osteolyses, severe cytopenias, or others) are found. (Table 14.5) (15).

Especially in patients with aggressive mast cell disorders, skin lesions are absent.

Therefore, it is of pivotal importance to know the subtype of systemic mastocytosis in these patients as soon as possible. In aggressive systemic mastocytosis, the serum tryptase level is usually higher than in patients with isolated bone marrow mastocytosis (often <20 ng/ml), a benign mast cell disease in which skin lesions are also absent.

In patients with an aggressive form of systemic mastocytosis, cytoreductive therapy might be recommended and used together with antimediator-type therapy (Table 14.6) (15). IFN-α, considered to affect the growth of early myeloid progenitor cells and to produce a major clinical response in about 15–20% of all patients with aggressive systemic mastocytosis has been mostly evaluated with or without a glucocorticoid (15). Cladribine can reduce the mast cell burden in patients with aggressive systemic mastocytosis, however, not all patients will respond. The use of targeted drugs in the treatment of patients with aggressive subtypes of systemic mastocytosis has been proposed such as Imatinib but it is of import to define the exact molecular defects that underly mastocytosis and the potential targets expressed in neoplastic cells (15). Several targets and altered genes (e.g., wild-type c-kit, c-kit Phe522Cys, or the FIPL1-PDGFRA fusion gene) are associated with a response to Imatinib, but other gene defects, such as the c-kit mutation Asp816Val = D816V, are associated with resistance to Imatinib (15). The major problem is that most patients with systemic mastocytosis exhibit c-kit D816V, so that Imatinib is not expected to be used widely to treat systemic mastocytosis. The ideal therapy or combination therapy to be used in patients with aggressive mastocytosis and mast cell leukemia has not yet been reported (15).

In summary, mastocytosis is a heterogeneous group of disorders of myelomastocytic progenitor cells and a great amount of information has been learned about neoplastic mast cells and disease variants (15). Using defined criteria, it is now possible to discriminate between mast disorders and other systemic diseases with reasonable certainty, even if mastocytosis shows an atypical presentation. In addition, much is now understood about disease-specific gene defects occurring in patients with mastocytosis and related disorders (15). Several altered genes and molecules have now been identified as potential therapeutic targets and these developments lead to the expectation of improved therapy in the near future (15).

Questions

1. The term used for cutaneous mastocytosis is:

   (a) Acute urticaria
   (b) Cutaneous papulosis
   (c) Urticaria pigmentosa

2. The major criteria for systemic mastocytosis includes multifocal mast cell collections of cells present in more than half of patients as:

   (a) 5 or more
   (b) 10 or more
   (c) 15 or more

3. In unexplained severe allergic or anaphylactoid reactions the following is suggested:

   (a) Serum tryptase
   (b) Repeat serum tryptase a few weeks later
   (c) Bone marrow examination, if systemic mastocytosis

(d) Systemic mastocytosis staging

(e) All the above

4. Name a current therapeutic agent to treat rapidly progressive aggressive systemic mastocytosis:

(a) Cyclophosphamide

(b) Intravenous gamma globulin

(c) Cladribine

(d) Anti-TNF

5. Mast cell collections associated with myelodysplastic syndromes include:

(a) Idiopathic thrombocytopenic purpura

(b) Acute leukemias

(c) myeloma

(d) (b) and (c)

Answers

1. (a)
2. (c)
3. (e)
4. (c)
5. (d)

References

1. Escribano L, Orfao A, Diaz-Agustin B, et al. Indolent systemic mast cell disease in adults: immunophenotypic characterization of bone marrow mast cells and its diagnostic implications. Blood 1998; 91:2731–2736.
2. Horny HP, Sotlar K, Valent P. Mastocytosis: state of the art. Pathobiology 2007; 74(2):121–132.
3. Valent P, Akin C, Escribano L, et al. Standards and standardization in mastocytosis: consensus statements on diagnostics, treatment recommendations and response criteria. Eur J Clin Invest 2007; 37(6):435–453.
4. Briley LD, Phillips CM. Cutaneous mastocytosis: A review focusing on the pediatric population. Clin Pediatr 2008; 47:757.
5. Schwartz LB, Metcalfe DD, Miller JS, Earl H, Sullivan T. Tryptase levels as an indicator of mast-cell activation in systemic anaphylaxis and mastocytosis. N Engl J Med 1987; 316(26):1622–1626.
6. Akin C, Kirshenbaum AS, Semere T, Worobec AS, Scott LM, Metcalfe DD. Analysis of the surface expression of c-kit and occurrence of the c-kit Asp816Val activating mutation in T cells, B cells, and myelomonocytic cells in patients with mastocytosis. Exp Hematol 2000; 28:140–147.
7. Buttner C, Henz BM, Welker P, Sepp NT, Grabbe J. Identification of activating c-kit mutations in adults-, but not in childhood-onset indolent mastocytosis: a possible explanation for divergent clinical behavior. J Invest Dermatol 1998; 111:1227–1231.

8. Rueff F, Placzek M, Przybilla B. Mastocytosis and hymenoptera venom allergy. Curr Opin Allergy Clin Immunol 2006; 6(4):284–288.
9. Brockow K, Jofer C, Behrendt H, Ring J. Anaphylaxis in patients with mastocytosis: a study on history, clinical features and risk factors in 120 patients. Allergy 2008; 63(2):226–232.
10. Dubois AE. Mastocytosis and hymenoptera allergy. Curr Opin Allergy Clin Immunol 2004; 4(4):291–295.
11. Haeberli G, Bronnimann M, Hunziker T, Muller U. Elevated basal serum tryptase and hymenoptera venom allergy: relation to severity of sting reactions and to safety and efficacy of venom immunotherapy. Clin Exp Allergy 2003; 33(9):1216–1220.
12. Rueff F, Wenderoth A, Przybilla B. Patients still reacting to a sting challenge while receiving conventional Hymenoptera venom immunotherapy are protected by increased venom doses. J Allergy Clin Immunol 2001; 108(6):1027–1032.
13. Florian S, Krauth MT, Simonitsch-Klupp I, et al. Indolent systemic mastocytosis with elevated serum tryptase, absence of skin lesions, and recurrent severe anaphylactoid episodes. Int Arch Allergy Immunol 2005; 136(3):273–280.
14. Frieri M, Linn N, Schweitzer M, Angadi C, et al. Lymphadenopathic mastocytosis with eosinophilia and biclonal gammopathy. J Allergy Clin Immunol 1990; 86:126–132.
15. Valent P, Sperr WR Schwartz LB, Horny, Hans-Peter. Diagnosis and classification of mast cell proliferative disorders: Delineation from immunologic diseases and non-mast cell hematopoietic neoplasms. J Allergy Clin Immunol 2004; 114:3–11.
16. Frieri M, Steinberg SC, Metcalfe DD. A controlled trial of the effects of oral disodium cromoglycate or the combination of chloropheniramine and cimetidine in the treatment of systemic mastocytosis. Am J Med 1985; 78:9–14.
17. Akin C. Review. Molecular diagnosis of mast cell disorders. A paper from the 2005 William Beaumont Hospital Symposium on Molecular Pathology. J Mol Diagn 2006; 8:412–419.
18. Frieri M, Papadopoulos NM, Kaliner MA, Metcalfe DD. An abnormal pre-beta lipoprotein in patients with systemic mastocytosis. Ann Intern Med 1982; 97:220–221.
19. Meggs WJ, Frieri M, Costello R, Metcalfe DD, Papadopoulos NM. Oligoclonal immunoglobulins in mastocytosis. Ann Intern Med 1985; 103:894.
20. Escribibano L. Akin C, Castelis M, Orfao A, Metcalfe DD. Mastocytosis: Current concepts in diagnosis and treatment. Ann Hematol 2002; 81:677–690.
21. Frieri M, Metcalfe DD. Analysis of the effect of mast cell granules on lymphocyte blastogenesis: Identification of heparin as a granule associated suppressor factor. J Immunol 1983; 131:1942–1948.
22. Frieri M, Claus M, Martinez S, Annunziato D, Kosuri S, Lin J. Fever, hemorrhagic bullae and gastritis in pediatric mastocytosis. Ann Allergy 1989; 63:179–183.
23. Rosenbaum RC, Frieri M, Metcalfe DD. Patterns of skeletal scintigraphy and their relationship to histamine levels in systemic mastocytosis. J Nucl Med 1984; 25:859–864.

Chapter 15
Allergic Bronchopulmonary Aspergillosis

Satoshi Yoshida

Abstract Allergic bronchopulmonary aspergillosis (ABPA) is a hypersensitivity response to *Aspergillus* antigens in the lung, which is an uncommon but serious respiratory condition characterized by chronic airway inflammation and airway damage resulting from persistent colonization by and sensitization to the fungus *Aspergillus fumigatus* (*A. fumigatus*). The first case of ABPA in the United States was identified more than 30 years ago, whereas the initial literature reported in the United Kingdom was in 1952. The prevalence of ABPA is as high as 1–2% of patients with persistent asthma if screening is carried out, though even higher rates have been reported. Especially in corticosteroid-dependent asthma patients, it has been reported that ABPA might be complicated as high as 7–14%. In cystic fibrosis, the prevalence of ABPA ranges from 2 to 15%. ABPA is sometimes recognized in patients with allergic fungal sinusitis, though such an association is unusual. Cases related to the presentation and management of ABPA are discussed later.

Keywords Allergic bronchopulmonary aspergillosis (ABPA)•Hyper-immunoglobulin E (IgE) • Syndrome pulmonary eosinophilia • Tenacious mucus plugging

Case 1

A 42-year-old woman presented to the outpatient clinic for evaluation with cough, difficulty breathing, and wheezing. Initially with the onset of symptoms, her family physician noted bibasilar rales and bilateral lower lobe infiltrates on chest radiograph and treated the patient with azithromycin 500 mg orally once daily for three days,

S. Yoshida (✉)
Department of Continuing Education, Harvard Medical School, Boston, MA, USA
e-mail: syoshida-fjt@umin.ac.jp

M. Mahmoudi (ed.), *Challenging Cases in Allergy and Immunology*,
DOI: 10.1007/978-1-60327-443-2_15,
© Humana Press, a part of Springer Science+Business Media, LLC 2009

but it was not effective. The patient was sent to the emergency department and was subsequently hospitalized and treated with intravenous prednisolone, 40 mg three times daily. These episodes were more frequent, with approximately five to six emergency department visits every year. The patient also had a pruritic erythematous maculopapular rash on her chest and extremities was treated with triamcinolone cream without relief.

The patient was diagnosed as having allergic rhinitis, asthma, and eczema since childhood at the age of 8 years. Her symptoms were seasonally exacerbated from November to April, which prevented her from attending school. She also had allergy to latex and multiple foods. A radioallergosorbent test performed 3 years previously was positive for dust mite hypersensitivity. Her medical history was significant for mitral valve prolapse, migraine, urticaria,and angioedema. She had smoked half a pack per day of cigarettes for approximately 20 years, and drinks alcohol socially. Medications included prednisolone, diphenhydramine, and hydroxyzine. Environmental control measures for dust mite were instituted. Her asthma medications included budesonide turbuhaler, two puffs twice a day; albuterol as needed. The patient described chest tightness and shortness of breath. No urinary complaints, nausea, vomiting, or diarrhea were described. The patient was alert and oriented. Her vital signs on admission were as follows: temperature, 99.5°F; blood pressure, 132/68 mmHg; pulse 66/min; and respiratory rate, 18/min. Weight and height were 150 lb and 64 in., respectively. Eye examination revealed no iritis. Tympanic membranes and nasal mucosa were normal. There was no lymphadenopathy, and chest examination revealed diffuse inspiratory and expiratory wheezing in all lung fields. Also bilateral basilar rales to midscapulae were noted on chest auscultation. S1 and S2 were audible in all four areas with no murmur. The abdomen was tender in the left hypochondrium and left flank without hepatosplenomegaly. Her skin had a diffuse maculopapular rash that was more pronounced on the chest and flexor surfaces of extremities. The overlying skin was normal, without scaling, cyanosis, or edema of the extremities. Joints were nontender without erythema or effusion.

Data

The complete blood cell count revealed the following: hemoglobin, 12.3 g/dL; hematocrit, 38%; total white blood cells count, 9,800/mm^3 with 78% neutrophils, 14.2% lymphocytes, and 0.5% eosinophils; platelets, 388,000/mm^3 with normal serum chemical analysis results; and erythrocyte sedimentation rate, 10 mm. Fluorescent antinuclear antibody and anti-DNA test results were negative. The total IgE level was 1,624 IU/mL; specific IgE for dust mite was class IV, but specific IgE for *Aspergillus fumigatus* (*A. fumigatus*) was class 0.

Results of spirometry after therapy and hospitalization include forced vital capacity (FVC), forced expiratory volume in 1 s (FEV1), FEV1/FVC ratio, and forced expiratory now between 25% and 75% within normal limits. The maximum voluntary ventilation was reduced. The slow vital capacity was also reduced. Following administration of bronchodilators, there was no significant response. The flow volume loops appeared normal; however, the effect was less than standard.

Imaging Studies

Chest radiograph showed diffuse alveolar and interstitial infiltrates most prominent in all lobes as shown in Fig. 15.1.

1. With the presented data, what is your diagnosis ?

   (a) Allergic asthma
   (b) Anergic bronchopulmonary aspergillosis (ABPA)
   (c) Allergic bronchopulmonary fusariosis (ABPF)
   (d) Invasive aspergillosis

Answer: 1. (b)

Considering the clinical course and, the work up

2. What is your diagnosis and why?

The final diagnosis of our patient's condition includes acute bronchospasm and allergic rhinitis. This patient is in accord with the criteria of ABPA as mentioned in Tables 15.1 (1) and 15.2 (2).

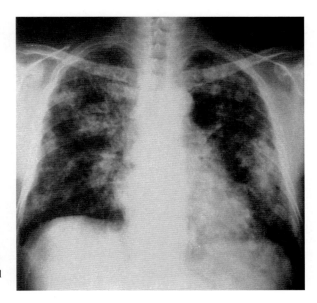

Fig. 15.1 Chest radiography: Diffuse alveolar and interstitial infiltrates most prominent in all lobes

Discussion

Classic criteria for the diagnosis of ABPA has been published by Rosenberg and colleagues in 1977 as mentioned in Table 15.1. Japanese allergist–immunologist or pulmonologist still usually use this criteria for the diagnosis of ABPA. Such cases will have other features as well, including chest roentgenographic infiltrates, peripheral blood eosinophilia in the absence of oral corticosteroids, precipitating antibodies to *A. fumigatus*, and production of mucus plugs containing *A. fumigatus*. In such cases, the allergist–immunologist or pulmonologist should have little difficulty with the diagnosis. Failure of the chest roentgenographic or chest CT infiltrates to clear over a 2-month period of prednisone therapy suggests noncompliance, another ABPA exacerbation, or possibly other diagnoses, such as cystic fibrosis. Of note, the prevalence of ABPA is higher in patients with cystic fibrosis than in patients with persistent asthma. Another criteria proposed for the diagnosis of ABPA in patients with asthma are presented in Table 15.2. Some patients who seem

Table 15.1 Criteria for the diagnosis of allergic bronchopulmonary aspergillosis

Primary
Episodic bronchial obstruction (asthma)
Periferal blood eosinophilia
Immediate skin reactivity to *Aspergillus* antigen
Precipitate skin reactivity to *Aspergillus* antigen
Elevated serum immunoglobulin E concentrations
History of pulmonary infiltrates (transient or fixed)
Central bronchiectasis
Secondary
Aspergillus fumigatus in sputum (by microscopic examination)
History of expectoration of brown plugs or flecks
Arthus reactivity (late skin reactivity) to *Aspergillus* antigens

Table 15.2 Criteria for the diagnosis of ABPA in patients with cystic fibrosis

From the ABPA Consensus Conference of the Cystic Fibrosis Foundation
Classic case criteria
Clinical deterioration (increased cough, wheezing, exercise intolerance, increased sputum, decrease in pulmonary function)
Immediate cutaneous reactivity to *Aspergillus* or presence of serum IgE-*A. fumigatus*
Total serum IgE concentration >1,000 kU/L
Precipitating antibodies to *A. fumigatus* or serum IgG-*A. fumigatus*
Abnormal chest roentgenogram (infiltrates, mucus plugging,or a change from earlier films)
Suggestions for screening on annual phlebotomy for ABPA
Maintain clinical suspicion for ABPA
Annual total serum IgE determination: If it is >500 kU/L, test for immediate cutaneous reactivity to *Aspergillus* or by an in vitro test for serum IgE-*A. fumigatus*.
If the total serum IgE is <500 kU/L, repeat if clinical suspicion is high

to have had no history of asthma or cystic fibrosis and then present with chest roentgenographic infiltrates and lobar collapse are found to have ABPA. Some patients with ABPA have had histories of intermittent mild asthma (exercise-induced bronchospasm) before their ABPA was diagnosed. Conversely, the asthma might have been persistent moderate or severe (corticosteroid-dependent).

ABPF is a mycosis caused by *Fusarium vasinfectum* in patients with asthma. The patient presents with a history and radiographic picture suggestive of ABPA but with negative ABPA serologic test results. The presence of a positive skin test result and precipitins against *F. vasinfectum*, high serum lgG and lgE antibody levels, and a decrease in total serum lgE levels with treatment suggest a diagnosis of ABPF. Acute bronchopulmonary mycosis caused by organisms other than *Aspergillus* is an important consideration in patients with findings suggestive of ABPA but negative serologic test results. ABPF is listed as a differential diagnosis to ABPA. Therefore, diagnostic tests were not performed in this patient.

Aspergillus are among the most common environmental molds, frequently present in decaying vegetation (compost heaps), on insulating materials, in air conditioning or heating vents, in operating pavilions and patient rooms, on hospital implements, and in airborne dust. Invasive infections are usually acquired by inhalation of spores or, occasionally, by direct invasion through damaged skin. Major risk factors include neutropenia, long-term high-dose corticosteroid therapy, organ transplantation (especially bone marrow transplantation), hereditary disorders of neutrophil function, such as chronic granulomatous disease, and, occasionally, acquired immunodeficiency distress syndrome (AIDS). *Aspergillus* tends to infect open spaces, such as pulmonary cavities from previous lung disease (e.g., bronchiectasis, tumor, tubercullosis), the sinuses, or ear canals (otomycosis). Such infections tend to be locally invasive and destructive, although systemic spread sometimes occurs, particularly in immunocompromised patients. *A. fumigatus* is the most common cause of invasive pulmonary disease; *A. flavus* most often causes invasive extrapulmonary disease. Focal infections sometimes form a fungus ball (aspergilloma), a characteristic growth of tangled masses of hyphae, with fibrin exudate and few inflammatory cells, typically encapsulated by fibrous tissue. A chronic form of invasive aspergillosis occasionally occurs, notably in patients with the hereditary phagocytic cell defect, chronic granulomatous disease. *Aspergillus* species can also cause endophthalmitis after trauma or surgery to the eye (or by hematogenous seeding) and infections of intravascular and intracardiac prostheses. Primary superficial aspergillosis is uncommon but may occur in burns; beneath occlusive dressings; after corneal trauma (keratitis); or in the sinuses, mouth, nose, or ear canal. Chronic pulmonary aspergillosis causes cough, often with hemoptysis and shortness of breath. Invasive pulmonary aspergillosis usually causes rapidly progressive, ultimately fatal respiratory failure if untreated. Extrapulmonary invasive aspergillosis begins with skin lesions, sinusitis, or pneumonia; may involve the liver, kidneys, brain, and other tissues; and is often rapidly fatal. Aspergillosis in the sinuses can form an aspergilloma, an allergic fungal sinusitis, or a chronic, slowly invasive granulomatous inflammation with fever, rhinitis, and headache. Necrosing cutaneous lesions may overlie the nose or sinuses, palatal or gingival ulcerations may be present, signs of cavernous sinus thrombosis may develop, and pulmonary or disseminated lesions may occur. Because *Aspergillus sp.* are common in the environment, positive sputum cultures may be due to environmental contamination or to noninvasive colonization in patients with chronic lung disease; positive cultures are significant mainly when obtained from patients with increased susceptibility due to immunosuppression or with high suspicion due to typical imaging findings. Conversely, sputum cultures from patients with aspergillomas or invasive pulmonary aspergillosis are often negative; cavities are often walled off from airways, and invasive disease progresses mainly by vascular invasion and tissue infarction.

Case 2

A 6-year-old girl was diagnosed with cystic fibrosis at the age of 8 months on the basis of failure to thrive, steatorrhea, and a positive sweat chloride determination of 97 mEq/L. She has been seen in our outpatient clinic four or five times a year. During the last 4 years, she remained well with mild pulmonary symptoms and no evidence of asthma. She had experienced a few episodes of infectious bronchitis without wheezing, which improved with oral antibiotic therapy. There was no history of production of brown sputum plugs, and she had never been treated with bronchodilators or oral or inhaled corticosteroids. At age 1, *Staphylococcus aureus* was cultured from her sputum. At age 2, *Pseudomonas aeruginosa* grew on her sputum culture without pulmonary involvement, and a 3-week course of intravenous antibiotic was given. Over the next three years, *S. aureus*, and sometimes *P. auerginosa*, were cultured from her sputum. *A. fumigatus* only grew twice at age 2 and 3. Her routine chest roentgenogram showed minor changes, such as increased lung markings and mild hyperinflation, without acute changes. On routine clinical examination, lung fields were clear to asuculatation.

Data

Routine laboratory evaluation always showed a peripheral eosinophil count less than 300 cells/mm³ (normal value: 70–440). Since June 2003, as part of the ABPA screening study, the patient was evaluated every 4 months with total serum IgE and IgE against *A. fumigatus* (IgE-Af) by CAP fluoro enzyme immuno assay (Pharmacia, Uppsala, Sweden); precipitins against *A. fumigatus* by means of the Ouchterlony technique; IgG, IgA, and IgM antibodies against *A. fumigatus* (IgG-Af, IgA-Af, IgM-Af) assessed by ELISA; peripheral eosinophil count; and immediate skin testing with *A. fumigatus*. In February 2005, when the patient was free of symptoms, laboratory data showed a blood eosinophil count of 320 cells/mm³, a total serum IgE of 52 kU/L (normal value <84 kU/L), and a negative IgE-Af (<0.35 kU/L). In August 2006, a left upper lobe infiltrate was seen on a routine chest roentgenogram. She had no symptoms, and clinical examination was normal. Sputum culture grew *S. aureus* and *Candida albicans*. Her total serum IgE increased to 170 kU/k, and she had positive assay results for IgE-Af (4.3 kU/L). All specific immunoglobulin classes to Af were increased. Three weeks later she had mild pulmonary wheezing on physical examination. Chest roentgenogram showed a persistence of pulmonary infiltrate. Precipitins to *A. fumigatus* and skin prick test responses to Af were positive. Total serum IgE was 162 kU/L, and a white blood cell count revealed 1,0800 cells/mm³ with 720 eosinophils/mm³. The patient was treated with oral trimethoprim/sulfamethoxazole for 3 weeks, inhaled bronchodilators, and vigorous chest physical therapy. In October 2007, the left upper lobe infiltrate improved, but on physical examoination revealed disseminated wheezing. Her eosmophil count increased to 1,240 cells/mm³, total serum IgE was 136 kU/L. IgE-Af was 7.6 kU/L, and all specific lmmunoglobulin classes to *A. fumigatus* remained elevated. Sputum samples contained 80% eosinophils.

Imaging Studies

Computed tomography (CT) scan with thin (1–2 mm) (HRCT; high resolution CT scan) was performed (Fig. 15.2). Proximal bronchiectasis is defined as being present when there are bronchi that are dilated in comparison with the caliber of an adjacent bronchial artery in the inner two thirds of the lung CT field. Bronchiectasis is described as cylindrical when the bronchus does not taper and is 1.5 to >3 times

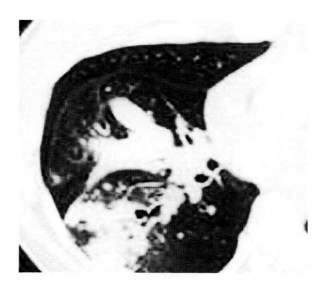

Fig. 15.2 Computed tomography scan described proximal bronchiectasis in ABPA

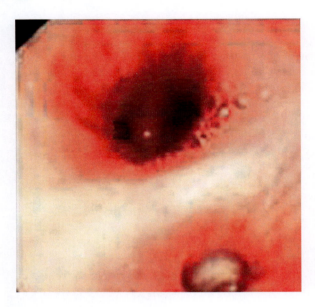

Fig. 15.3 Picture of broncho-fiberscopy described mucoid impaction in the patient with ABPA

the caliber of diameter of an adjacent artery. Bronchiectasis can also be varicoid or cystic. Ring shadows on chest roentgenograms are 1–2 cm in diameter; they represent dilated bronchi seen in an en face orientation. When the same dilated bronchus is visualized in a tangential (coronal) plane, it is called a parallel-line shadow. These findings are consistent with bronchiectasis. Some of the other findings include mucus plugs or mucoid impactions, bronchial wall thickening as occurs in asthma, atelectasis, lobar or whole lung collapse, pulmonary fibrosis, and cavities with or without air-fluid levels. Mucus plugs was shown in the picture of bronchoscopy in Fig. 15.3.

1. With the presented data what is your diagnosis?

    (a) Allergic asthma
    (b) Vocal cord disfunction
    (c) Anergic bronchopulmonary aspergillosis (ABPA)
    (d) Transient hypogammaglobulinemia

Answer: (c)

Considering the differential diaganosis

2. What is your diagnosis and why?

Despite the total low IgE levels, the clinical, radiologic, and immunologic data suggested the diagnosis of ABPA (see discussion below).

Discussion

Proposed criteria for the diagnosis of ABPA in patients with cystic fibrosis are presented in Table 15.3(3), which is based on the work of a Consensus Conference of the Cystic Fibrosis Foundation.

ABPA is characterized by stages of exacerbation demonstrating reversible airflow obstruction, pulmonary infiltrates, peripheral eosinophilia, immediate skin reactivity to *A. fumigatus* extract, total serum IgE more than 1,000 ng/mL, and the presence of precipitins against *A. fumigatus*. Additional criteria are proximal bronchiectasis and significant elevated levels of IgE-Af and IgG-Af. During exacerbations of ABPA, the high antigen load resulting from fungal growth causes a vigorous polyclonal antibody response, resulting in high IgG, IgA, and IgM titers against *A. fumigatus*. When complete clinical symptoms and radiographic and laboratory findings are present, diagnosis of ABPA does not represent a problem. Although elevated total serum IgE has been considered essential for diagnosis of ABPA, an acute clinical ABPA without an elevated total serum IgE level has been reported in a 20-year-old woman with cyctic fibrosis with clinical asthma and pulmonary infiltrates (4). In our patient, at the time of pulmonary infiltration, although total serum IgE levels were below values reported in ABPA, there was an increase greater than 100% over the baseline IgE levels, and she also had an increase in all serum immunoglobulin classes against *A. fumigatus*, eosinophilia in blood and sputum, immediate skin prick test response to *A. fumigatus*, and presence of precipitins to *A. fumigatus*. The low total serum IgE levels in this child might be due to early diagnosis and treatment. Elevated levels might only occur if the process becomes chronic or recurrent, and perhaps some episodes of ABPA with low IgE levels are not diagnosed. In this case, total serum IgE titers might not be useful in follow-up, and additional clinical, radiologic, and laboratory (IgE-Af, IgG-Af and IgA-Af) criteria should be used and periodically monitored.

Table 15.3 Criteria for the diagnosis of ABPA in patients with asthma

Criteria for ABPA-central bronchiectasis/minimal essential criteria
    Asthma/Yes
       Central bronchiectasis (inner two thirds of chest CT field)/Yes
       Immediate cutaneous reactivity to *Aspergillus* species or *A. fumigatus*/Yes
       Total serum IgE concentration >417 kU/L (1,000 ng/mL)/Yes
       Elevated serum IgE: *A. fumigatus* and or IgG: *A. fumigatus*/Yes
       Chest roentgenographic infiltrates/No
       Serum precipitating antibodies to *A. fumigatus*/No
Criteria for the diagnosis of ABPA-seropositive
    Asthma/Yes
       Immediate cutaneous reactivity to *Aspergillus* species or *A. fumigatus*/Yes
       Total serum IgE concentration > 417 kU/L (1,000 ng/mL)/Yes
       Elevated serum IgE: *A. fumigatus* and or IgG-A. *fumigatus*/Yes
       Chest roentgenographic infiltrates/No

The syndrome of vocal cord dysfunction mimicking asthma in which less severe laryngeal obstruction can produce a sensation of dyspnea similar to that of asthma has been reported by Christopher et al. (5). Vocal cord abnormalities can be triggered by allergen provocation and gastroesophageal reflux disease. Examination was offered to the patient, but she desired to have this procedure performed elsewhere.

Transient hypogammaglobulinemia of infancy is a temporary decrease in serum IgG and sometimes IgA and other Ig isotypes to levels below age-appropriate normal values. In transient hypogammaglobulinemia, IgG levels continue to be low after the physiologic fall in maternal IgG at around age 3–6 months. This condition rarely leads to significant infections and is not thought to be a true immunodeficiency. Diagnosis is by serum Ig measurements and demonstration that antibody production in response to vaccine antigens (e.g., tetanus, diphtheria) is normal. Thus, this condition can be distinguished from permanent forms of hypogammaglobulinemia, in which specific antibodies to vaccine antigens are not produced. This condition may persist for months to few years but usually resolves.

Questions

A 38-year-old woman with a history of mild persistent asthma presents for evaluation of worsening asthma symptoms over the past 3 months. She reports nocturnal symptoms three times per week and daytime symptoms five times per week, on her current regimen of fluticasone metered-dose inhaler, 220 µg twice daily. She uses her albuterol metered-dose inhaler every 3–4 h for shortness of breath and difficulty in breathing. She has received courses of oral prednisolone on two occasions over the past 3 months with improvement in these symptoms. Her pulmonary function tests reveal a moderate obstructive pattern. Aeroallergen skin-prick tests are positive to several weeds and molds including *A. fumigatus*. Total serum IgE is 750 kU/L.

1. What additional findings are required to meet the minimal essential criteria for the diagnosis of ABPA?

    (a) Central bronchiectasis noted on chest CT scan
    (b) Chest roentgenographic infiltrates
    (c) Sputum cultures positive for *A. fumigatus*
    (d) Elevated serum eosinophilia
    (e) Expectoration of mucous plugs

2. What is your diagnosis and why?

    (a) Invasive aspergillosis
    (b) Anergic bronchopulmonary aspergillosis
    (c) Cystic fibrosis
    (d) Eosinophilic pneumonia

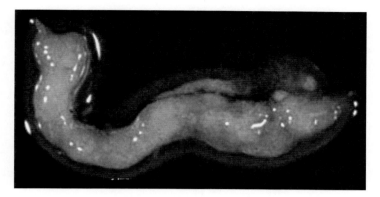

Fig. 15.4   Brown mucous plugs in induced sputum

This patient is in accord with the criteria of ABPA as mentioned in Tables 15.1 and 15.2. ABPA commonly presents in asthmatic patients whose clinical manifestations progress from mild asthma to asthma requiring steroids. Occasionally, ABPA and asthma may present concomitantly. Symptoms of episodic bronchospasm with progression to a chronic cough productive of brown mucous plugs (Fig. 15.4), hemoptysis, chest pain, and recurrent pulmonary infiltrates are frequent markers of the disease. Intermittent fevers, peripheral and sputum eosinophilia, and bronchopulmonary lesions often are noted on evaluation. Radiographs may show "gloved finger shadows" of mucoid impaction with fleeting pulmonary infiltrates from bronchial plugging. CT may reveal central bronchiectasis in the inner two-thirds of the lung with predominantly upper lung field involvement (6). Bronchial wall thickening, atelectasis, lung collapse, pulmonary fibrosis, and cavitary lesions also may be noted on radiographic examination. Typically, total serum IgE and precipitating *Aspergillus* antibodies are elevated and sputum cultures reveal fungus. Immediate cutaneous hypersensitivity to *Aspergillus* species is nearly universal, and atopy has been well associated with the disease. Differential diagnosis includes asthma, pulmonary infiltration with eosinophilia syndromes, helminthic lung disease, and other hypersensitivity pneurnonitis syndromes. Interestingly, yeast and fungi other than *Aspergillus* have been reported to cause a similar pattern of allergic bronchopulmonary disease, also known as allergic bronchopulmonary mycosis. ABPA associated with allergic *Aspergillus* sinusitis has also been reported (7).

Cystic fibrosis is the most common life-shortening genetic disease in the white population. In the USA, it occurs in about 1/3,300 white births, 1/15,300 black births, and 1/32,000 Asian-American births. Because of improved treatment and life expectancy, 40% of patients are adults. Diagnosis is suggested by characteristic clinical features and confirmed by a sweat test or identification of two known cystic fibrosis mutations. Diagnosis is usually confirmed in infancy or early childhood, but up to 10% of patients escape detection until adolescence or early adulthood. The only reliable sweat test is the quantitative pilocarpine iontophoresis test: localized sweating is stimulated pharmacologically with pilocarpine; the amount of sweat is measured, and its Cl concentration is determined. In patients with a suggestive clinical picture or a positive family history, a Cl concentration of >60 mEq/L confirms the diagnosis. In infants, a Cl concentration of >30 mEq/L is highly suggestive of cystic fibrosis. False-negative results are rare (about 1:1,000 patients with cystic fibrosis have sweat Cl <50 mEq/L) but may occur in the presence of edema and hypoproteinemia or with collection of inadequate quantities of sweat. False-positive results are usually related to technical errors. Transient elevation of sweat Cl concentration can occur in association with psychosocial deprivation (child abuse, neglect) and in patients with anorexia nervosa. Although results are valid after the first 24 h of life, an adequate sweat sample (>75 mg on filter paper or >15 μL in microbore tubing) may be difficult to obtain before 3 and 4 weeks of age. Although the sweat Cl concentration normally increases slightly with age, the test is still valid in adults.

Prevalence and incidence of chronic eosinophilic pneumonia are unknown. Etiology is suspected to be an allergic diathesis. Most patients are nonsmokers. Patients often present with fulminant illness characterized by cough, fever, progressive breathlessness, weight loss, wheezing, and night sweats. Asthma accompanies or precedes the illness in >50% of cases. Diagnosis requires exclusion of infectious causes and is based on clinical presentation, blood tests, and chest X-ray. Peripheral blood eosinophilia, a very high erythrocyte sedimentation rate, iron deficiency anemia, and thrombocytosis are all frequently found. Chest X-ray findings of bilateral peripheral or pleural-based opacities (present in about 60% of cases), most commonly in the middle and upper lung zones, is described as the "photographic negative" of pulmonary edema and is virtually pathognomonic (although seen in <25% of patients). A similar pattern is identified on CT in virtually all cases. Bronchoalveolar lavage eosinophilia >40% is suggestive of eosinophilic pneumonia; serial bronchoalveolar lavage examinations may help document the course of disease. Biopsy demonstrates interstitial and alveolar eosinophils and histiocytes, including multinucleated giant cells, and bronchiolitis obliterans organizing pneumonia.

Chronic pulmonary aspergillosis causes cough, often with hemoptysis and shortness of breath. Invasive pulmonary aspergillosis usually causes rapidly progressive, ultimately fatal respiratory failure if untreated. Extrapulmonary invasive aspergillosis begins with skin lesions, sinusitis, or pneumonia; may involve the liver, kidneys, brain, and other tissues; and is often rapidly fatal. Aspergillosis in the sinuses can form an aspergilloma, an allergic fungal sinusitis, or a chronic, slowly invasive granulomatous inflammation with fever, rhinitis, and headache. Necrosing cutaneous lesions may overlie the nose or sinuses, palatal or gingival ulcerations may be present, signs of cavernous sinus thrombosis may develop, and pulmonary or disseminated lesions may occur.

A 9-year-old boy who had suffered from reactive airway disease since 5 months of age had undergone pulmonary function tests at age 6 and was diagnosed as having airway hyperreactivity. He then received regular treatment with inhaled steroids, which was lately replaced by fluticasone 250 μg/salmeterol 50 μg twice a day. Before treatment, pulmonary function tests showed bronchial hyperreactivity with severe obstruction, partially reversible. For this case, blood tests showed total IgE levels of 466 kU/L, radioallergosorbent test (IgE-RAST) specific IgE was 8.20 U/mL against *A. fumigatus*, and normal levels of IgA, IgG, and IgM, and peripheral blood eosinophils of 15.2%, respectively. Skin tests were positive for *A. fumigatus*. Sweat tests were normal. The chest radiograph showed marked diffuse peribronchial cuffing with hyperinnation and infiltrates. We also performen high-resolution CT. This patient is a representative cases of severe unstable asthma with frequent acute exacerbations, which were detected by clinical status and pulmonary function tests and for which they received systemic steroids.

3. What finding should be useful to confirm the diagnosis for this patient?

   (a) Increasing of sputum eosinophils
   (b) Charcot-Leyden crystals in induced sputum
   (c) Fungus ball in chest radiography
   (d) α1-antitrypsin deficiency

4. What finding should be useful of the examination with high-resolution CT?

   (a) Perihilar bronchieclasis
   (b) Segmental infiltration
   (c) Fibrotic changes
   (d) Bilateral hilar lymphadenopathy

The diagnosis is suspected in patients with asthma with recurrent asthma exacerbations, migratory or nonresolving infiltrates on chest X-ray (often due to atelectasis from mucoid plugging and bronchial obstruction), evidence of bronchiectasis on imaging studies, sputum cultures positive for *A. fumigatus*, or notable peripheral eosinophilia. Bronchoscopy with bronchial biopsy and washing plays a pivotal role in detecting ABPA. The presence of "allergic" mucin might be overlooked in the small biopsy fragments obtained by bronchoscopy. Charcot–Leyden crystals and scattered hyphae would be observed in the patients with ABPA, which is sometimes useful for the diagnosis of ABPA.

Increasing of sputum eosinophils is commonly shown in allergic airway diseases including bronchial asthma, which is not specific for ABPA. A chronic form of invasive aspergillosis occasionally occurs, notably in patients with the hereditary phagocytic cell defect, chronic granulomatous disease. *Aspergillus sp*. can also cause endophthalmitis after trauma or surgery to the eye (or by hematogenous seeding) and infections of intravascular and intracardiac prostheses. Primary superficial aspergillosis is uncommon but may occur in burns; beneath occlusive dressings; after corneal trauma (keratitis); or in the sinuses, mouth, nose, or ear canal. *Aspergillus* tends to infect open spaces, such as pulmonary cavities from previous lung disease (e.g., bronchiectasis, tumor, tuberculosis), the sinuses, or ear canals (otomycosis). Such infections tend to be locally invasive and destructive, although systemic spread sometimes occurs, particularly in immunocompromised patients. *A. fumigatus* is the most common cause of invasive pulmonary disease; *Aspergillus flavus* most often causes invasive extrapulmonary disease. Focal infections sometimes form a fungus ball (aspergilloma), a characteristic growth of tangled masses of hyphae, with fibrin exudate and few inflammatory cells, typically encapsulated by fibrous tissue.

Findings suggestive of but nonspecific for the disease include presence in sputum of Aspergillus mycelia, eosinophils, and/or Charcot–Leyden crystals (elongated eosinophilic bodies formed from eosinophilic granules. Fig. 15.5). Giemsa-stained or Grocott-stained induced sputum disclosed A. *fumigatus* hyphae (shown in Fig. 15.6) and more than 50% eosinophils in the cell counts. Sometimes denatured eosinophils would be shown as Fig. 15.7. Also, induced sputum containing denatured eosinophils

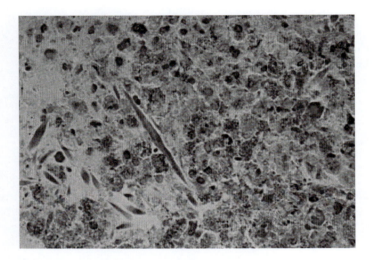

Fig. 15.5 Charcot-Leyden crystals in Grocott-stained induced sputum

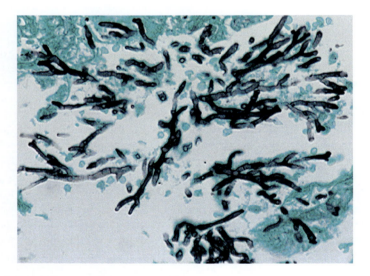

Fig. 15.6 *Aspergillus fumigatus* hyphae in Giemsa-stained induced sputum

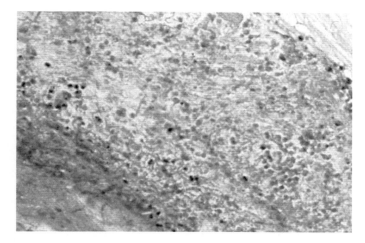

Fig. 15.7 Degenerated eosinophils in induced sputum in the patients with ABPA

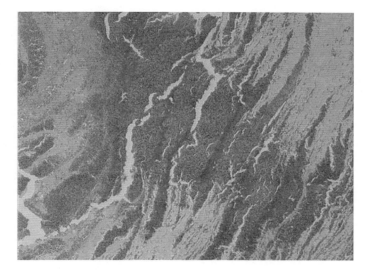

Fig. 15.8 Fir-tree structure cocsist with denatured eosinophils in H–E-stained induced sputum

appear as "fir-tree structure" (Fig. 15.8). Analysis of sputum formation is useful for the diagnosis of ABPA.

α1-Antitrypsin is a neutrophil elastase inhibitor (an antiprotease), the major function of which is to protect the lungs from protease-mediated tissue destruction. Most α1-antitrypsin is synthesized by hepatocytes and monocytes and passively diffuses through the circulation into the lungs; some is secondarily produced by alveolar macrophages and epithelial cells. The protein conformation (and, hence, functionality) and quantity of circulating α1-antitrypsin are determined by codominant expression of parental alleles;>90 different alleles have been identified and described by protease inhibitor phenotype. In the lung, α1-antitrypsin deficiency increases neutrophil elastase activity, which facilitates tissue destruction leading to emphysema (especially in smokers, because cigarette smoke also increases protease activity). α1-Antitrypsin deficiency accounts to account for 1–2% of all cases of COPD. α1-Antitrypsin deficiency most commonly causes early emphysema; symptoms and signs of lung involvement occur earlier in smokers than in nonsmokers but in both cases are rare before age 25. α1-Antitrypsin deficiency is congenital and is lack of a primary lung antiprotease, α1-antitrypsin, which leads to increased protease-mediated tissue destruction and emphysema in adults. Hepatic accumulation of abnormal α1-antitrypsin can cause liver disease in both children and adults. Serum α1-antitrypsin level <11 µmol/L (<80 mg/dL) confirms the diagnosis. Treatment is smoking cessation, bronchodilators, early treatment of infection, and, in selected cases, α1-antitrypsin replacement. Severe liver disease may require transplantation. *Pseudomonas* prognosis is related mainly to degree of lung impairment.

A 38-year-old woman had a chronic productive cough and dyspnea on exertion for 6 years. She had had episodic seasonal asthma and rhinitis since infancy. During childhood she had at least annual hospitalizations for exacerbations of asthma occasionally associated with respiratory infections. At the age of 25 years, she developed gradual onset of a daily cough poductive of up to one-half cup of purulent sputum per day and dyspnea on exertion. Positive features on physical examination were moderate clubbing and nailbed cyanosis of fingers and toes. Chest examination showed intercostal muscle retraction and inspiratory rales. The hematocrit level was 42.40, the white cell count was 6,200/mm^3 with 480 neutrophils and 120 eosinophils. IgG, IgM, and IgA concentrations, rheumatoid factor, antinuclear factor, α1-Antitrypsin level, and sweat chlorides were normal. The serum IgE level was 3,420 ng/mL (normal values less than 1,000 ng/mL). Serum precipitating anlibodies against *A. fumigatus* were present. Immediate cutaneous tests to common inhalant antigens including *A. fumigatus* were positive. Specific IgE and IgG against *A. fumigatus* were elevated. In arterial blood, the pH was 7.41, PO$_2$ was 71 Torr, and PCO$_2$ was 37 Torr. The chest radiography showed multiple centrally located parenchymal lucencies, widely scattered small patchy infiltrates, and tenting of the right side of the diaphragm. Lung tomograms showed bilateral perihilar thickened linear markings wilh rounded and oblong areas of lucency consistent with central bronchiectasis. Pulmonary function studies showed severe expiratory obstruction, slight restriction, diminished diffusion capacity, and moderate air trapping. Leukocyte function studies including endotoxin-stimulated nitroblue tetrazolium assay, endotoxin-activated chemotaxis, polymorphonuclear random movement, and hexose monophosphate shunt activity were normal. Phagocytosis and intracellular killing at 30 min of *S. aureus* were slightly decreased, but intracenular killing at 120 min was normal.

5. What is the cause of pulmonary infiltration?

   (a) Bacterial pneumonia
   (b) Infiltration of *Aspergillus*
   (c) Immunological cell infiltration
   (d) Granulomatous formations

6. What is the appropriate therapy for this patient?

   (a) Antibiotic therapy
   (b) Mechanical ventilation
   (c) Antifungal therapy
   (d) Corticosteroid therapy

The current recommended approach is presented in Table 15.4. As the disease is a manifestation of a hypersensitivity reaction rather than an infection, treatment is aimed at immune modulation. The administration of oral prednisone to patients with ABPA is associated with the improvement of asthma, and the presence of pulmonary infiltrates and eosinophilia, with reduction in serum levels of IgE, and probably reduced progression of bronchiectasis. The optimal dose is unknown, but 0.5 mg/kg/day is recommended, followed by a gradual taper and adjustment based on the patient's condition. The long-term use of corticosteroids is often necessary, but carries risk, including the development of invasive *Aspergillus* infection. Therefore, the antifungal agent itraconazole was tested in patients with ABPA as an adjunctive, steroid-sparing agent in two randomized placebo-controlled studies.

Table 15.4 Suggestions for initial treatment of ABPA

1. For new ABPA infiltrates, administer prednisone 0.5 mg/kg/day for 1–2 weeks, then on alternate days for 6–8 weeks. Then attempt to discontinue prednisone by tapering by 5–10 mg every 2 weeks.
2. Repeat the total serum IgE concentration in 6–8 weeks, then every 8 weeks for 1 year to determine the range of IgE concentrations. Increases of 100% over baseline can signify a silent ABPA exacerbation.
3. Repeat the chest roentgenogram or CT of the lung after 4–8 weeks to demonstrate that infiltrates have cleared.
4. Consider environmental sources of fungi (e.g., moldy basements, leaking roofs, water damage in walls) and recommend remediation.
5. Monitor pulmonary function tests.
6. If the patient cannot be tapered off prednisone despite optimal anti-asthma treatment and avoidance measures, then he or she has evolved into stage IV (corticosteroid-dependent asthma). Try to manage with alternate-day prednisone as opposed to daily prednisolone.
7. New ABPA infiltrates may be identified by:
   a. Cough, wheeze, or dyspnea with sputum production
   b. Unexplained declines in expiratory flow rates
   c. Sharp (>100%) increases in total serum IgE concentration
   d. Absent symptoms but new infiltrates on chest roentgenograms or chest CT examinations.
8. Diagnose and manage concomitant conditions such as allergic rhinitis, sinusitis, and gastro-esophageal reflux disease.

The dose was 20 mg daily for another 16 weeks. Both studies spanned 16 weeks of treatment and showed reduced levels of markers of systemic immune activation (serum IgE level and eosinophil count). The study by Wark et al. (8) also showed reduced levels of markers of airway inflammation in induced sputum. Neither study showed significant changes in lung function, although Wark and colleagues showed that subjects receiving itraconazole experienced fewer exacerbations of disease requiring increased doses of corticosteroids. Therefore, although itraconazole appears to be promising as adjunctive treatment for patients with ABPA, long-term trials are needed to assess the clinical efficacy and safety in patients in different disease severity strata. There have been no randomized controlled trials to evaluate the use of antifungal therapies in patients with ABPA complicating cystic fibrosis. Optional effective antifungal agent for ABPA might be fluconazole, according to our clinical experiences. In addition, American College of Chest Physicians proposed a new guideline for the treatment of the patients with chronic cough due to bronchiectasis including ABPA.

With early diagnosis and treatment, ABPA can enter a remission stage, a recurrent exacerbation stage, or perhaps a corticosteroid-dependent asthma stage. Patients who have end-stage fibrocavitary lung disease often present in that stage without having been identified and treated previously. The other modalities for management of asthma should be instituted, and patients should be encouraged not to be overly pessimistic. The goal is to avoid progressive loss of lung function and maintain good respiratory status, which is achievable for many patients.

Staging of ABPA is also important in management of this disease. The five stages, shown in Table 15.5, proposed by Patterson et al. remain useful (9). These stages are not phases of a disease, and in each case the physician should attempt to determine the stage that is present. The stages are presented in Table 15.4. Most patients who have classic findings and current chest roentgenographic or CT infiltrates are in stage III (recurrent exacerbation). Other patients with current infiltrates are in stage IV (corticosteroid-dependent asthma) or possibly stage I (acute) for first-time recognized infiltrates. High doses of inhaled corticosteroids have not prevented the emergence of infiltrates. Similarly, despite its widespread administration, the antifungal agent itraconazole has not prevented new infiltrates consistently. Patients who are in stage I or stage III with acute infiltrates should respond to prednisone administration, with clearing of the chest roentgenographic or CT infiltrates over 1–2 months, and they should become less symptomatic (reduced dyspnea and

Table 15.5 Stages of ABPA

Stage	Description	Radiographic infiltrates	Total serum IgE
I	Acute	Lobes or middle lobe	Sharply elevated
II	Remission	No infiltrate and patient off prednisone for >6 mo	Elevated or normal
III	Exacerbation	Upper lobes or middle lobe	Sharply elevated
IV	Corticosteroid-dependent asthma	Often without infiltrates, but intermittent infiltrates might occur	Elevated or normal
V	End stage	Fibrotic, bullous, or cavitary lesions	Might be normal

cough and improved spirometry results). Total serum IgE, if obtained serially, will decline by at least 35% over 6 weeks. One should not attempt to administer prednisone indefinitely in an attempt to reduce the total serum IgE concentration to the normal range. Unless the patient enters stage II (remission) or stage V (end stage), it is doubtful that the total serum IgE concentration will return to normal ranges. Conversely, knowing the ranges of total serum IgE when there are no chest roentgenographic infiltrates will establish a baseline from which increases of 100% or greater can alert one to an exacerbation. Patients with fibrocavitary ABPA (stage V) can have extensive bronchiectasis resembling end-stage cystic fibrosis. Infiltrates can be from *P. aeruginosa* or *S. aureus* pneumonias or from rare species that have colonized the bronchi. Response to prednisone is limited, and additional modalities, such as bronchial hygiene, coughing- or sputum-assist devices, inhaled RNAase, and anti-pseudomonal antibiotic coverage might be required. An earlier diagnosis of ABPA will result in fewer stage-V patients. Noncompliant patients who refuse to take prednisone for infiltrates might develop a greater number of bronchiectatic areas that can eventually lead to stage V ABPA with a poor prognosis. Similarly, delays in diagnosis of ABPA are known to have resulted in patients' presenting in stage V.

Answers: 1. (a); 2. (b); 3. (b); 4. (a); 5. (c); 6. (d)

References

1. Rosenberg M, Patterson R, Mintzer R, Cooper BJ, Roberts M, Harris KE. Clinical and immunologic criteria for the diagnosis of allergic bronchopulmonary aspergillosis. Ann Intern Med. 1977; **86**(4):405.
2. Greenberger PA, Patterson R. Allergic bronchopulmonary aspergillosis and the evaluation of the patient with asthma. J Allergy Clin Immunol. 1988; **81**:646.
3. Proceedings of the Cystic Fibrosis Foundation ABPA Consensus Conference; Jun 12–13; Bethesda, MD, USA, 2001.
4. Schwartz RH, Hollick GE. Allergic bronchopulmonary aspergillosis with low serum immunoglobulin E. J Allergy Clin Immunol 1981; **68**:290–4.
5. Christopher KL, Wood RP II, Eckert RC. Vocal cord dysfillction presenling as asthma. N Engl J Med 1998; **308**:1566–70.
6. Ward S, Heyneman L, Lee MJ, et al. Accuracy of CT in the diagnosis of allergic bronchopulmonary aspergillosis in asthmatic patients. AJR Am J Roentgenol. 1999; **173**:937.
7. Sher TH, Schwartz HJ. Allergic aspergmus sinusitis with concurrent allergic bronchopulmonary aspergillus: Report of a case. J Allergy Clin Immunol. 1988; **81**:844–6.
8. Wark P, Hensley M, Saltos, N. Anti-inflammatory effect of itraconazole in stable allergic bronchopulmonary aspergillosis: a randomized controlled trial. J Allergy Clin Immunol. 2003; **111**:952.
9. Patterson R, Greenberger PA, Radin RC. Allergic bronchopulmonary aspergillosis: Staging as an aid to management. Ann Intern Med. 1982; **96**:286.

Chapter 16
HIV/AIDS and Complications

David Lim and Peter Jensen

Abstract In the setting of human immunodeficiency virus (HIV) and acquired immune deficiency syndrome (AIDS), two well-characterized syndromes can present with fevers, rash, headache, and other nonspecific complaints that may mimic an allergic or immune system-mediated reaction. Both the HIV specialist and non-HIV health care provider need to recognize these syndromes to initiate effective treatment and prevent further complications. Here we present a case of acute HIV syndrome with a severe oral ulcer. Our second case highlights an individual presenting with abacavir hypersensitivity reaction in an otherwise healthy HIV patient.

Keywords HIV • AIDS • HIV complications • Abacavir hypersensitivity

Case I

A 55-year-old Turkish man presented with the chief complaint of mouth pain. Ten days ago, he developed subjective fevers, sore throat, headache and a runny nose. He also had a rash described as small red spots on his chest and arms but this dissipated within the first week of symptoms. One week ago he developed painful oral ulcer on the back of his left throat. He describes it as small, white in appearance and very painful with drinking, chewing, or swallowing. He endorses extreme fatigue, malaise, and some mild joint pain mostly in his right hand and right knee. He denies any recent sick contacts, international travel, or exposures to animals. He obtains his yearly influenza shot. He is divorced with two adult children who live elsewhere. He works as an interstate truck driver constantly traveling across the United States.

D. Lim (✉) and P. Jensen
Division of Infectious Diseases, J. David Gladstone Institute of Virology and Immunology,
360: The Positive Care Center, University of California, San Francisco, San Francisco,
CA, USA
e-mail: david.lim@ucsf.edu

M. Mahmoudi (ed.), *Challenging Cases in Allergy and Immunology*,
DOI: 10.1007/978-1-60327-443-2_16,
© Humana Press, a part of Springer Science + Business Media, LLC 2009

Past Medical History: hypertension, unknown cardiac arrhythmia requiring ablation
   procedure in 2006, former heavy alcohol use – now sober over 10 years
Allergies: no known drug allergies
Medications: aspirin 325 mg daily by mouth, lisinopril 40 mg daily by mouth
Social History: formerly paid female commercial sex workers for intercourse
   10-years ago shortly after divorce (did not use barrier protection), denies any
   current female partners over the last year; smokes a half pack of cigarettes daily
   for the last 30 years, denies intravenous drug use, occasional "uppers" to stay
   aware while driving
Family History: father with adult onset diabetes, mother with hypertension
Review of Systems: no visual acuity loss, mild nausea but no vomiting;
   3 weeks ago patient had 8 h of profuse watery diarrhea less than 30 min after
   eating funny tasting sushi at a roadside café in Arizona (states fellow truck drivers
   also has same diarrhea attack); no chest pain, palpitations, shortness of breath or
   dyspnea on exertion; no arthralgias; no pain on urination or penile discharge

Physical Exam

Vitals: max temperature 38.5°C, heart rate 80 beats per minute, blood pressure
145/90 mmHg, respiratory rate 14 breaths per minute
   General: nontoxic appearing, no acute distress, obese, alert, and oriented
   Head, ears, eyes, nose, and throat: anicteric sclerae, mild rhinorrhea, oropharynx
with single, shallow ulcerations roughly 0.5–1 cm in diameter with white, nonre-
movable surface on left posterior pharynx; erythematous posterior pharynx without
exudates, bilateral anterior and posterior lymphadenopathy
   Heart: regular rate and rhythm with no murmurs, rubs or gallops
   Lungs: clear to auscultation bilaterally to lung bases
   Abdomen: soft, nontender, nondistended, bowel sounds present
   Extremities: no edema, warm and well-perfused, 2+ peripheral pulses; right
hand and knee joints with no swelling, erythema but mild pain to touch - intact range
of motion
   Genitourinary Exam: glans penis with shallow ulceration on right dorsal surface
about 0.5 cm in diameter with mild surrounding erythema and mild tenderness to
palpation; no penile exudates, no anal lesions, no testicular swelling
   Skin: diffuse acne upon upper torso and back; no erythema, petechiae, macules,
or papules
   Neurological exams: cranial nerves II through XII intact; no focal findings

Data

See Table 16.1.

Table 16.1 Initial laboratory workup

White cell count	7,100 cells/µL (nl: 3,400–10,000)
Hematocrit	38% (nl: 41–53%)
Platelets	260,000 per µL (nl: 140,000–450,000)
Sodium	134 mM (nl: 134–143)
Potassium	3.6 mM (nl: 3.4–4.9)
Chloride	98 mM (nl: 98–107)
Bicarbonate	31 mM (nl: 23–32)
Blood urea nitrogen	5 mg/dL (nl: 8–23)
Creatinine	0.7 mg/dL (nl: 0.6–1.2)
Glucose	95 mg/dL (nl: 70–199)
Aspartate aminotransferase	32 U/L (nl: 16–41)
Alanine aminotransferase	35 U/L (nl: 12–59)
Alkaline phosphatase	117 U/L (nl: 29–111)
EBV VCA IgM/IgG	Negative/positive
CMV IgM/IgG	Negative/positive
Monospot test	Negative
HIV serology	Negative
Urine toxicology screen	*Positive for amphetamines*; negative for barbiturates, benzodiazepines, cannabis, cocaine, ethanol and opiates

Images

Image of oral ulcer (see Fig. 16.1)

Impressions

With the Presented Data What Is Your Working Diagnosis?

This 55-year-old, divorced truck driver presents with mild fever, fatigue, arthralgias, acne, oral ulcers and a penile ulcer. At first glance, he appears to arrive with an infectious mononucleosis syndrome. His negative IgM serologies for EBV (Epstein Barr Virus) and CMV (cytomegalo virus) make acute, active infection with these viruses unlikely. The positive IgG titers only show that he has been exposed to EBV and CMV in the past. Interestingly, he describes a half day bout of diarrhea immediately after ingesting raw fish a few weeks ago. The rapid onset and resolution of the seafood-associated diarrhea 3 weeks prior is not consistent with bacterial gastroenteritis but more consistent with scombroid food poisoning or histamine-like, toxin-mediated diarrhea. Therefore, a postinfectious, autoinflammatory syndrome is not likely. Although oral ulcerations are more commonly observed with sexually transmitted infections, this patient denies current behavior for such exposures. In addition, he also has a negative HIV-1 serology. Therefore, the initial impression was

Fig. 16.1 Single small ulcer on left posterior pharynx (Images courtesy: AIDS Images Library http://www. aids-images.ch)

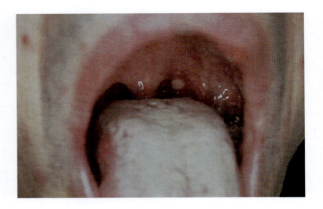

that this represented a noninfectious etiology and we propose *Behcet's Syndrome* as the cause of this patient's illness.

Differential Diagnosis

Sexually Transmitted Diseases (non-HIV)

Fevers, mild rash, malaise, and an oral and penile ulcer are all consistent with syphilis or herpetic virus infection (herpes simplex virus 1 or 2). One key feature, however, for syphilis is that ulceration or the chancre is usually painless, which does not fit with our patient's oral or penile lesion (1). Fever, pharyngitis, and intraoral herpetic lesions are usually associated with primary HSV-1 infections. Lesions are usually multiple, however, and/the patient denies recent contact history. Recurrence of HSV-1 usually localizes along the vermilion border of the lips and not the posterior pharynx also making this less likely. Gonorrhea is not associated with oral ulcers and when present in the oropharynx, usually presents with an exudative phayngitis with cervical lymphadenopathy.

HIV

Acute HIV syndrome may present with fever, fatigue, a diffuse maculopapular rash, headache, lymphadenopathy, pharyngitis, and oral lesions, all of which are consistent with our patient. However, at first glance, his behavioral history does not reveal overt risk factors for HIV – no reported intravenous drug use or recent unprotected intercourse (with women). Although his HIV serology is negative, seroconversion may be delayed for as long as six months after infection, though typically occurring within six weeks. Therefore a negative HIV test in our patient does not exclude this diagnosis.

Advanced HIV infection and AIDS (acquired immunodeficiency syndrome as defined by CD4 count less than 200 cells per mL or presence of opportunistic infection) is associated with painful oral, and esophageal aphthous ulcerations. This is an indolent process progressing over weeks to months. The underlying etiology of these lesions is unclear but is thought to be secondary to loss of cellular immunity.

Behcet's Sydrome

This is a multisystem inflammatory disease with a predisposition for people from Asia or the Eastern Mediterranean region. Patients present with recurrent oral and genital ulcers, recurrent anterior chamber eye inflammation, pathergy (pustule formation on skin after needle prick) and occasionally acne. Our patient fulfills many of these criteria except he does not describe recurrence of symptoms. Therefore, while Behcet's was proposed as the likely diagnosis, further history for recurrence of symptoms would clinically confirm this diagnosis.

Adult Still's Disease

This is an inflammatory disorder with daily fevers greater than 39°C for at least one week, arthritis and an evanescent, salmon-colored, maculopapular rash over the trunk or extremities during febrile episodes. Laboratory values include leukocytosis (greater than 10,000 cells per μL) and at least 80% granulocytes. Sore throat, lymphadenopathy, and an enlarged liver or spleen can be present. Contrary to these criteria, our patient had only a mild fever (only 38.5), no leukocytosis and one episode of macular rash that is no longer present. Therefore, he fails to fulfill criteria for adult Still's disease.

Workup

Upon further questioning about the positive urine toxicology screen for amphetamines, the patient admitted to periodic inhalation of crystal methamphetamines to help him remain awake while driving his truck. He also disclosed engaging in unprotected receptive and insertive oral and anal intercourse with other male truck drivers at rest stops in the context of shared crystal methamphetamine use. The patient identifies his sexual orientation as "closet" bisexual and states that a sexual encounter with another man led to his divorce over 10 years ago. He does state an HIV test performed 3 months ago was negative. This new history prompted extensive STD testing, HIV testing with qualitative nucleic acid amplification, and CD4 lymphocyte quantification (Table 16.2).

Table 16.2 Additional laboratory testing

Gonorrhea and chlamydia nucleic acid PCR amplification (urine and pharyngeal swab)	Negative
Serum RPR	Negative
Herpes simplex virus 1 and 2 direct fluorescent antibody test of oral and penile ulcer swabs	Negative
Viral cultures from oral and penile ulcer swabs	Negative
Hepatitis B surface antigen	Negative
Hepatitis B surface and core antibodies	Both positive
Hepatitis C antibody	Negative
CD4 T cells (absolute)	182 cells per mL (nl: 410–1,590)
HIV RNA detection	Positive
Chest X-ray	No infiltrates, effusions or masses
Electrocardiogram	Normal sinus rhythm

What Is Your Final Diagnosis and Why?

This is acute HIV Syndrome given the low CD4 count and new positive qualitative nucleic acid amplification test result. Of note, his hepatitis B virus (HBV) serologies are consistent with exposure and not immunization since his core antibody is positive. There is no active HBV replication since surface antigen is negative.

Discussion

Brief History

Acute HIV syndrome was recognized early in the HIV epidemic initially named as AIDS-related complex (ARC) usually presenting as our patient did with fever, rash, malaise, and numerous other nonspecific symptoms (described later). The syndrome is very suggestive of a mononucleosis syndrome and has been misdiagnosed as such. As diagnostic techniques have improved, so have our abilities to recognize this syndrome earlier in infection. Treatment during this very early stage of HIV infection, however, is an ongoing area of investigation.

Signs and Symptoms

Acute HIV syndrome usually occurs 1–4 weeks after transmission associated with a dramatic but transient rise in viral count and drop in CD4 T helper lymphocytes. Usual symptoms include fever, rash (diffuse maculopapular viral exanthems usually on the face and trunk), nonexudative pharyngitis, arthralgias/myalgias, and oral/genital ulcers. Symptoms can also include: oral thrush that is persistent and poor to respond to antifungals, recurrent herpes zoster diarrhea, and peripheral neuropathy. The greater the severity of symptoms, the greater the degree of HIV viremia and more rapid the disease progression (2).

Pathophysiology

Acute retroviral syndrome is believed to result from both the severe, inflammatory systemic antiviral response as well as targeted CD4 depletion by HIV, itself. Because of the acute immunodeficiency, opportunistic infections particularly oral candidrasis and reactivation herpes zoster can occur. The transient immune suppression in early HIV, however, usually does not lead to *Pneusmocystits jivorecki* pneumonia, cryptococcal meningitis or Kaposi's sarcoma as seen in later disease.

Workup

As noted earlier, the majority of HIV-1 serologies turn positive in 6 (average of 4 weeks) weeks. Almost all serologies of acute HIV turn positive by 6 months. Routine HIV-1 serology testing for all patients between the ages of 13 and 64 is now recommended by the CDC (3). Annual testing is recommended for patients with high risk to contract HIV as deemed by an evaluating physician. All pregnant women should be screened for HIV. The earliest the current enzyme-linked immunoassay (ELISA) (used for initial HIV serology screening) can detect acute infection is 12 days postexposure if a patient has robust HIV antibody production. Therefore, if suspicion for acute HIV syndrome is high, nucleic acid amplification testing is recommended with APTIMA qualitative HIV RNA testing as the only FDA-approved test for diagnosis. Quantitative HIV RNA testing can be used with the caveat that a higher rate of false negative tests occur when compared with the APTIMA test.

Management/Treatment

Studies are currently ongoing investigating the long-term benefits of early intervention with highly active anti-retroviral therapy (HAART) for patients presenting with acute HIV. Pregnant women presenting with a new diagnosis of HIV regardless of acute presentation should be started on HAART. All patients should have an HIV genotype obtained and then referred to an HIV specialist for assistance with treatment regimens for pregnant patients and perhaps, referral to clinical trials for others. Patients should be advised to remain sexually abstinent or to always use barrier protection, if engaging in sexual activity.

Questions

1. Which of the following symptoms is NOT associated with acute HIV syndrome?

   (a) Fever
   (b) Diffuse maculopapular rash of face and trunk
   (c) Exudative phayngitis

(d) Arthralgias and myalgias

(e) Painful oral ulcer(s)

2. All of the following statements are true regarding CDC recommended guidelines for HIV serology testing and treatment EXCEPT:

(a) All patients between the ages of 13 and 64 should be screened once for HIV.

(b) Patients deemed high risk by an evaluating physician for HIV should be screened annually.

(c) If initial serology screening is negative but suspicion for acute HIV syndrome remains high, diagnostic HIV nucleic acid amplification testing should be performed.

(d) Pregnant women who are newly diagnosed with HIV should refrain from antiretroviral therapy until their CD4 count falls below 350 cells per mL.

(e) It is currently unclear whether immediate antiretroviral therapy has long-term benefits for patients presenting with acute HIV.

3. All of the following conditions can present with painful oral ulceration EXCEPT:

(a) Oral gonorrhea

(b) Acute HIV syndrome

(c) Behcet's Syndrome

(d) Primary HSV-1 infection

(e) Aphthous ulcers

4. After HIV-1 transmission, the AVERAGE time for the HIV enzyme-linked immunoassay (ELISA) to turn positive is:

(a) 40 h

(b) 4 days

(c) 12 days

(d) 40 days

(e) 4 weeks

5. Which of the following is true regarding management of a patient diagnosed with acute HIV?

(a) If pregnant, the patient should immediately be started on triple drug therapy that includes efavirenz to prevent transmission of HIV to the fetus.

(b) Triple drug therapy with a boosted protease inhibitor should immediately be initiated to preserve CD4 count and reduce setpoint HIV viral load.

(c) HIV genotyping should be performed and patient should be referred to an HIV specialist for possible enrollment into study investigating utility of early antiretroviral therapy for acute HIV.

(d) Patient should immediately start PCP (*Pneumocystis jiroveci* pneumonia) prophylaxis with trimethoprim/sulfamethoxazole (Bactrim or Septra).

(e) If patient decides to engage in sexual activity, then he or she should take antiretroviral therapy prior to activity to reduce risk of HIV transmission.

Answers: 1. (c); 2. (d); 3. (a); 4. (e); 5. (c)

Case 2

A 36-year-old, Caucasian man, diagnosed with HIV in 1995, presented with the chief complaint of malaise. Five days ago he developed subjective fevers, chills, nausea, vomiting, diarrhea, and progression of a diffuse erythematous maculopapular rash. He also endorsed sore throat, headache, and general malaise. His HIV was suppressed on a regimen of nelfinavir (Viracept), a protease inhibitor, lamivudine or 3TC (Epivir) and stavudine or d4T (Zerit), the latter two both nucleoside HIV reverse transcriptase inhibitors. He stated his CD4 count has been stable and viral load undetectable for years. About 1 week ago he noticed slight chills followed two days later by a rash on his trunk described as red, scaly, and warm to touch with no discrete borders, lesions, or pustules. This progressed over the next few days to cover his arms, legs, and neck with some extension to his face. Soon his symptoms progressed to subjective fevers, shaking chills, headache, sore throat, and muscle cramps. He saw his HIV provider who recommended emergency room evaluation. Of note, 4 weeks ago, his antiretrovirals were changed to a new regimen, which the patient cannot currently recall.

Past Medical History: HIV with unknown CD4 nadir and no opportunistic infections; depression and former polysubstance abuse (crystal methamphetamine and cocaine)

Allergies: no known previous drug reactions

Medications: currently on unknown regimen of antiretroviral medications

Social History: engages in unprotected receptive and insertive oral sex with other men; over five different partners in last month; occasional alcohol; no tobacco use or current illicit drug use

Family History: no significant history

Review of Systems: no photophobia, no oral ulcers, no thrush, no cough, occasional palpitations over last week, no nausea or vomiting, no diarrhea, no active symptoms of depression

Physical Exam

Vitals: max temperature 39.4°C, heart rate 108 beats per minute, blood pressure 130/80 mmHg, respiratory rate 18 breaths per minute

General: ill-appearing, in mild discomfort; well nourished man; alert and oriented

Head, ears, eyes, nose, and throat: anicteric sclerae but injected conjunctivae; oropharynx with beefy red mucosal membranes, erythematous pharynx but no exudates, neck supple; no lymphadenopathy

Heart: tachycardic, regular rate and rhythm with no murmurs, rubs, or gallops

Lungs: slight inpiratory crackles at left posterior base but otherwise clear

Abdomen: soft, nontender, nondistended, bowel sounds present

Extremities: no edema, warm and well perfused, 2+ peripheral pulses

Skin: diffuse maculopapular erythematous, somewhat scaly rash without discrete borders on trunk, abdomen, back, neck, upper arms and legs; skin warm to touch but with no exudates or open ulcers or tenderness to touch (see Images) Palms and soles with no evidence of rash.

Neurological exam: cranial nerves II through XII intact; 5/5 strength throughout; intact reflexes and sensation

Data

See Table 16.3.

Images

See Fig. 16.2.

Impressions

With the Presented Data What Is Your Working Diagnosis?

This HIV-seropositive individual with reportedly stable CD4 T cell count and undetectable viral load presents with fever, rash, nausea, vomiting, and mild transaminitis. He has had multiple unprotected sexual encounters over the last month making him high-risk for sexually transmitted diseases. Given the diffuse eruption of his

Table 16.3 Initial laboratory workup

White cell count	6,000 cells per μL (nl: 3,400–10,000)
Hematocrit	42% (nl: 41–53%)
Platelets	160,000 per μL (nl: 140,000–450,000)
Sodium	140 mM (nl: 134–143)
Potassium	4.1 mM (nl: 3.4–4.9)
Chloride	105 mM (nl: 98–107)
Bicarbonate	25 mM (nl: 23–32)
Blood urea nitrogen	10 mg/dL (nl: 8–23)
Creatinine	0.8 mg/dL (nl: 0.6–1.2)
Glucose	84 mg/dL (nl: 70–199)
Aspartate aminotransferase	291 U/L (nl: 16–41)
Alanine aminotransferase	208 U/L (nl: 12–59)
Alkaline phosphatase	128 U/L (nl: 29–111)
Urine toxin screen	Negative for amphetamines, barbiturates, benzodiazepines, cannabis, cocaine, ethanol, and opiates

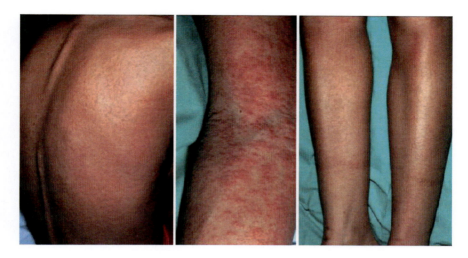

Fig. 16.2 Diffuse maculopapular, erythematous, scaly rash without discrete borders. (Images courtesy: AIDS Images Library http://www.aids-images.ch)

maculopapular rash, we are foremost suspicious of *secondary syphilis*. The absence of rash on his palms or soles does not rule-out this infection.

Differential Diagnosis

The following additional conditions warrant further consideration and potential workup:

Viral Syndrome

Influenza, parainfluenza, respiratory syncytial virus, and acute HIV can all present with fever, nausea, vomiting, and transaminitis. The only atypical feature for our patient would be his diffuse macluopapular rash, which is more often associated with acute HIV than the other viral syndromes. The incidence of acute, superinfection with HIV in a previously HIV-seropositive individual is rare. This, however, is rare and only reported in patients who are not taking antiretroviral medications (4).

Other Infections

The patient's unprotected sexual practice raises the possibility of other sexually transmitted diseases such as, herpes simplex virus, gonorrhea, chlamydia, hepatitis B, hepatitis C, and human papilloma virus.

Sweet's Syndrome

This is an acute febrile neutrophilic dermatosis that usually affects the back, neck, arms, and face. Rash usually appears in form of small red nodules shortly after presentation of a fever or upper respiratory infection. This soon, however, develops into coalescing plaques that are painful to touch and sometimes blister which our patient did not have. The exact cause of Sweet's syndrome is unknown but is seen in response to certain triggers including infections (viral or bacterial), acute myelogenous leukemia, inflammatory bowel disease, bowel or breast cancer, rheumatoid arthritis or certain medications such as NSAIDS (nonsteroidal antiinflammatory drugs).

Immune Reconstitution Inflammatory Syndrome (IRIS)

This is observed in HIV-seropositive patients who have a recently restored immune system after the initiation of anti-retroviral therapy. The hyperreactive immune system can be responsive to latent infections (e.g., tuberculosis, CMV retinintis, JC virus in progressive multifocal leukoencephalopathy, herpetic viruses including HSV and VZV, Cryptococcosis, *Pneumocystis jirovecii*) or chronic, noninfectious conditions (e.g., rheumatoid arthritis, systemic lupus erythematosis, sarcoidosis). The syndrome is associated with a recently restored CD4 count or dramatically reduced HIV serum viral load with paradoxical worsening in clinical status over the subsequent weeks to months. Our patient has had a restored immune system for years, however, making IRIS unlikely.

Vasculitis

Some forms of vasculitis that affect small and medium size vessels can present as fever and rash. In particular, syndromes such as Wegeners' granulomatosis, mixed cryoglobulinemia (from hepatitis C), polyarteritis nodosa, Churg-Strauss, and hypersensitivity vasculitis can cause rash that usually presents as palpable purpura or diffuse petechiae.

Drug Hypersensitivity

NSAIDs, antibiotics, and anti-retroviral drugs are common causes of skin rashes, particularly in patients with HIV. Skin reactions can range from urticaria, macular exanthems, eczematous fixed drug eruptions, erythema multiforme, Stevens-Johnson Syndrome to toxic epidermal necrolysis. This patient denies any over the counter medications or recent antibiotic use. He is, however, taking new antiretroviral medications. It is imperative to determine the exact regimen and exact doses he is currently taking.

Workup

After speaking to the patient's HIV provider, it was determined that he replaced the lamivudine and stavudine with Epzicom, a combination tablet of abacavir and lamivudine. The patient continued with the Viracept. Upon further history from the patient, he associated chills and worsening of his rash roughly 1 or 2 h after his daily Epzicom dose. This prompted testing for the major histocompatiblity complex allele, HLA-B*5701 (Table 16.4).

What Is Your Final Diagnosis and Why?

The final diagnosis is abacavir hypersensitivity reaction. The nonspecific syndrome of fever, maculopapular rash, nausea, vomiting, and transaminitis temporally associated with abacavir administration clinically raises the suspicion of adverse drug reaction. The patient's serum RPR was negative making secondary syphilis highly unlikely. The positive result for HLA-B*5701 further supports the diagnosis of abacavir hypersensitivity. HLA-B*5701 testing is now standard of care for pre-abacavir treatment screening as discussed later.

Discussion

Brief History

Abacavir is a guanasine nucleoside reverse transcriptase inhibitor effective against HIV. There are few known drug-drug interactions with abacavir as well as few long-term toxicity effects. The major drawback of abacavir use has been its associated

Table 16.4 Additional laboratory testing

Gonorrhea and chlamydia nucleic acid PCR amplification (urine and pharyngeal swab)	Negative
Serum RPR	Negative
Herpes simplex virus 1 and 2 direct fluorescent antibody test of oral and penile ulcer swabs	Negative
Viral cultures from oral and penile ulcer swabs	Negative
Hepatitis B surface antigen	Negative
Hepatitis B surface and core antibodies	Both positive
Hepatitis C antibody	Negative
CD4 T cells (absolute)	182 cells per mL (nml 410 – 1,590)
HIV RNA detection	Positive
Chest X-ray	No infiltrates, effusions, or masses
Electrocardiogram	Normal sinus rhythm

hypersensitivity reaction, which affects between 5 and 8% of patients within the first 6 weeks of therapy (5). The major histocompatibility allele HLA-B*5701 was found to be associated with abacavir hypersensitivity. This led to further studies showing the prevention of abacavir hypersensitivity with prescreening of patients for HLA-B*5701 before initiation of abacavir (6). Such testing is now recommended by the US Department of Health and Human Services (7). HLA-B*5701 has a prevalence of 8% within Caucasians compared with a prevalence of 1% in Sub-Saharan Africans (8).

Signs and Symptoms

Nonspecific, multiorgan involvement can manifest as fever, diffuse maculopapular rash, sore throat, gastrointestinal symptoms (nausea, vomiting, diarrhea), malaise, tachypnea, and nonspecific respiratory complaints (cough, shortness of breath). Other less common symptoms include: myalgia, arthralgia, headache, pruritis, hypotension, and phayngitis. Since none of these symptoms are specific for abacavir hypersensitivity, providers must remain vigilant soon after starting ABC. Laboratory findings can reveal mild transaminitis, an elevated erythrocyte sedimentation rate (ESR), and perhaps mild leukocytosis but again, these are relatively nonspecific.

Pathophysiology

It is postulated that ABC is metabolized by cytoplasmic alcohol dehydrogenase to a reactive compound that haptenates an unknown protein. This protein is processed within the cell to then bind HLA-B*5701. Display of this complex then triggers robust CD8+ cell response and subsequent cytokine cascade (9).

Workup

Abacavir hypersensitivity should always be suspected. In any patient who has recently initiated ABC (within the last few weeks to months) and who presents with nonspecific signs and symptoms of fever, rash, malaise/fatigue, and nausea/vomiting, Prescreening for HLA-B*5701 should be performed to avoid abacavir hypersensitivity. Some centers in limited studies have explored the use of skin patch testing to confirm abacavir hypersensitivity but this is limited to study protocols only.

Management/Treatment

Once abacavir hypersensitivity is suspected then all ABC should be stopped and patient given supportive care. Currently, no role for corticosteroids has been proven.

Most symptoms resolve within 72 h. Importantly, the patient should carry the label for abacavir allergy for life and should never be rechallenged with abacavir as this has been associated with development of Stevens-Johnson syndrome. Coformulations of HIV medications such as Epzicom (abacavir and lamivudine) or Trizivir (abacavir, AZT, and lamivudine) can obscure a patient's medication list. Therefore, it is imperative for both patient and provider always to know exactly each medication being administered in combination tablets to avoid future, complications.

Questions

1. Which of the following is NOT associated with abacavir-hypersensitivity?

   (a) Dysuria
   (b) Fever
   (c) Pruritis
   (d) Headache
   (e) Rash

2. Screening for which gene will avoid abacavir hypersensitivity?

   (a) HLA-B*27
   (b) HLA-DR3
   (c) CCR5
   (d) CD4
   (e) HLA-B*5701

3. Abacavir hypersensitivity occurs

   (a) Only when taken with other antiretroviral medications
   (b) Usually within the first 2 weeks of starting medications
   (c) Only in Caucasian patients
   (d) In less than 1% of patients (prior to genetic prescreening)
   (e) Usually within the first 4–6 weeks of starting medications

4. Management includes all of the following EXCEPT:

   (a) Discontinuation of abacavir
   (b) Symptomatic and supportive care
   (c) Use of corticosteroids
   (d) Early recognition
   (e) Designating patient with abacavir allergy for life

5. All the following medical conditions may mimic abacavir hypersensitivity EXCEPT:

   (a) Syphilis
   (b) MRSA folliculitis

(c) Sweet's syndrome

(d) Acute HIV

(e) Other adverse drug reactions (e.g., NSAIDS)

Answers: 1. (a); 2. (e); 3. (e); 4. (c); 5. (b)

References

1. Veraldi, S., Lunardon, L., Persico, M.C., Francia, C., & Bottini, S., Multiple aphthoid syphilitic chancres of the oral cavity. *Int J STD AIDS* **19**(7), 486–487 (2008).
2. Kelley, C.F., Barbour, J.D., & Hecht, F.M., The relation between symptoms, viral load, and viral load set point in primary HIV infection. *J Acquir Immune Defic Syndr* **45**(4), 445–448 (2007).
3. Branson, B.M. et al., Revised recommendations for HIV testing of adults, adolescents, and pregnant women in health-care settings. *MMWR Recomm Rep* 55 (RR-14), 1–17; quiz CE11–14 (2006).
4. Sidat, M.M. et al., Incidence of putative HIV superinfection and sexual practices among HIV-infected men who have sex with men. *Sex Health* **5**(1), 61–67 (2008).
5. Hughes, C.A. et al., Abacavir hypersensitivity reaction: an update. *Ann Pharmacother* **42**(3), 387–396 (2008).
6. Mallal, S. et al., HLA-B*5701 screening for hypersensitivity to abacavir. *N Engl J Med* **358**(6), 568–579 (2008).
7. HHS, Guidelines for the use of antiretroviral agents in HIV-1 infected adults and adolescents. *Department of Health and Human Services* (January, 29), 1–128; Available at http://www.aidsinfo.nih.gov/ContentFiles/AdultandAdolescentGL.pdf (2008).
8. Phillips, E.J., Genetic screening to prevent abacavir hypersensitivity reaction: are we there yet? *Clin Infect Dis* **43**(1), 103–105 (2006).
9. Martin, A.M. et al., Predisposition to abacavir hypersensitivity conferred by HLA-B*5701 and a haplotypic Hsp70-Hom variant. *Proc Natl Acad Sci USA* **101**(12), 4180–4185 (2004).

Chapter 17
Disorders of Immune Regulation

Amy L. Marks and Haig Tcheurekdjian

Abstract Immune system homeostasis is tightly maintained by regulatory mechanisms that allow for the destruction of pathologic microorganisms while preventing pathologic inflammation. Disruption of these regulatory mechanisms can lead to immunodeficiency and uncontrolled inflammation as seen in hyper-IgE syndrome and in immunodysregulation, polyendocrinopathy, enteropathy, X-linked syndrome. The discovery of monogenic defects in these disorders has led to a greater understanding of these complex disorders and of the mechanisms underlying immune system regulation.

Keywords Hyper-IgE syndrome • IPEX syndrome • Immune dysregulation

Case 1

The patient is a 13-year-old male referred for the evaluation of recurrent infections. He was the product of a full-term gestation and was born without any complications. Within the first week of life, he developed eczema which became progressively worse during his first few years of life. Aggressive skin care with moisturization and topical corticosteroid use was moderately effective, and food avoidance based on allergen skin testing was not beneficial. The patient developed a number of superinfections of his eczema requiring periodic systemic antimicrobial therapy. He also developed periodic superficial abscesses requiring incision and drainage. When performed, the cultures of the abscess contents grew methicillin sensitive *Staphylococcus aureus*.

A.L. Marks and H. Tcheurekdjian (✉)
Allergy/Immunology Associates, Inc, 1611 South Green Road, Suite 231, South Euclid, OH 44121, USA
e-mail: haig.tcheurekdjian@gmail.com

M. Mahmoudi (ed.), *Challenging Cases in Allergy and Immunology*,
DOI: 10.1007/978-1-60327-443-2_17,
© Humana Press, a part of Springer Science+Business Media, LLC 2009

During the first 2 years of life the patient had an average of five episodes of otitis media per year, one of which required parenteral antimicrobials for therapy after treatment failure with multiple oral antimicrobials. At 6 years of age, he developed a pneumonia which required hospitalization and parenteral antimicrobials for therapy. He was hospitalized for pneumonia again at 10 years of age after failing outpatient therapy. Sputum culture at that time grew *S. aureus*.

Current medications include albuterol metered-dose inhaler as needed for dyspnea, topical triamcinolone 0.1% ointment for eczema, and levofloxacin for a pneumonia that failed to respond to amoxicillin/clavulanate.

The patient's past medical history is significant for the extraction of multiple primary teeth due to the lack of deciduation after the eruption of his secondary teeth. He also suffered an ulnar fracture after falling off of a couch earlier this year.

Family history is significant for atopic dermatitis in a younger sibling and discoid lupus in his mother. There is no family history of recurrent infections.

On physical examination, the patient is comfortable and cheerful. HEENT examination is significant for slight facial asymmetry and a broad nasal bridge. Pulmonary examination reveals decreased breath sounds in the right lower lung fields posteriorly. There is hyperresonance in this same area upon percussion. Skin examination shows atopic dermatitis of moderate severity affecting most aspects of his body. The remainder of the physical examination is unremarkable.

Initial laboratory evaluation (Table 17.1) is remarkable for a slight eosinophilia and an elevated total serum IgE level. The remainder of the laboratory evaluation, including evaluation of humoral immunity, is unremarkable.

Computed tomography of the chest shows a large cystic structure consistent with a pneumatocele in the right hemithorax (Fig. 17.1).

With the Presented Data, What Is Your Working Diagnosis?

This patient's history and evaluation is highly suggestive of hyper-IgE syndrome. This syndrome has classically been defined by the presence of the following triad of findings (a) recurrent Staphylococcal abscesses, (b) pneumatoceles, and (c) elevated serum IgE levels. This patient possesses all of these features plus other features commonly seen in hyper-IgE syndrome including eczema, delayed shedding of primary teeth, and fractures after minor trauma.

Recurrent deep-seated Staphylococcal infections are also a feature of chronic granulomatous disease (CGD). Patients with CGD have defects in those enzymes that produce the oxidative burst used to destroy organisms engulfed by phagocytes. The oxidative burst is required for the destruction of only a handful of organisms, including *S. aureus*; therefore, patients with CGD are highly susceptible to infections from *S. aureus*. CGD can be inherited in either an X-linked or autosomal recessive manner. With the X-linked form of the disease, female carriers of the abnormal gene have a higher incidence of lupus with which this patient's mother has been diagnosed.

Table 17.1 Initial laboratory evaluation for case 1

Laboratory test	Result	Reference range
Complete blood count		
White blood cells	9,300/mm³	3,000–13,000/mm³
Hemoglobin (g/dl)	12.0	11–18
Platelets	215,000/mm³	140,000–450,000/mm³
Neutrophils	5,100/mm³	2,500–7,000/mm³
Lymphocytes	3,250/mm³	1,700–3,500/mm³
Monocytes	90/mm³	200–600/mm³
Eosinophils	860/mm³	100–300/mm³
Immunoglobulins		
IgG (mg/dl)	895	759–1,549
IgA (mg/dl)	120	58–358
IgM (mg/dl)	96	35–239
IgE (IU/ml)	3,260	2–170
Anti-tetanus toxoid IgG (IU/ml)	2.4	<0.1
Anti-pneumococcal IgG		
Serotype 2 (μg/ml)	7.3	<1.4
Serotype 9V (μg/ml)	5.1	<1.4
Serotype 12F (μg/ml)	1.6	<1.4
Serotype 20 (μg/ml)	2.7	<1.4
Lymphocyte phenotyping		
CD3	2,270/mm³ (70%)	800–3,500/mm³ (52–78%)
CD4	1,545/mm³ (48%)	400–2,100/mm³ (25–48%)
CD8	715/mm³ (22%)	200–1,200/mm³ (9–35%)
CD19	570/mm³ (17%)	200–600/mm³ (8–24%)
CD16/56	410/mm³ (13%)	70–1,200/mm³ (6–27%)

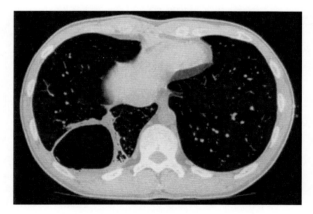

Fig. 17.1 Computed tomography of the chest for Patient #1. There is a large pneumatocele in the right lower lobe. Reproduced from (1), with kind permission of Springer Science and Business Media

The presence of an elevated serum IgE level is nonspecific and can be seen in a number of other primary immunodeficiency states including Wiskott–Aldrich syndrome and Omenn syndrome. Wiskott–Aldrich syndrome is characterized primarily by the presence of eczema, recurrent infections, thrombocytopenia, and bleeding. Although the patient possesses the first two features, lack of the latter two features makes this diagnosis unlikely. Omenn syndrome is a form of severe combined immunodeficiency associated with elevated IgE levels. This is not the cause of this patient's symptoms because Omenn syndrome invariably leads to death during infancy if not treated by stem cell transplantation.

Atopic disorders such as eczema and asthma are frequently associated with elevated IgE levels, and these levels can exceed 40,000. Although the patient does have eczema, his history of severe, recurrent, deep-seated infections indicates that an underlying immune deficiency is also present.

Work-Up

A flow cytometric assessment of neutrophil oxidative burst capacity with the use of dihydrorhodamine was obtained. In this assay, neutrophils are exposed to the chemical dihydrorhodamine which is phagocytosed when the neutrophils are activated. If the oxidative burst mechanism is intact, the dihydrorhodamine is reduced to rhodamine which is strongly fluorescent, and this fluorescence is detected by the flow cytometer. If the neutrophils have a defective oxidative burst mechanism, rhodamine is not produced, and the flow cytometer detects these abnormal neutrophils as nonfluorescent cells. The results in this patient were normal (Fig. 17.2).

For further evaluation of the patient, the presence of T helper (Th) 1, Th2, and Th17 cells in the peripheral blood was quantified which revealed a complete absence of Th17 cells. Subsequently, sequencing of the signal transducer and activator of transcription 3 (STAT3) gene was performed which revealed a missense mutation in the DNA binding domain of STAT3.

What Is Your Diagnosis and Why?

Based on the clinical presentation, absence of Th17 cells, and mutation in the STAT3 gene, this patient's diagnosis is hyper-IgE syndrome.

Case 2

The patient is a 2-year-old male who presents for the evaluation of multiple immunologic disorders seemingly unrelated. He was the product of a full term gestation and was born without any complications. Within the first weeks of life he developed widespread, difficult to control eczema. He also suffered from chronic oral candidiasis. Anemia and thrombocytopenia developed at 4 weeks of age, and autoantibodies were detected on the surface of red cells, neutrophils, and platelets. Multiple infusions of both red cells and platelets were required over the course of several months.

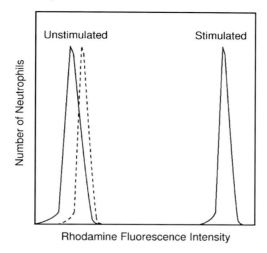

Fig. 17.2 Neutrophil oxidative burst capacity for Patient #1. When stimulated, the patient's neutrophils (*solid lines*) show normal oxidation of dihydrorhodamine to rhodamine as evidenced by a shift in the rhodamine fluorescence intensity to the right. The *dotted lines* demonstrate the shift that would be expected in neutrophils from an individual with chronic granulomatous disease which could not generate an oxidative burst

At 1 month of age the patient developed a persistent secretory diarrhea. Both infectious and hormonal causes of diarrhea were excluded, yet his clinical condition progressively worsened. By 8 months of age the patient had severe failure to thrive. The patient was subsequently diagnosed with insulin-dependent diabetes mellitus and hypothyroidism. At 18 months of age he started having symptoms of asthma such as nighttime coughing and wheezing and was started on controller medications.

The patient's severe gastrointestinal dysfunction and failure to thrive led to the placement of a gastrostomy tube to increase caloric intake. Infectious causes, eosinophilic gastritis, food allergy, and celiac disease were all ruled out with numerous stool cultures, elimination diets, as well as endoscopies with tissue biopsies. Biopsies of the esophagus were normal. Biopsies of the gastric mucosa, small intestines, and large intestines demonstrated chronic and diffuse gastritis and colitis without evidence of ulceration or exudate. The results of the duodenal biopsies were of the most diagnostic significance with the evidence of diffuse chronic enteritis with partial to near total villous atrophy consistent with the diagnosis of autoimmune enteritis (Fig. 17.3). Biopsies on repeated endoscopies yielded similar results, but on occasion suggested eosinophilic gastroenteritis. Despite dietary changes and total parenteral alimentation, there was very little improvement in his condition. Ultimately, the patient was placed on cyclosporine A intravenously. The diarrhea markedly improved with a decrease in the amount of stool volume and normalization of his stool electrolytes.

On physical examination the patient is comfortable but appears malnourished and cachectic. HEENT examination reveals oral candidiasis. Skin examination

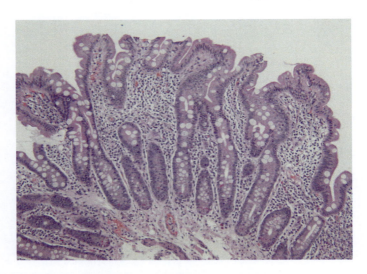

Fig. 17.3 Duodenal biopsy sample for Patient # 2. This demonstrates duodenal mucosa with diffuse chronic enteritis with near complete villous atrophy and glandular elongation. There are diffuse infiltrates of lymphocytes and plasma cells. These finding are consistent with the diagnosis of autoimmune enteritis. Photograph courtesy of Beverly B. Dahms

Table 17.2 Initial laboratory evaluation for case 2

Laboratory test	Result	Reference range
Complete blood count		
White blood cells	8,470/mm^3	4,000–12,000/mm^3
Hemoglobin (g/dl)	9.0	11–14
Platelets	475,000/mm^3	150,000–450,000/mm^3
Neutrophils	6,100/mm^3	1,400–6,600/mm^3
Lymphocytes	1,140/mm^3	1,500–5,500/mm^3
Monocytes	550/mm^3	100–600/mm^3
Eosinophils	680/mm^3	50–200/mm^3
Immunoglobulins		
IgG (mg/dl)	900	430–1,109
IgA (mg/dl)	125	15–142
IgM (mg/dl)	99	19–146
IgE (IU/ml)	32,000	2–120
Lymphocyte phenotyping		
CD3	890/mm^3 (78%)	1,180–6,960/mm^3 (59–87%)
CD4	565/mm^3 (50%)	650–3,650/mm^3 (29–57%)
CD8	320/mm^3 (28%)	160–1,200/mm^3 (7–31%)
CD19	220/mm^3 (19%)	150–1,520/mm^3 (6–19%)
CD16/56	30/mm^3 (3%)	0.2–1,440/mm^3 (0–18%)

shows widespread atopic dermatitis of moderate severity and a severe candidal diaper rash. The remainder of his physical examination is normal.

The patient's current medications include levothyroxine, nystatin oral suspension, subcutaneous insulin, inhaled corticosteroids, and multiple immunosuppressants including azathioprine and mycophenolate mofetil.

The initial laboratory evaluation is detailed in Table 17.2. Anti-pneumococcal and anti-tetanus toxoid IgG levels were present at protective levels. Lymphocyte proliferation assays to mitogens and antigens were normal.

With the Presented Data, What Is Your Working Diagnosis?

The differential diagnosis for this patient is broad due to the numerous abnormalities affecting multiple organ systems. Considerations include infections as well as genetic and congenital disorders. The latter disorders include Wiskott–Aldrich syndrome, Omenn syndrome, autoimmune lymphoproliferative syndrome (ALPS), autoimmune polyenocrinopathy-candidiasis-ecotdermal dystrophy syndrome (APECED), neonatal diabetes, pancreatic agenesis, and autoimmune enteropathy, among others.

Individuals with Wiskott–Aldrich syndrome and Omenn syndrome present with severe rashes, recurrent infections, and elevated IgE levels. However, the lack of thrombocytopenia and bleeding makes Wiskott–Aldrich syndrome an unlikely diagnosis for this patient. Likewise, Omenn syndrome is also unlikely because, as noted in Case 1, it is a form of severe combined immunodeficiency which invariably leads to death in infancy if a successful stem cell transplantation is not performed.

ALPS presents early in life with autoimmune phenomena including hemolytic anemia similar to that of this patient. However, patients with this syndrome also have striking lymphadenopathy and hepatosplenomegaly. Immunologically, ALPS is characterized by defective lymphocyte apoptosis that leads to the accumulation of nonmalignant lymphocytes. These long-lived lymphocytes lose their surface CD3 and CD4 leading to an abnormally large number of circulating CD4$^-$ CD8$^-$ T lymphocytes bearing $\alpha\beta$ T cell receptors. The patient in question did not have evidence of lymphadenopathy or hepatosplenomegally, and he had normal numbers of CD4$^-$ CD8$^-$ T lymphocytes, indicating that he did not have ALPS.

APECED is a rare autosomal recessive disorder caused by mutations in the autoimmune regulator (AIRE) gene. AIRE is a regulator of transcription with a key role in preventing the production of autoimmune T cells during thymic education. Defects in the AIRE protein lead to immune dysregulation with the primary clinical manifestation being autoimmune endocrinologic disorders. As with the current case, APECED patients present with chronic mucocutaneous candidiasis plus endocrine organ dysfunction leading to such disorders as diabetes mellitus, hypothyroidism, hypogonadism, adrenocortical failure, and hypoparathyroidism.

The concern for neonatal diabetes was evident in this patient due to the early onset of persistent hyperglycemia which required insulin for management. Neonatal diabetes mellitus often is a transient process which resolves spontaneously during infancy. These patients present with weight loss, volume depletion, and hyperglycemia frequently without ketoacidosis, but they do not present with the other autoimmune phenomena or with severe gastroenteritis as seen in our patient. Infants with permanent neonatal diabetes occasionally have pancreatic agenesis which this patient does not have evidence of.

The presence of numerous, seemingly unrelated inflammatory disorders in this patient is highly suggestive of immunodysregulation, polyendocrinopathy, enteropathy, X-linked (IPEX) syndrome. The spectrum of clinical disorders seen in individuals with IPEX syndrome includes autoimmune destruction of endocrine organs (leading to early onset insulin-dependent diabetes mellitus, hypothyroidism, and hypoparathyroidism), autoimmune enteropathy, eczema, autoimmune cytopenias, and failure to thrive. In the most severe forms of IPEX syndrome, symptoms present in the first several months of life. Immunologically, this disorder is characterized by the complete absence of CD4$^+$CD25$^+$ regulatory T cells (T$_{Regs}$) expressing the transcription factor Forkhead Box P3 (FOXP3). These cells are key regulators of the immune system, and their absence leads to the IPEX syndrome's hallmark immunodysregulation.

Work-Up

The patient's presentation and initial evaluation leads to a high index of suspicion for IPEX syndrome and APECED. The presence of IPEX syndrome was evaluated for first with the quantification of CD4$^+$CD25$^+$FOXP3$^+$T$_{Regs}$ which were found to be completely absent (Fig. 17.4). The FOXP3 gene was then sequenced which revealed a mutation affecting the DNA binding site of the protein.

What Is Your Diagnosis and Why?

Based on the clinical presentation, absence of CD4$^+$CD25$^+$FOXP3$^+$T$_{Regs}$, and mutation in the FOXP3 gene, this patient's diagnosis is IPEX syndrome.

Discussion

The human immune system's primary role is to protect against the myriad of pathogens to which individuals are naturally exposed. These pathogens are constantly evolving in order to evade recognition and destruction, therefore, the immune system has also evolved into a highly complex and rapidly adaptable system that can quickly combat microorganisms even as they try to avoid detection. The plasticity inherent in the immune system requires that it remain under strict regulatory control because inadvertent activation of the immune system can lead to unchecked inflammation and destruction of healthy tissue.

One of the primary methods by which the immune system's homeostasis is maintained is by tightly controlling those mechanisms that lead to activation of immune cells. Activation signals received by immune cells frequently culminate in the activation of transcription factors that modify gene transcription and cellular function. Mutations in these transcription factors lead to alterations in cellular function

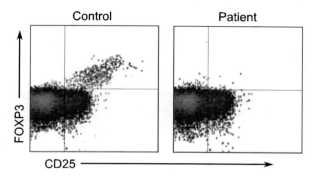

Fig. 17.4 FOXP3 expression for Patient #2. CD4⁺ T cells from the patient show no FOXP3 expression as compared to a control patient's cells which show normal FOXP3 staining

and subsequent dysregulation of immune function. This dysregulation can manifest in a number of ways including a heightened susceptibility to infections and the development of systemic inflammatory disorders as is seen in hyper-IgE syndrome and IPEX syndrome.

The monogenic transcription factor mutations seen in both hyper-IgE syndrome and IPEX syndrome lead to the absence of specific CD4⁺ T cell subtypes that are important in maintaining immune system homeostasis. CD4⁺ T cells are generally subdivided into T helper (Th) cells and regulatory T cells with abnormalities in the Th compartment being found in hyper-IgE syndrome and abnormalities in the regulatory compartment being found in IPEX syndrome.

Th cells are comprised of Th1, Th2, and Th17 cells, each of which produce distinct cytokines and promote different types of immune responses. For example, Th1 cells are prominent in promoting cellular immune responses against viruses, Th2 cells promote allergic inflammation, and Th17 cells promote immune responses against many pathogens. Dysfunctional STAT3 in hyper-IgE syndrome leads to an absence of Th17 cells.

Regulatory T cells are important mediators of immune responses and act to prevent pathologic inflammation. Expression of the transcription factor FOXP3 identifies a unique group of regulatory T cells (CD4⁺CD25⁺FOXP3⁺T$_{\text{Regs}}$) that help prevent autoimmune and allergic inflammation. The absence of FOXP3 in IPEX syndrome leads to an absence of these CD4⁺CD25⁺FOXP3⁺T$_{\text{Regs}}$.

Hyper-IgE Syndrome

Hyper-IgE syndrome is a rare disorder first described over 50 years ago. It was initially called Job's syndrome because the recurrent boils experienced by the patients were similar in description to the severe boils suffered by the biblical figure Job.

This disorder has traditionally been defined by the triad of elevated serum IgE levels, recurrent Staphylococcal abscesses, and pneumatocele formation secondary to Staphylococcal pneumonias. It is now recognized that these individuals have a number of other findings including severe eczema, recurrent candidiasis, delayed shedding of primary teeth, fractures after minor trauma due to osteopenia, eosinophilia, asymmetric and coarse facies, and hyperextensible joints (2). These findings are present to varying degrees in individuals with the disorder, but essentially all patients have elevated IgE levels, Staphylococcal abscesses, and eczema.

Hyper-IgE syndrome is primarily a sporadic disease with some cohorts showing an autosomal dominant inheritance pattern. An even rarer autosomal recessive form of the disease has also been described, but this appears to be a distinct clinical entity.

The presentation of the patient in Case 1 is typical for hyper-IgE syndrome. Eczema begins very early in infancy frequently followed by the development of recurrent soft tissue abscesses. Delayed deciduation of the primary teeth is noted around school age when the permanent teeth begin to erupt. The coarse, asymmetric facies tends to become more noticeable during adolescence. Staphylococcal pneumonias and other deep-seated Staphylococcal infections can occur at any age.

The underlying abnormality in most cases of hyper-IgE syndrome is abnormal STAT3 function (3, 4). STAT proteins are transcription factors that along with Janus kinases (JAK) form an important signal transduction mechanism known as the JAK-STAT signaling pathway (Fig. 17.5). Activation of surface receptors by their ligand leads to phosphorylation of these receptors and their subsequent aggregation. STAT proteins are then recruited to these receptor aggregates and are themselves phosphorylated by JAK. These phosphorylated STAT proteins then dimerize and

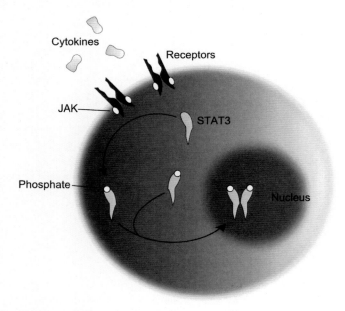

Fig. 17.5 JAK-STAT3 signaling pathway. Binding of cytokines to their receptors leads to phosphorylation of the intracellular component of the receptor by JAK. The receptors then aggregate, and STAT3 is recruited to the site of aggregation. STAT3 subsequently becomes phosphorylated by JAK, dimerizes, and then enters the nucleus to bind to target DNA sites

enter the nucleus to bind to their DNA targets, thereby altering the transcription of a multitude of genes.

STAT3 mutations in hyper-IgE syndrome create STAT3 proteins that cannot bind to their DNA targets. This leads to a breakdown of the JAK-STAT3 signaling pathway whereby activation of surface receptors in the JAK-STAT3 signaling pathway does not lead to the natural endpoint – altered target gene transcription. The lack of STAT3 function leads to the complete absence of Th17 cells, indicating that the presence of Th17 cells are imperative for the prevention of the clinical abnormalities seen in hyper-IgE syndrome (5).

Th17 cells have been demonstrated to be necessary for the eradication of certain pathogens, and their absence may be the cause of the recurrent infections seen in individuals with hyper-IgE syndrome. Furthermore, Th17 cells have an important role in osteogenesis in murine models which may explain why individuals with hyper-IgE syndrome develop osteopenia and dental abnormalities.

The diagnosis of hyper-IgE syndrome is based on identification of the noted clinical abnormalities in the presence of an elevated IgE level. Although extremely elevated IgE levels were previously thought to be necessary to make the diagnosis, it is now apparent that many individuals with hyper-IgE syndrome may have near normal or even normal IgE levels. The diagnosis may be confirmed by the absence Th17 cells in the peripheral blood or mutations in the STAT3 gene. STAT3 gene sequencing is available commercially while quantification of Th17 cells is currently only available on a research basis.

There is no curative therapy for hyper-IgE syndrome; therefore, therapy involves the prevention of infections and management of associated clinical abnormalities. All subjects should be placed on daily anti-Staphylococcal prophylaxis such as trimethoprim-sulfamethoxazole, and anti-fungal prophylaxis should be strongly considered since many patients die from invasive fungal disease. Intravenous immunoglobulin therapy has been helpful in some cases. All presumed infectious illnesses should be aggressively investigated with identification of a causative organism, if possible, in order to institute pathogen-specific therapy. Pneumatocele resection may be necessary if these become superinfected.

All children with the disorder should have regular dental examinations so that their primary teeth can be extracted if they do not naturally exfoliate during the eruption of the permanent teeth. Eczema care should be according to standard guidelines, but care should be taken not to unnecessarily restrict foods thought to be contributing to the eczema based on positive skin tests or food-specific serum IgE levels. In our experience, these patients have frequent false positive skin and serum test results.

Immunodysregulation, Polyendocrinopathy, Enteropathy, X-linked Syndrome

The recognition that severe diarrhea associated with various inflammatory and autoimmune disorders was a distinct clinical entity that could be inherited in an X-linked fashion was first made in 1982. In this initial report, a kindred of eight males spanning three generations had various combinations of intractable diarrhea, eczema, hemolytic anemia, thrombocytopenia, diabetes mellitus, thyroid disease, and infections. After identification of other kindreds with similar clinical features, this syndrome complex was given the name Immunodysregulation, Polyend ocrinopathy, Enteropathy, X-linked Syndrome, which is more commonly known as IPEX syndrome.

The clinical presentation of the patient in Case 2 is representative of how many patients with IPEX syndrome present. The most common findings are intractable diarrhea secondary to autoimmune enteritis and insulin-dependent diabetes mellitus which begin early infancy. Other findings include eczema, autoimmune hematologic cytopenias, hypothyroidism, lymphadenopathy, and hepatosplenomegally. The results of routine immunologic studies can be variable but are usually normal except for the frequent finding of elevated serum IgE levels. Recurrent infections are sometimes seen in IPEX syndrome, but these are usually secondary to the immunosuppressive therapies required to treat the disorder rather than an underlying inability to defend against pathogens.

As more individuals with IPEX syndrome were identified, it soon became apparent that these individuals shared many of immunologic characteristics with a murine model of immunodysregulation known as scurfy (6). The immunologic abnormalities in mouse scurfy were secondary to mutations in the transcription factor FOXP3, therefore, the homologous gene in humans was sequenced leading to the discovery that IPEX syndrome in humans was caused by mutations in FOXP3 (7).

FOXP3 is a master regulator of cellular function. Like other transcription factors, FOXP3 binds to the promoter region of numerous genes altering their transcription, but FOXP3 also directly interacts with and impedes the activity of other transcription factors, such as nuclear factor of activated T cells (NFAT) and nuclear factor kappa-B (NFκB), which are key players in cytokine production and other immune system functions.

Furthermore, FOXP3 is absolutely necessary for the generation of $CD4^+CD25^+FOXP3^+T_{Regs}$, therefore, these T_{Regs} are completely absent in IPEX syndrome. $CD4^+CD25^+FOXP3^+T_{Regs}$ play an essential role in maintaining immune system homeostasis and regulating immune tolerance by a number of mechanisms including suppressing the proliferation of lymphocytes, altering cytokine production by target lymphocytes and dendritic cells, and killing of target lymphocytes. Because T_{Regs} play an important role in the suppression of pathologic immune responses, their dysfunction leads to the development of numerous disease processes including allergic and autoimmune diseases. The complete lack of $CD4^+CD25^+FOXP3^+T_{Regs}$ in IPEX syndrome leads to the wholesale immunodysregulation seen in this syndrome which causes the severe allergic and autoimmune phenotype seen in affected individuals.

The diagnosis of IPEX syndrome is based on the recognition of a compatible clinical phenotype usually in early infancy. The presence of an X-linked inheritance pattern or the early death of males on the maternal side of the family is helpful in making the diagnosis. The diagnosis is confirmed by the lack of intracellular FOXP3 staining in any T cells and the identification of a mutation in the FOXP3 gene. These assays are currently available on a commercial basis from a small number of laboratories.

The mainstay of therapy in IPEX syndrome is immunosuppressive therapy to limit the extent of autoimmune and inflammatory tissue destruction. Any number of immunosuppressive therapies have been attempted (such as cyclosporine A, corticosteroids, tacrolimus, azathioprine, etc.), but the choice of specific medications should be tailored to the individual patient. Appropriate nutritional support is imperative and may include enteral feeding through a gastrostomy tube or parenteral nutrition. Other therapies are based on the individual disorders experienced by each individual, such as thyroid replacement therapy in hypothyroid patients.

The clinical response to the above therapies is frequently poor with patients frequently dying in infancy or early childhood, therefore, stem cell transplantation has been attempted as a curative therapy. A number of investigators have reported reversal of autoimmune pathologies and significant clinical improvement after transplantation. Early attempts at transplantation were associated with an unacceptably high mortality rate from transplantation-related complications such as infection and hemophagocytic syndrome. More recently, there have been a number of successful stem cell transplantations with good outcomes at up to 30 months posttransplantation (8, 9). This indicates that early stem cell transplantation may become the standard of care for IPEX syndrome since the disorder is otherwise usually associated with the fatality in early childhood. Longer follow-up data on transplanted patients is necessary before the role of transplantation in the therapy of IPEX syndrome is fully established.

Conclusion

Immune system homeostasis is tightly maintained by regulatory mechanisms that allow for the destruction of pathologic microorganisms while preventing pathologic inflammation. Disruption of these regulatory mechanisms can lead to immunodeficiency and uncontrolled inflammation as seen in hyper-IgE syndrome and IPEX syndrome. Ongoing research is further elucidating the roles of the mutated transcription factors that underlie the immunodysregulation seen in hyper-IgE syndrome and IPEX syndrome, and this may allow for the development of more effective therapies for affected individuals.

Questions

1. Hyper-IgE syndrome is traditionally defined by which of the following triads?

   (a) Recurrent Staphylococcal abscesses, bronchiectasis, and elevated IgE levels
   (b) Recurrent Streptococcus abscesses, pneumatoceles, and elevated IgE levels

(c) Recurrent pneumonia, bronchiectasis, and elevated IgE levels

(d) Recurrent Staphylococcal abscesses, pneumatoceles, and elevated IgE levels

2. A patient with a history of delayed shedding of the primary teeth, severe eczema, and recurrent abscesses is likely to have a history of which of the following conditions?

(a) Bone cysts

(b) Fractures following a minor trauma

(c) Autoimmune enteritis

(d) Thrombocytopenia

3. Hyper IgE syndrome can be characterized by which of the following molecular abnormalities?

(a) Mutation in the transcription factor FOXP3

(b) Mutation in the DNA binding domain of STAT3

(c) Absence of Th17 cells

(d) Both (a) and (c)

(e) Both (b) and (c)

4. The main features of IPEX syndrome can be described by which of the following?

(a) X-linked syndrome, bronchiectasis, enteropathy, and immunodeficiency

(b) X-linked syndrome, polyendocrinopathy, immune dysregulation, and eczema

(c) X-linked syndrome, polyendocrinopathy, immune dysregulation, and enteropathy

(d) X-linked syndrome, pneumonia, enteropathy, and immunodeficiency

5. IPEX syndrome is characterized by which of the following molecular abnormalities?

(a) Mutation in the transcription factor FOXP3

(b) Mutation in the DNA binding domain of STAT3

(c) Absence of CD25

(d) Both (a) and (c)

(e) None of the above

Answer Key: 1. (d); 2. (b); 3. (e); 4. (c); 5. (a).

References

1. Kobashi Y, Yoshida K, Miyashita N, et al. (2005) Infectious bulla of the lung caused by Mycobacterium intracellular. J Infect Chemother **11**, 293–6.
2. Grimbacher B, HollandSM, GallinJI, et al. (1999) Hyper-IgE syndrome with recurrent infections – and autosomal dominant multisystem disorder. N Engl J Med **340**, 692–702.

3. Holland SM, DeLeoFR, Elloumi HZ, et al. (2007) STAT3 mutations in the hyper-IgE syndrome. N Engl J Med **357**, 1–12.
4. Minegishi Y, Saito M, Tsuchiya S, et al. (2007) Dominant-negative mutations in the DNA-binding domain of STAT 3 cause hyper-IgE syndrome. Nature **448**, 1058–62.
5. Milner JD, BrenchleyJM, LaurenceA, et al. (2008) Impaired Th17 cell differentiation in subjects with autosomal dominant hyper-IgE syndrome. Nature **452**, 773–6.
6. Wildin RS, RamsdellF, PeakeJ, et al. (2001) X-linked neonatal diabetes mellitus, enteropathy and endocrinopathy syndrome is the human equivalent of mouse scurfy. Nat Genet **27**, 18–20.
7. Bennett CL, RamsdellCJ, BrunkowME, et al. (2001) The immune dysregulation, polyendo-crinopathy, enteropathy, X-linked syndrome (IPEX) is caused by mutations of FOXP3. Nat Genet **27**, 20–1.
8. Rao A, Kamani N, Filipovich A, et al. (2007) Successful bone marrow transplantation for IPEX syndrome after reduced-intensity conditioning. Blood **109**, 383–5.
9. Zhan H, Sinclair J, Adams S, et al. (2008) Immune reconstitution and recovery of FOXP3 (Forkhead Box P3)-expressing T cells after transplantation for IPEX (immune dysregulation, polyendocrinopathy, enteropathy, X-linked) syndrome. Pediatrics **121**, e998–1002.

Chapter 18
Autoimmune Diseases

Marcy B. Bolster

Abstract Autoimmune diseases are characterized by autoantibody formation and visceral involvement that is often of an inflammatory nature. Rheumatoid arthritis (RA) is a classic immune complex disease characterized by antibody formation and inflammatory arthritis. Extra-articular manifestations of RA may also occur. Systemic sclerosis (scleroderma, SSc) is another autoimmune disease and includes autoantibody formation as well as visceral involvement; however, the visceral manifestations in SSc relate to excessive collagen deposition and/or a vasculopathy. Internal organ inflammatory changes are typically seen in other autoimmune diseases; however, these do not typically occur in SSc.

Keywords Autoimmune diseases • Rheumatoid arthritits • Systemic sclerosis

Case 1

A 36-year-old woman presents to her primary care physician with an 8-week history of painful swelling in her wrists, hands, and ankles. She reports that her symptoms began in her feet and ankles and subsequently involved her wrists and hands. Her symptoms are worse upon awakening and she notes marked stiffness in her hands for the first 3 h of the day. She reports that her feet feel as though she is "walking on rocks" when she first wakes up. She denies back pain or other joint symptoms. She has also noted occasional tingling in her fingertips for the past 3 weeks. The patient works as a temporary pool nurse at the hospital and has experienced great difficulty with working in the early morning shift. She has taken ibuprofen 400 mg three times daily with only minimal relief.

M.B. Bolster (✉)
Director, Rheumatology Fellowship Training Program, Medical University of South Carolina, Charleston, SC, USA
e-mail: bolsterm@musc.edu

M. Mahmoudi (ed.), *Challenging Cases in Allergy and Immunology*,
DOI: 10.1007/978-1-60327-443-2_18,
© Humana Press, a part of Springer Science+Business Media, LLC 2009

Her past medical history is significant for a 3-day hospitalization 3 months ago for aseptic meningitis, which was diagnosed based on clinical presentation as well as cerebrospinal fluid pleocytosis and elevated protein. Her hospital course was uncomplicated. She has two children of age 7 and 4 years. Her 4-year-old daughter had a viral illness characterized by fever, facial rash, rhinitis, and cough 4–5 months ago. Her family history is notable for a paternal uncle with Crohn's disease. Her only medication is ibuprofen. She has no known allergies.

She denies fever, oral or genital ulcers, shortness of breath, chest pain, gastro-esophageal reflux, nausea, vomiting, diarrhea, Raynaud phenomenon, history of inflammatory eye disease, or skin rash. She does report a longstanding history of developing a skin rash with sun exposure.

On physical examination she is afebrile and vital signs are within normal limits. HEENT examination reveals anicteric sclerae, no oral lesions or ulcers, and no cervical or submandibular lymphadenopathy. Lung, cardiac, and abdominal exami-nations are unremarkable. The skin is without rash, including examination of the scalp, umbilicus, and gluteal cleft. Musculoskeletal examination reveals synovitis of bilateral first through fifth proximal interphalangeal (PIP) joints, bilateral first and fifth metacarpophalangeal (MCP) joints, and bilateral wrists (Fig. 18.1). There is reduced extension and flexion of bilateral wrists. There is also synovitis of the right ankle and tenderness of the metatarsophalangeal (MTP) joints to compression. Bilateral ankles demonstrate stiffness with range of motion. The remainder of the joint examination is unremarkable. Neurologic examination reveals a positive Tinel's sign bilaterally; otherwise, motor, sensory, reflex, and cranial nerve testing is unremarkable.

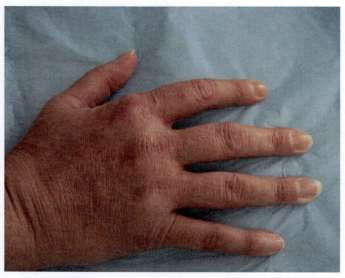

Fig. 18.1 Clinical photograph of the patient demonstrating synovitis of the right wrist, PIP, and MCP joints

With the Presented History and Physical Examination Findings, What Is Your Working Diagnosis?

This patient presents with an 8-week history of additive, symmetrical polyarthritis of small and medium joints. She provides a history of longstanding photosensitivity. She has a history of a diagnosed viral illness 3 months ago (aseptic meningitis). She is a healthcare worker and a mother, and thus has the potential for other viral exposures. She has a family history of Crohn's disease, which can be associated with the development of a seronegative spondyloarthropathy.

Differential Diagnosis

The differential diagnosis at this point should include postviral sequela of arthritis (as relates to the recent episode of aseptic meningitis) termed a reactive arthritis, Parvovirus B19-associated arthritis, Hepatitis C arthropathy, acute Hepatitis B arthritis, HIV, rheumatoid arthritis (RA), systemic lupus erythematosus (SLE), and one of the seronegative spondyloarthropathies, including psoriatic arthritis, ankylosing spondylitis this, or inflammatory bowel disease associated arthritis.

Evaluation

Laboratory testing should include a CBC, CMP, and urinalysis as well as other specific autoimmune and viral serologies. In this case, laboratory results reveal a normal or negative CBC, CMP, urinalysis, HIV, Hepatitis B sAg, and Hepatitis C antibody. Additionally, an anti-DNA antibody, anti-Smith antibody, C3, C4, and Parvovirus B19 IgM levels are negative or normal. Parvovirus B19 IgG is positive. Additional positive lab testing includes an antinuclear antibody (ANA) 1:320, speckled, rheumatoid factor (RF) 199 IU/mL, anticyclic citrullinated peptide (anti-CCP) antibody 88 U/mL, and Hepatitis B surface antibody. The erythrocyte sedimentation rate (ESR) is 50 mm/h. A radiograph of the sacroiliac joints is normal. A radiograph of the hands reveals periarticular osteopenia and erosive changes at the MCP and PIP joints.

What Is Your Diagnosis and Why?

This patient has a typical presentation of rheumatoid arthritis (RA) and she meets the American Rheumatism Association (ARA) 1987 criteria for the diagnosis of RA (1) (see Table 18.1). Specifically, she presents with a greater than 6-week history of a symmetrical polyarthritis involving the small joints of the hands, as

Table 18.1 The 1987 American Rheumatology Association (ARA) criteria for rheumatoid arthritis (1)

Morning stiffness lasting >1 h
Arthritis in three or more joint areas observed by a physician, occurring simultaneously, and present for >6-weeks duration
Arthritis of the hand joints including wrists, proximal interphalangeal joints, and metacarpophalangeal joints and present for >6 weeks
Symmetric arthritis for >6 weeks
Rheumatoid nodules present as defined by subcutaneous nodules located over boney prominences
Rheumatoid factor positive
Radiographic changes of erosions on hand films

well as other joints. This patient has prolonged morning stiffness. Lab testing reveals a positive RF and there are erosions visualized on hand radiographs.

There are clearly many other considerations in the differential diagnosis for this patient; however, RA is the best diagnosis to confirm at this time. The development of an inflammatory arthritis in a young woman should always place SLE into the differential diagnosis. Additionally, this patient has a history of photosensitivity, which is one other criterion for the diagnosis of SLE. In order to confirm a diagnosis of SLE, four criteria are needed (see Chap. 19). Further review of the records from the recent hospitalization to confirm that the central nervous system (CNS) process was in fact attributable to a viral meningitis would also be of consideration since CNS involvement is one of the manifestations of SLE. CNS disease in SLE can manifest as cerebritis, aseptic meningitis (particularly in patients taking nonsteroidal anti-inflammatory agents), or cerebrovascular accident. This patient did not have other positive serologies characteristic of SLE, aside from the positive ANA. The positive ANA may well be associated with the presentation of RA since many patients with RA will have a positive ANA, particularly early in the disease. It would not be unreasonable, however, to monitor this patient for other manifestations of SLE, as many rheumatic diseases may have overlap features with other connective tissue diseases.

Many viral illnesses are associated with the development of an inflammatory polyarthritis including Parvovirus B19, acute Hepatitis B infection, acute or chronic Hepatitis C infection, and HIV infection. This patient has a child who likely may have had a recent Parvovirus B19 infection. The patient's symptoms, however, began 2–3 months after her daughter's illness. Classically, the postviral sequela of arthritis associated with Parvovirus B19 occurs within 1–2 weeks of the illness, or of viral exposure, with an overall duration typically of 6 weeks. The patient's presentation with arthritis is thus at a later time than would be expected if due to Parvovirus infection. To lend further support to the fact that this likely is not a Parvovirus B19 infection is that her serologies demonstrate a prior exposure to Parvovirus B19 (positive Parvovirus B19 IgG antibody) without evidence of acute or recent exposure (negative IgM antibody to Parvovirus B19). The patient also has a documented personal history of a viral infection as she had a recent hospitalization for aseptic meningitis. It is also possible that she could have developed a postviral arthritis; however, the time course, both in terms of interval and duration, is somewhat prolonged over what would have been expected. A postviral synovitis typically presents within the first 1–2 weeks following viral exposure and classically resolves within 6–8 weeks.

As a health care worker, consideration must be given to viral exposures including Hepatitis B, Hepatitis C, and HIV. Hepatitis B can be associated with an acute arthritis syndrome and this may present prior to the patient's development of transaminase elevation and/or of icterus. This patient's serologies for Hepatitis B indicate prior exposure or immunization. Hepatitis C can present with an additive inflammatory polyarthritis involving the small joints of the hands and feet, and this may be difficult to clinically distinguish from RA. However, Hepatitis C causes a nonerosive arthropathy. A positive RF commonly occurs in Hepatitis C due to the chronic inflammatory nature of the disease; however, the positive anti-CCP antibody, highly specific for RA, is not found in Hepatitis C infection. Thus, this patient has a clinical presentation that could be consistent with Hepatitis C arthropathy; however, the presence of the anti-CCP antibody and radiographic evidence of erosions make this an unlikely diagnosis.

HIV arthropathy can present as an inflammatory synovitis of the small joints of the hands and feet and should be of consideration in this patient's case; however, the HIV testing is negative, making this an unlikely diagnosis.

The patient has a family history of Crohn disease, which raises the suspicion for a seronegative spondyloarthropathy. The seronegative spondyloarthropathies are most often associated with a positive HLA-B27 and include ankylosing spondylitis, inflammatory bowel disease, psoriatic arthritis, and reactive arthritis. Behcet disease can also be associated with sacroiliitis. This patient does not have symptoms or findings of sacroiliitis, evidence of psoriasis, or history suggestive of inflammatory bowel disease. A reactive arthritis can occur following a bacterial infection such as with a bacterial enterocolitis or after a sexually transmitted disease of the genitourinary tract, and be associated with sacroiliitis and peripheral oligoarticular arthritis. This patient does not have a history suggestive of these. Although skin and gastrointestinal manifestations of the seronegative spondyloarthropathies are not currently present, the arthritis associated with psoriasis or with inflammatory bowel disease may present many years prior to the onset of skin or gastrointestinal disease, respectively. HLA-B27 testing is, in fact, negative in this case. Although it cannot be definitively stated that this patient's presentation is not due to an early stage of a seronegative spondyloarthropathy, this patient has classic findings of RA and meets criteria for RA. Although a symmetrical peripheral synovitis may occur in a seronegative spondyloarthropathy, it would be highly unusual to have such a presentation in the absence of back pain, sacroiliitis, signs and symptoms of Crohn disease, or psoriasis, and to have a negative HLA-B27.

It is worth mentioning that Behcet disease may be manifested by aseptic meningitis. Other clinical features of Behcet disease include oral and genital ulcers, uveitis, arthritis (usually an asymmetric oligoarticular presentation), erythema nodosum, and the more severe manifestations of vascular aneurysms and CNS vasculitis. Although this patient had a recent episode of aseptic meningitis, she does not have features otherwise typical of Behcet disease. She does have classic features and findings of RA.

Discussion

RA is an autoimmune disease characterized by an inflammatory, symmetrical polyarthritis. RA is a very common form of arthritis and has been estimated to occur in approximately 1% of the US population. It more commonly occurs in women, with a 3:1 predilection for women compared with men (2). Its incidence is estimated at 0.75 per 1,000 adults per year (3).

The clinical presentation of a patient with RA includes a symmetrical, polyarticular, inflammatory arthritis typically involving the small joints of the hands and feet in association with prolonged morning stiffness that has been present for at least 6 weeks in duration. Patients may also have subcutaneous nodules typically located on the extensor surfaces of the arms or at the Achilles tendons.

Laboratory testing demonstrates a positive rheumatoid factor (RF) in 85% of patients at the time of presentation. Many patients may also have a positive ANA. The anti-CCP antibody is highly specific for RA, and if present in combination with a positive RF, it has a 95% specificity for the diagnosis of RA (4). The presence of anti-CCP antibody is associated with a poorer prognosis including an increased likelihood for the development of erosive disease. Radiographic changes most commonly occur in the hands and feet and include periarticular osteopenia and marginal erosions, which are evident on plain films. Ultrasound and MRI are modalities that are also being used to evaluate for the presence of synovitis and/or early erosive changes (5).

There is good evidence that treatment for RA should be instituted early, and that early aggressive management reduces inflammation and pain, loss of function, as well as progressive, erosive, deforming arthritis (American College of Rheumatology subcommittee on Rheumatoid Arthritis Guidelines, 2002) (6). The ACR recommendations are such that disease-modifying antirheumatic drug (DMARD) therapy should be initiated within the first 3 months of symptom onset (Table 18.2). In appropriate patients the first line of treatment would be methotrexate, and if the patient does not obtain an adequate clinical response, then additional DMARD therapy should be considered. This may include the addition of hydroxychloroquine and sulfasalazine (triple therapy), or leflunomide, or tumor necrosis factor alpha (TNF-alpha) antagonists. Glucocorticoids can be used as short-term anti-inflammatory agents to help gain rapid symptomatic relief for the patient; however, the dosage should be reduced quickly and discontinued as soon as possible in order to avoid toxicities associated with glucocorticoid use. The early referral to the rheumatologist of the patient with RA plays a key role in the management of these patients so that early, aggressive therapy may be initiated.

Table 18.2 Disease-modifying antirheumatic drugs (DMARDs) used in treating patients with RA

Methotrexate
Hydroxychloroquine
Sulfasalazine
Leflunomide
Cyclosporine
Azathioprine
Etanercept
Adalimumab
Infliximab
Abatacept
Rituximab

Case 2

A 25-year-old woman presents to her primary care physician with an 8-month history of skin changes involving her fingers, hands, forearms, and face. She also reports a 6-month history of gastroesophageal reflux symptoms. She has noted an increased level of fatigue for the past 2 months and she reports dyspnea on exertion with climbing steps in her home.

She was last seen by this physician 18 months ago when she noted a 2-year history of sensitivity of her hands such that her fingertips would turn blue with exposure to cold. There were no skin changes or other symptoms at that time and she was otherwise well. Her primary care physician performed lab testing at that visit 2 years ago, and she was noted to have a negative or normal CBC, comprehensive metabolic panel (CMP), urinalysis, ESR, and RF. An ANA was 1:640 nucleolar.

Her past medical history is otherwise unremarkable. Family history is noncontributory. She takes famotidine 20 mg as needed for gastroesophageal reflux with some relief.

On review of systems, she denies chest pain, nausea, vomiting, constipation, photosensitivity, oral ulcers, or joint swelling. She has had some joint pain in her knees.

On physical examination, she is afebrile. Her blood pressure is 118/72, pulse 78, and respiratory rate 20. Skin examination reveals thickening over the fingers, hands, forearms, and face. There are telangiectasias on her face, palms, and chest. Digital pits are not present. HEENT, cardiac, lung, and abdominal examinations are unremarkable. There is no lower extremity edema. Musculoskeletal examination reveals tendon friction rubs at the left knee and right wrist. All joints have full range of motion and there is no joint swelling present. Neurologic examination is intact.

With the History and Examination Presented, What Is Your Working Diagnosis?

This patient presents with a 3–4-year history of Raynaud phenomenon and the recent development of skin thickening, gastroesophageal reflux symptoms, and dyspnea on exertion. Her examination reveals skin thickening typical of limited cutaneous systemic sclerosis (SSc) with skin changes noted distal to the elbows and knees only. Diffuse cutaneous involvement is defined by skin changes in a proximal distribution, including skin changes proximal to the elbows and knees and also potentially involving the trunk. Facial involvement may occur with either limited or diffuse cutaneous disease. Of note, however, patients with SSc may have progression of their skin disease within the first 2 years following the onset of skin findings, such that it is premature, in this patient, to diagnose her with limited cutaneous SSc, formerly termed CREST (*c*alcinosis, *R*aynaud phenomenon, *e*sophageal dysmotility, *s*clerodactyly, *t*elangiectasia) syndrome. The duration of her skin changes is too brief to be assured that she will not have more proximal progression of skin thickening. Additionally, the presence of tendon friction rubs is predictive of the development of diffuse cutaneous disease (7). Thus, in summary, this patient has limited cutaneous involvement of systemic sclerosis; however, the duration of her findings falls within the first 2 years of disease onset, thus progression of her skin disease may occur. In fact, skin disease progression is likely to occur as predicted by the presence of the tendon friction rubs. She also meets ACR criteria for the diagnosis of systemic sclerosis (Table 18.3) (8) since she fulfills one major criterion.

Differential Diagnosis

The differential diagnosis at this time includes systemic sclerosis as the most likely explanation of her symptoms and signs. This patient has a classic presentation of SSc. Of consideration in the differential diagnosis is whether she has limited or diffuse cutaneous disease, as previously discussed. Other fibrosing skin conditions to consider, though are much less likely, include eosinophilic fasciitis, scleromyxedema, scleredema, and nephrogenic fibrosing dermopathy.

Evaluation

Further evaluation is warranted. Laboratory testing should include a CBC, BMP, and urinalysis. Visceral involvement in SSc may be associated with lab abnormalities, thus routine lab testing, as described, is advisable. Early signs of scleroderma renal

Table 18.3 ACR criteria for systemic sclerosis (scleroderma, SSc) (8)

Major criterion
Proximal skin thickening (proximal to the metacarpophalangeal joints)
Minor criteria
Sclerodactyly
Digital pitting scars
Bibasilar pulmonary fibrosis

SSc diagnosis is confirmed with the presence of one major criterion or two minor criteria crisis, in addition to new onset hypertension, may include microangiopathic hemolytic anemia, thrombocytopenia, proteinuria, and microscopic hematuria. Renal insufficiency also occurs in scleroderma renal crisis, and the worsening of renal function may be detected as small as a 20–30% change from a normal creatinine level and should raise concern. Patients with scleroderma renal crisis or those with occult gastrointestinal blood loss may present with anemia. Additional serologic testing should include an anti-Scl-70 antibody and anti-RNA-polymerase III antibody. The anti-Scl-70-antibody is associated with an increased risk of developing diffuse cutaneous SSc and interstitial lung disease (ILD) (9) and anti-RNA- polymerase III antibody is associated with diffuse cutaneous skin disease and scleroderma renal crisis. An anticentromere antibody is most often associated with limited cutaneous SSc (9). Further evaluation of this patient's complaint of dyspnea is also warranted.

The laboratory testing reveals a normal CBC, BMP, and urinalysis. The anti-Scl-70 antibody is 212 units (normal < 99 units). A chest radiograph is normal. Pulmonary function testing (PFT) is performed and the patient's forced vital capacity (FVC) is 65% predicted and diffusion capacity (DLCO) is 68% predicted. The FEV1 and FEV1/FVC are normal. An echocardiogram reveals a normal left ventricular ejection fraction, normal right ventricular pressures and volumes, normal valvular function, and no pericardial effusion.

Diagnosis

This patient has limited cutaneous SSc at the time of this presentation. She reported initial symptoms of Raynaud phenomenon 3–4 years before, and during her previous work-up, she was found to have a positive ANA in a nucleolar pattern on immunofluorescence. Raynaud phenomenon may occur as a primary or secondary condition. The presence of a positive ANA and/or nailfold capillary changes, using widefield microscopy, are predictive of the development of a connective tissue disease in a patient with Raynaud phenomenon (10, 11). An ANA in a nucleolar pattern is most likely to be found in patients with SSc (11). Thus, it was predictable at the time of her prior office visit that she was at risk for developing a connective tissue disease, and SSc was of high consideration.

The patient has evidence at the current time of limited cutaneous systemic sclerosis; however, she has indicators present that are predictive of the development of diffuse cutaneous disease, including tendon friction rubs, positive anti-Scl-70 antibody, and knowing that her disease duration is of less than 2 years. Patients with either limited or diffuse cutaneous SSc are at risk of developing ILD; however, ILD occurs more commonly in those patients with diffuse skin disease. The positive anti-Scl-70 antibody is also predictive of the development of ILD. Patients are at highest risk for the development of ILD within the first 4 years of disease duration (12).

Patients with SSc and ILD typically present with a restrictive pattern on PFT. It is not uncommon for these patients to have a paucity of physical findings, though bibasilar late crackles could also be a characteristic physical examination finding. A normal chest radiograph is also reasonably common. This patient does demonstrate a restrictive pattern on PFTs with a reduced FVC. The DLCO is also reduced and it is proportionately reduced to the lung volume loss. A disproportionate reduction in DLCO, as compared with lung volumes, can be suggestive of pulmonary vascular disease (13). Additionally, early in the course of ILD the DLCO can be the first abnormal finding. Nevertheless, in this patient the lung volume (FVC) and DLCO are proportionately reduced suggestive of an interstitial process. Further testing with a high-resolution computed tomography (HRCT) scan of the chest is warranted in order to evaluate for ILD as well as for the presence of ground glass opacification, indicative of alveolitis.

Discussion

Systemic sclerosis (SSc) is a disease characterized by microvascular injury, excessive tissue fibrosis, and autoimmunity. The etiology of the disease is unknown. The peak age of onset is 30–50 years and there is a female predominance. SSc does not occur more commonly in African-American patients; however, the severity of disease is greater in African-American patients.

Sytemic sclerosis has broad visceral involvement including the skin, vasculature, gastrointestinal tract, lungs, kidneys, heart, and musculoskeletal system. It is also associated with autoimmunity, and patients typically have a positive ANA. The most specific immunofluorescence patterns of the ANA in SSc are nucleolar and centromere. An anti-centromere antibody most often occurs in patients with limited cutaneous SSc (9). Other autoantibodies occurring in patients with diffuse cutaneous SSc include a positive anti-Scl-70 antibody and a positive RNA polymerase III antibody, the former being associated with an increased risk of developing ILD, and the latter associated with an increased risk of scleroderma renal crisis.

The skin manifestations of SSc include skin thickening, digital pits, telangiectasias, and digital ulcerations. The characteristic skin changes typically begin with thickening of the skin on the fingers and hands and progress more proximally. Limited cutaneous skin changes involve the skin distal to the elbows and/or knees and may involve the fingers, hands, forearms, feet, and lower legs. Diffuse cutaneous involvement includes regions proximal to the elbows and/or knees. Thickening of the skin on the face can occur in either limited or diffuse cutaneous disease. Digital pits are the result of ischemic tissue injury of the fingers as a result of Raynaud phenomenon and occur on the fingertips. Digital pits are one of the diagnostic criteria for SSc (Table 18.3). Telangiectasias occur on the fingers, palms, chest, face, and oral mucosa. Skin ulcerations, most typically involving the fingers, occur due to Raynaud phenomenon.

Nearly all patients with SSc have cold sensitivity of their hands – Raynaud phenomenon. Additionally, larger vessel involvement may occur and contribute to the presence of ischemic digital ulcers, such as involvement of the ulnar arteries. The ischemic insult to the digits occurs as a result of vasospasm as well as due to vascular narrowing from intimal proliferation and adventitial fibrosis. Poorly healing digital ulcers can develop in patients with SSc who may benefit from vasodilator therapy, aspirin, digital sympathectomy, or arterial bypass. Antibiotics may be required if the digital ulcers become infected.

Nearly all patients with SSc will have gastrointestinal involvement (GI) and this may include all or part of the GI tract. Gastroesophageal reflux is the most common GI manifestation and may be associated with the development of esophageal strictures or Barrett's esophagus. Dysmotility is also characteristic of GI tract involvement and may include delayed gastric emptying, small bowel bacterial overgrowth, intestinal pseudo-obstruction, and rectal incontinence. Malabsorption may also occur. The GI manifestations are treated symptomatically and include H2-blocker therapy, proton pump inhibitors, promotility agents, and rotating antibiotics for bacterial overgrowth. In patients with intestinal pseudo-obstruction, the management is nonsurgical and includes bowel rest, decompression from above and below, IV fluids, possible parenteral nutrition, and careful use of opiate pain medications.

Lung disease is the major cause of morbidity and mortality in patients with SSc. The two most common forms of lung disease in SSc include ILD and pulmonary vascular disease [pulmonary artery hypertension (PAH)]. ILD can occur in patients with limited or diffuse cutaneous disease, but is more common in patients with diffuse skin involvement. Patients with ILD will present with dyspnea and perhaps a dry cough. PFT will reveal a restrictive pattern with reduced lung volumes. An early finding may be a reduction in diffusion capacity (DLCO) even before the loss of lung volumes occur. The chest radiograph may be normal or may demonstrate basilar fibrosis. A high-resolution CT scan will show ground glass opacification (alveolitis) and interstitial fibrosis. There is evidence to suggest that patients with SSc and ILD have a benefit from treatment with daily oral cyclophosphamide (14). The Scleroderma Lung Study also demonstrated that the HRCT scan of the chest is an adequate investigative tool to evaluate for alveolitis (14). A bronchoalveolar lavage is not warranted unless an infectious etiology of lung symptoms is being considered. Similarly, an open lung or videoscopic lung biopsy is not needed to document the presence of ILD and alveolitis in association with SSc.

Isolated PAH may occur in patients with limited cutaneous SSc, or PAH may occur secondary to underlying ILD or heart disease including valvular heart disease or diastolic dysfunction. Patients with PAH will present with dyspnea, fatigue, and/or rarely with syncope. An isolated reduction in the DLCO on PFTs is characteristic of PAH (13). PAH can be detected by echocardiogram; however, right heart catheterization is required for management of patients with vasodilator therapy. Vasodilator therapy may include prostacyclin, endothelin-receptor antagonists, and phosphodiesterase type V inhibitors. Other therapies include supplemental oxygen and warfarin.

Renal disease in SSc is not of an inflammatory nature as might be seen in other autoimmune diseases. Scleroderma renal crisis is heralded by an elevation of the patient's blood pressure and is associated with microangiopathy. Laboratory abnormalities include a hemolytic anemia (non-Coombs), thrombocytopenia, and elevation of serum creatinine. The urinalysis may reveal proteinuria and microscopic hematuria. The pathologic changes in scleroderma renal crisis are similar to those seen in hypertensive emergency and are characterized by intimal hyperplasia and fibrinoid necrosis of vessel walls. Treatment with angiotensin-converting enzyme (ACE) inhibitors has markedly affected the morbidity and mortality associated with this disease manifestation. ACE inhibitors are the drug of choice and should be continued even if the renal insufficiency worsens and/or the patient requires dialysis. Improved renal function with ACE inhibitors may occur months after the progression of the renal insufficiency. Angiotensin receptor blocking agents have not had the same consistent success in the treatment of scleroderma renal crisis.

Cardiac involvement occurs frequently in patients with SSc as found on postmortem examination; however, it is much less likely to be clinically apparent. Cardiac manifestations include conduction abnormalities, diastolic dysfunction, and cardiomyopathy. Rarely, large pericardial effusions will occur. If clinically detected, treatment of cardiac manifestations should be focused on appropriate clinical management as in any other patient with similar cardiac abnormalities.

Musculoskeletal involvement is very common in patients with SSc and may include arthralgia, inflammatory arthritis, flexion contractures due to skin thickening, and tendon friction rubs. Tendon friction rubs occur in patients with diffuse skin involvement or are indicative of the likelihood of a patient with limited skin involvement progressing to have diffuse skin thickening. Proximal muscle weakness may occur in SSc and may be due to a bland myopathy of SSc or due to an overlap with polymyositis. Treatment of the musculoskeletal manifestations includes analgesia for the arthralgia, physical and occupational therapy to avoid flexion contractures, and immunosuppression for inflammatory joint or muscle involvement.

The management of patients with SSc is focused on the particular visceral manifestation. Immunosuppression with glucocorticoids is rarely indicated since SSc is typically not an inflammatory disorder. There are instances of inflammatory manifestations of disease that warrant glucocorticoids, such as inflammatory arthritis or inflammatory myopathy. Glucocorticoids are used in the lowest doses possible and for the briefest possible time due to the association of the development of normotensive renal crisis in patients with SSc who have been treated with high doses of glucocorticoids (15). There is not a known effective disease modifying agent, thus immunosuppression with steroid-sparing agents is rarely indicated.

Questions

1. A 24-year-old woman presents with a 3-month history of pain and swelling in her PIP and MCP joints bilaterally. She has morning stiffness lasting 3 h. Examination reveals synovitis of the PIPs and MCPs as well as bilateral knee effusions. Lab testing reveals a normal or negative CBC, CMP, ANA, and urinalysis. The ESR is 62 mm/h. The RF is 77 IU/mL and the anti-CCP antibody is 132 U/mL. X-rays of the hands and feet are without erosions.

What feature of her disease is most predictive of the future development of joint erosions on X-ray?

(a) Elevated ESR
(b) Her age
(c) Negative ANA
(d) Positive RF
(e) Positive anti-CCP antibody

Correct answer: (e)

2. A 55-year-old man has a 10-year history of RA. He has been maintained on methotrexate 15 mg orally each week and folic acid 1 mg orally daily. He has been doing well. Examination reveals no evidence of synovitis. There are no deformities. He has a small left olecranon subcutaneous nodule. The remainder of his physical examination is unremarkable. Lab testing in the past revealed a RF 188 IU/mL and an anti-CCP antibody 98 U/mL. Lab monitoring on a regular basis for methotrexate toxicity has been within normal range.

Which of the following is the most common extra-articular feature of disease associated with RA?

(a) Aortic insufficiency
(b) PAH
(c) Pleural effusion
(d) Erythema nodosum
(e) Mononeuritis multiplex

Correct answer: (c)

3. A 48-year-old man with a 5-year history of RA presents to his primary care physician with acute sinusitis. He reports that his arthritis has been well controlled on his usual regimen of methotrexate 15 mg orally per week and folic acid 1 mg orally daily.

Which antibiotic choice for treating the acute sinusitis is associated with a potential drug interaction and should be avoided?

(a) Trimethoprim/sulfamethoxazole
(b) Amoxicillin/clavulanate
(c) Azithromycin
(d) Cefuroxime
(e) Ciprofloxacin

Correct answer: (a)

4. The highest mortality risk in patients with RA is due to which one of the following conditions?

(a) ILD
(b) Aortic stenosis
(c) Coronary artery disease
(d) Lymphoma
(e) Breast cancer

Correct answer: (c)

5. A 64-year-old man with a 10-year history of RA presents to his primary care physician with a 2-day complaint of a red, painful right eye. His vision seems blurred and it is difficult for him to keep his eye open due to discomfort associated with light exposure. He denies fever. His arthritis has been well controlled. He reports no other symptoms. His medications include methotrexate 20 mg orally weekly, folic acid 1 mg orally daily, and hydroxychloroquine 400 mg orally daily. On examination, he is afebrile and his vital signs are normal. HEENT examination reveals a red, injected right eye. The remainder of the examination is unremarkable.

Which of the following is a potential association of this extra-articular manifestation of disease?

   (a) Dural sinus thrombosis
   (b) Corneal melt
   (c) Retinal vein thrombosis
   (d) Ophthalmic artery thrombosis
   (e) Acute angle glaucoma

Correct answer: (b)

6. A 25-year-old woman presents to her primary care physician with a 2-year history of cold sensitivity of her hands. She describes that her fingertips turn white with exposure to cold. She has no other symptoms. She takes no medications. She denies tobacco or alcohol use. Examination reveals normal vital signs. There are no skin changes. The remainder of the physical examination is unremarkable.

Which of the following lab abnormalities is most predictive of her future development of a connective tissue disease?

   (a) ANA 1:640
   (b) RF 212 IU/mL
   (c) C3 65 mg/dL
   (d) ESR 20 mm/h
   (e) Platelet count 414 K/μL

Correct answer: (a)

7. A 45-year-old woman with a 4-year history of diffuse cutaneous systemic sclerosis presents to the emergency department with complaint of a 2-day history of severe headache. She denies blurred vision and fever. She has no other complaints. She has no other significant medical history. She takes omeprazole 20 mg daily and nifedipine XL 60 mg daily. She denies tobacco and alcohol use. Examination reveals her to be afebrile. Blood pressure is 200/120, pulse 92, and respiratory rate 18. Funduscopic examination is unremarkable. Lungs are clear. Cardiovascular exam reveals a normal S1 and S2 with a positive S4. There is no S3 and there are no murmurs. There is no lower extremity edema. Skin exam reveals no digital ulcers. There is skin thickening over the fingers, hands, forearms, face, chest, and abdomen.

Lab testing reveals an EKG with normal sinus rhythm without abnormality.
WBC: 7.8 K/mL
Hemoglobin: 9.2 g/dL
Platelets: 102 K/mL
Creatinine: 1.2 mg/dL
Urinalysis 2 + protein, 0 RBCs, 0 WBCs

What is the next step in her management?

- ○   Admit to the hospital for renal biopsy
- ○   Initiate lisinopril 10 mg and ask her to follow up with her phyisican in one week
- ○   Initiate captopril 6.25 mg and admit to the hospital
- ○   Increase the Procardia XL and ask her to follow up with her physician in one week
- ○   Increase the Procardia XL and schedule a captopril renal scan

Correct answer: (c)

8. A 26-year-old woman with diffuse cutaneous SSc presents to the emergency department with a 1-week history of abdominal pain. She has nausea and vomiting and has obstipation. She has no other pertinent medical history. She takes lansoprazole. She is afebrile; blood pressure is 125/80 and HR is 105. Abdominal exam reveals absent bowel sounds and is distended. The abdomen is tympanic to percussion and there is diffuse tenderness without palpable masses or organomegaly. Pelvic exam is unremarkable. An abdominal film reveals dilated loops of small and large bowel and pneumatos is intestinales is visualized. Laboratory testing reveals a normal CMP except the BUN is 40 mg/dL and creatinine is 0.8 mg/dL. The CBC is normal. Urinalysis and urine pregnancy tests are negative. Lipase and amylase are normal.

The next step in this patient's management should be:

(a) General surgery consult
(b) Insertion of a nasogastric and rectal tube
(c) Abdominal ultrasound
(d) Central access for total parenteral nutrition

Correct answer: (b)

9. A 45-year-old woman with a 20-year history of limited cutaneous SSc presents to her primary care physician for an annual exam. She reports a 6-month history of increased fatigue and dyspnea on exertion. She is no longer able to carry her laundry basket upstairs. Her Raynaud phenomenon and GER symptoms are well controlled on amlodipine 10 mg daily and lansoprazole 30 mg daily, respectively. On physical examination, she is afebrile; blood pressure is 100/60, pulse 95, and respiratory rate 18. Lungs are clear to auscultation. Cardiovascular exam reveals a regular rate and rhythm with a normal S1. The second heart sound has a prominent P2 component. There is no lower extremity edema. Sclerodactyly is present; however, there are no digital ulcers. A chest X-ray reveals no parenchymal disease.

The most likely finding in the work-up of her dyspnea is as follows:

(a) Ground glass opacification on high-resolution CT scan of the chest
(b) Forced vital capacity 68% predicted
(c) Diffusion capacity 56% predicted
(d) Pericardial effusion on echocardiogram

Correct answer: (c)

10. Which of the following findings is most predictive that a patient with limited cutaneous SSc will progress to develop diffuse skin changes?

(a) Tendon friction rubs
(b) Digital pits
(c) Positive anti-centromere antibody
(d) Atrial fibrillation
(e) Telangiectasias

Correct answer: (a)

References

1. Lawrence, R.C., et al., *Estimates of the prevalence of arthritis and selected musculoskeletal disorders in the United States.* Arthritis Rheum. 1998. **41**(5): pp. 778–99.
2. MacGregor, A.J., et al., *Rheumatology*, Fourth edn, M. Hochberg (ed.). Elsevier, Philadelphia, PA. 2008, pp.755–61.
3. Doran, M.F., et al., *Trends in incidence and mortality in rheumatoid arthritis in Rochester, Minnesota, over a forty-year period.* Arthritis Rheum. 2002. **46**(3): pp. 625–31.
4. Vallbracht, I. and K. Helmke, *Additional diagnostic and clinical value of anti-cyclic citrullinated peptide antibodies compared with rheumatoid factor isotypes in rheumatoid arthritis.* Autoimmun Rev. 2005. **4**(6): pp. 389–94.
5. McQueen, F.M. and M. Ostergaard, *Established rheumatoid arthritis – New imaging modalities.* Best Pract Res Clin Rheumatol, 2007. **21**(5): pp. 841–56.
6. Combe, B. *Early rheumatoid arthritis: Strategies for prevention and management.* Best Pract Res Clin Rheumatol, 2007. **21**: pp. 27–42.
7. Steen, V.D. and T.A. Medsger, Jr., *The palpable tendon friction rub: An important physical examination finding in patients with systemic sclerosis.* Arthritis Rheum, 1997. **40**(6): pp. 1146–51.
8. Masi, A.T., G.P. Rodnan, and T.A. Medsger, Jr., et al., *Preliminary criteria for the classification of systemic sclerosis (scleroderma).* Arthritis Rheum, 1980. **23**: pp. 581–90.
9. Steen, V.D., D.L. Powell, and T.A. Medsger, Jr., *Clinical correlations and prognosis based on serum autoantibodies in patients with systemic sclerosis.* Arthritis Rheum, 1988. **31**(2): pp. 196–203.
10. Blockmans, D., G. Beyens, and R. Verhaeghe, *Predictive value of nailfold capillaroscopy in the diagnosis of connective tissue diseases.* Clin Rheum, 1996. **15**(2): pp. 148–53.
11. Reimer, G., et al., *Correlates between autoantibodies to nucleolar antigens and clinical features in patients with systemic sclerosis (scleroderma).* Arthritis Rheum, 1988. **31**(4): pp. 525–32.
12. Steen, V.D., et al., *Severe restrictive lung disease in systemic sclerosis.* Arthritis Rheum, 1994. **37**(9): pp. 1283–9.

13. Steen, V.D., et al., *Isolated diffusing capacity reduction in systemic sclerosis*. Arthritis Rheum, 1992. **35**(7): pp. 765–70.

14. Tashkin, D.P., et al., *Cyclophosphamide versus placebo in scleroderma lung disease*. N Engl J Med, 2006. **354**(25): pp. 2655–66.

15. Steen, V.D. and T.A. Medsger, Jr., *Case-control study of corticosteroids and other drugs that either precipitate or protect from the development of scleroderma renal crisis*. Arthritis Rheum, 1998. **41**(9): pp. 1613–19.

Chapter 19
Immune-Mediated Rheumatic Diseases

H. Michael Belmont

Abstract Systemic lupus erythematosus (SLE) is the prototypical human, autoimmune disease and is characterized by immune dysregulation, production of autoantibodies, generation of circulating immune complexes, and activation of the complement system. SLE is notable for unpredictable exacerbations and remissions with a predilection for clinical involvement of joint, skin, kidney, brain, serosa, lung, heart, hematological system, and gastrointestinal tract (Wallace, The clinical presentation of systemic lupus erythematosus. In: Wallace D and Hahn B, Eds. Dubois' Lupus Erythematosus, Lippincott Williams & Wilkins, Hagerstown, MD, 2006, pp. 621–628) (Table 19.1). The pathological hallmark of SLE is recurrent, widespread, and diverse vascular lesions including both inflammatory and thrombotic vasculopathy, the latter most often occurring in the setting of antiphospholipid antibodies. Cases related to the presentation and management of SLE are discussed (Belmont and Abramson, Arthritis and Rheumatism 39:9–23, 1996).

Keywords Systemic lupus erythematosus • Antiphospholipid syndrome • Glomerulonephritis

Case 1

A 28-year-old African-American female with a 3-year history of a connective tissue disease presents with bilateral pedal edema. The patient was diagnosed 2 years previously with systemic lupus erythematosus (SLE) based on the presence of fever, discoid lesion, chronic cutaneous lupus skin lesions, Raynaud's phenomenon, polyarthritis, positive antinuclear antibody (ANA), and positive dsDNA (1). The patient had been managed with recommendation to avoid prolonged, unopposed

H.M. Belmont (✉)
Division of Rheumatology, Department of Medicine, NYU Hospital for Joint Diseases,
301 East 17th Street, New York, NY 10003, USA
e-mail: michael.belmont@nyumc.org

M. Mahmoudi (ed.), *Challenging Cases in Allergy and Immunology*,
DOI: 10.1007/978-1-60327-443-2_19,
© Humana Press, a part of Springer Science+Business Media, LLC 2009

Table 19.1 Major clinical manifestations of systemic lupus erythematosus by organ system

Constitutional	Fever, weight loss, malaise, and fatigue
Musculoskeletal	Myalgia, arthralgia, deforming non-erosive arthritis (Jaccoud's arthropathy), erosive arthritis [RA-like (rare)] myositis
Mucocutaneous	Acute cutaneous lupus (malar rash), subacute cutaneous lupus (annular rash), chronic cutaneous lupus (discoid lupus), painless oral and nasal ulcers, urticaria, tumid lupus, bullous lupus
Cardiopulmonary	Pericarditis, myocarditis, valvulitis, pleuritis, pneumonitis, pulmonary hypertension
Hematologic	Anemia of chronic disease, autoimmune hemolytic anemia, autoimmune thrombocytopenia purpura, Evan's syndrome, leukopenia, lymphopenia, TTP, hypercoagulable state in setting of antiphospholipid antibodies
Neuropsychiatric	Acute confusional state, organic mental syndrome, organic affective disorder, seizures, cerebrovascular accident, cranial neuropathy, mononeuritis multiplex, transverse myelitis
Vasculitic (rare)	Cutaneous vasculitis, coronary vasculitis, dysenteric vasculitis, intracerebral vasculitis (very rare)
Renal	Nephrotic syndrome, glomerulonephritis, azotemia, hypertension, end stage renal disease
Gastrointestinal	Medical peritonitis, pancreatitis (rare), non-specific hepatitis, esophageal dysfunction (rare)

(e.g. no sunscreen) sun exposure and hydroxychloroquine 200 mg bid. Three weeks before admission, the patient had upper respiratory infection with coryza, nonproductive cough, and mild pharyngeal pain. Two weeks earlier, she had accompanied her family to the beach and had used sunscreen and a wide-brim hat. She now had increasing joint pain and significant bilateral pedal edema accompanied by a 5-lb weight gain. On examination, the patient had a blood pressure of 130/80, normal heart rate, and normal respiratory rate. She was a well-developed, well-nourished black female in no distress. Skin exam revealed inactive discoid skin lesions involving the forehead and right helix. Head, ears, eyes, nose, and throat exam revealed no oral ulcers. The lungs are clear to auscultation. The cardiac exam was without murmur. The abdomen was soft and nontender. Extremity exam revealed 3+ bilateral pitting edema. Joint exam revealed no active synovitis. There was mild digital cyanosis, but no digital ulcerations or infarcts. Neurological exam revealed no focal weakness.

Laboratory Data

Laboratory studies revealed a normal CBC except for a total lymphocyte count of 900, sedimentation rate was 60, CRP was 1 mg/dl, BUN was 28, and creatinine was 1.1. The serum albumin was 3.9 and the cholesterol was 268. The U/A revealed 3+ protein and 2+ blood. Urine microscopy revealed 5–10 white blood cells per high power field. The dsDNA was positive at 60 units (normal less than 10 units). The C3 was 58 and the C4 was 5.6. ASO titer mildly elevated at 280.

Working Diagnosis

The patient's history of lupus and presentation of nephrotic syndrome is consistent with an episode of lupus glomerulonephritis.

Differential Diagnosis

1. Lupus with membranous glomerulonephritis
2. Lupus with proliferative glomerulonephritis
3. Lupus with minimal change disease
4. SLE with secondary antiphospholipid antibody syndrome and thrombotic glomerulopathy
5. Scleroderma renal crisis
6. Acute poststreptococcal glomerulonephritis

Final Diagnosis

The patient's clinical presentation is most consistent with nephrotic syndrome as a manifestation of immune-mediated inflammatory disease affecting the glomerular capillary in a patient with SLE. This clinical presentation is consistent with lupus glomerulonephritis most likely WHO Class IV membranous type. The patient has preexisting lupus and presents with a classic nephrotic syndrome accompanied by proteinuria, edema, and hypercholesterolemia. The absence of significant hypertension, active urinary sediment (e.g., red blood cells), or hypertension mitigates against proliferative lupus nephritis. The absence of strong serological evidence for recent poststreptococcal exposure makes acute poststreptococcal glomerulonephritis unlikely. The lack of significant hypertension accompanied by microangiopathic hemolytic anemia makes scleroderma renal crisis untenable. The thrombotic glomeropathy that can occur in the setting of lupus with significant antiphospholipid syndrome (APS) is also unlikely given the normal platelet count and the otherwise classic presentation of lupus membranous nephropathy with nephrotic syndrome. SLE with secondary APS can be excluded, moreover, by negative testing for lupus anticoagulant, IgG and IgM anticardiolipin antibodies, and VDRL.

Discussion

The diagnosis of lupus rests upon the combination of the history, physical examination, and laboratory tests. The sensitivity and specificity of antinuclear antibodies depends in part upon the assay system used, and this is an important fact to keep in mind when analyzing ANAs measured in an individual patient. ANAs are found in over 95% of patients with lupus with the Hep-2 assay, in which human tissue is used as the substrate. Disease-specific autoantibodies like those directed against dsDNA, or extractable nuclear antigens like the Smith antibody (anti-Smith), are more specific than the ANA, and can assist the clinician in making a diagnosis of lupus, but their absence does not negate the diagnosis. High levels of dsDNA antibodies can antedate the development of lupus nephritis, and evidence of renal dysfunction should be carefully searched for when high amounts of dsDNA antibodies are found. Serum complements, in particular C3, C4, and CHSO, may be depressed in active lupus, and should also be monitored when diagnosing and managing a patient with lupus. How measurements in the dsDNA antibodies and complements correlate with specific disease manifestations should be determined for each individual patient, since elevated dsDNA and depressed serum complements in an individual patient may not be associated with disease flare.

In lupus, organ injury results from inflammatory vasculopathy best modeled by vasculitis or by the Shwartzman phenomenon, or thrombotic vasculopathy seen with the APS (2). Antibody-mediated injury in SLE is thought to play a role in the pathogenesis of autoimmune hemolytic anemia (the antigen is red blood cell RhD), idiopathic thrombocytopenic purpura (the antigen is platelet glycoprotein IIb/IIIa), and thrombotic thrombocytopenic purpura (the antigen is von Willebrand F cleaving protease also know as ADAMTS-13). Self-antigens recognized by autoantibodies in SLE associated with the APS and neuropsychiatric lupus include negatively charged phospholipid–protein complexes and ribosomal P (a neuronal antigen), respectively. The specific pathogenic mechanism by which these autoantibodies and immune complexes containing self-antigens are induced remains unclear.

Renal involvement in SLE is a common disease manifestation and a strong predictor of poor outcome. The prevalence of renal disease in eight large cohort studies involving 2,649 SLE patients ranged from 31 to 65%. A recent study analyzed the annual incidence of nephritis in 384 lupus patients followed at the Johns Hopkins Medical Center from 1992 to 1994. The 1-year incidence of acute renal disease was 10%. The general consensus is that 50% of lupus patients will develop clinically relevant nephritis at some time in the course of their illness.

Most patients develop nephritis early in their disease. It is uncommon to have the original onset of renal disease more than 10 years after the appearance of SLE. Although SLE is nine times more common in women than men; a greater percentage of male patients may develop renal disease. Asians, African-Caribbean, and African-Americans may develop nephritis more frequently than other ethnic groups. Outcomes and response to therapy may be affected by race, with African-American patients being predisposed to aggressive and treatment-resistant nephritis. Presence of certain human leukocyte antigen (HLA) types has been associated with an increased risk of developing nephritis, with HLA-DR2 and HLA-B8 being more frequently associated with the development of lupus renal disease than HLA-DR4. Polymorphisms of Fc receptors for IgG were recently identified in African-Americans and Caucasians in Europe as a risk factor for lupus renal disease, implicating defective handling of circulating immune complexes in the development of renal disease.

A detailed discussion of the immunopathogenesis of lupus nephritis is beyond the scope of this article. An understanding of the basic etiology, however, is relevant. SLE is characterized by autoantibody production, the generation of immune complexes, and episodic, uncontrolled complement activation. Autoantibodies in SLE are T cell dependent and their expression requires T cell signaling of autoreactive B cell clones. At least three potentially overlapping, immunopathogenic mechanisms capable of producing renal injury are supported by experimental data. First, circulating immune complexes consisting chiefly of DNA and anti-DNA antibodies are deposited in the kidney. Resulting complement activation and chemotaxis of neutrophils lead to a local inflammatory process. Second, in situ formation of antigen and antibody complexes may similarly lead to complement activation and leucocyte-mediated injury. Third, antibodies against specific cellular targets may produce renal injury. For example, antibodies, such as anti-ribosomal P, may bind to cytoplasmic antigens that have been translocated to the cell membrane, with subsequent penetration and disruption of cellular function.

Lupus renal disease can also be defined pathologically. Material obtained by renal biopsy is evaluated by light microscopy, immunofluorescence, and electron microscopy. The World Health Organization (WHO) has described a classification of lupus renal disease as follows:

- Class I: normal histology
- Class II-A (mesangial): normal histology on light microscopy but mesangial immune complex deposition evident on electron microscopy
- Class II-B (mesangial): immune complex deposits plus mesangial proliferation on light microscopy
- Class III (focal proliferative): peripheral capillary loop proliferation in a segmental distribution involving <50% of the glomeruli
- Class IV (diffuse proliferative): peripheral capillary loop proliferation in a global distribution and involving >50% of the glomeruli involved
- Class V (membranous): diffuse glomerular basement membrane thickening
- Class VI (chronic glomerulosclerosis): chronic sclerosis without inflammation (Table 19.2)

More recently the National Institutes of Health have developed activity and chronicity indices for lupus renal disease. High chronicity scores are associated with poor outcome and a lack of response to immunosuppression. High activity scores indices are associated with poor outcomes, but may be reversible, especially with aggressive treatment. There has been some concern regarding reliability of the indices as well as their reproducibility in the community setting. Patients with severe active and chronic histological changes, however, should be viewed as being, at increased risk for renal insufficiency.

The distribution and quantity of electron microscopic for immune complexes are also of prognostic and therapeutic significance. WHO Class II and Class V diseases are associated with mesangial and subepithelial location of electron dense deposits, respectively. Proliferative nephritis (WHO Class III and Class IV) is associated with subendothelial deposits.

Table 19.2 WHO classification

Class	Light microscopy	Electron microscopy	Clinical features
I (Normal)	Normal	Normal	Negative
II-A (Mesangial)	Normal	Mesangial deposits	Negative
II-B (Mesangial)	Mesangial hypercellularity	Mesangial deposits	Proteinuria <1 g/24 h; RBC 5–15/HPF
III (Focal proliferative)	Segmental endocapillary hypercellularity involving <50% of the glomeruli	Subendothelial deposits	Proteinuria <2 g/24 h; RBC 5-15/HPF
IV (Diffuse proliferative)	Global endocapillary hypercellularity involving >50% of the glomeruli	Subendothelial deposits	Proteinuria 2–20 g/24 h; RBC > 20/HPF
V (Membranous)	Glomerular basement thickening	Subepithelial depotis	Proteinuria 3.5–20 g/24 h; no hematuria
VI (Chronic glomerulosclerosis)	Sclerosis without inflammation	Deposits may be absent	Hypertension; renal failure

Although clearly not without exception, there is a correlation between the pathological type of lupus renal disease and the aforementioned clinical features. Obviously, patients with normal renal biopsies have normal diagnostic and blood tests. However, it should be mentioned that there are patients with so-called silent lupus nephritis who have normal urinalyses, absence of proteinuria, and normal serum creatinine levels, but who, on renal biopsy, have anywhere from mesangial to proliferative nephritis. Fortunately, it has not been demonstrated that progressive loss of renal function in these cases occurs silently, that is to say without the appearance of a perturbed urinary sediment and albuminuria.

Mesangial lupus nephritis (WHO class II) is accompanied by normal diagnostic findings or with a mild degree of proteinuria but typically without hypertension or abnormal urinary sediment. Focal and diffuse proliferative lupus glomerulonephritis (WHO class III and class IV, respectively) are often associated with the worst prognosis for kidney survival and can be accompanied by nephrotic syndrome, significant hypertension, and abnormal urine sediment. Membranous lupus nephritis (WHO class V) often presents with proteinuria, moderate to high grade, but usually normal urinary sediment in the absence of hypertension.

In summary, mesangial lupus nephropathy is generally associated with an excellent prognosis, whereas proliferative lupus nephropathy, especially the diffuse variant; is often characterized by hypertension, red blood cell casts, and significant deterioration of renal function. Nephrotic syndrome in the absence of hypertension, active urinary sediment, or significant hypocomplementemia suggests the membranous variant of lupus nephropathy. Membranous nephropathy generally is associated with a good prognosis and relative preservation of renal function. However, in the presence of persistent nephrotic range proteinuria, membranous lupus nephropathy can, in fact, lead to loss of renal function and end stage renal disease (ESRD).

Standard management of lupus often requires sunscreen, anti-inflammatory agents and for relief of cutaneous and articular manifestations, anti-malarials, specifically hydroxychloroquine. Immunosuppressive agents are also used to treat various disease manifestations, and to minimize the use of steroids. "Lupus nephritis," one of the most serious manifestations of lupus, is associated with a number of different histologies, including disease isolated to the mesangium, focal or diffuse proliferative glomerulonephritis, focal sclerosis, and membranous glomerulonephritis. The treatment of diffuse proliferative glomerulonephritis seen with lupus often consists of corticosteroids and cyclophosphamide. Controversy remains regarding the treatment approach to patients' initial episode of clinical proliferative glomerulonephritis. Additionally, uncertainty remains in the matter of need, choice, and duration of maintenance therapy to minimize risk of renal relapse, progression of renal scarring, and ESRD (3).

Studies at the National Institute of Health (NIH) were the first to establish the superiority of cyclophosphamide plus prednisone compared to prednisone alone for the treatment of lupus nephritis. Additionally, the NIH studied the relative efficacy of long course cyclophosphamide (i.e., 14 treatments over 2.5 years) vs. short course cyclophosphamide (six monthly treatments) vs. pulses of methylprednisolone alone for the treatment of lupus nephritis. These studies demonstrated that either long or short course cyclophosphamide was superior to methylprednisolone alone in preserving renal function, and that longer courses of cyclophosphamide were less often associated with renal relapse than short course (10% vs. 50%). Finally, the NIH studied the safety and efficacy of pulses of methylprednisolone vs. pulses of cyclophosphamide vs. combination pulses of methylprednisolone and cyclophosphamide (4). Here, again, the treatment arms with cyclophosphamide were superior to those with methylprednisolone alone. Furthermore, the combination of methylprednisolone and cyclophosphamide was most often associated with a remission of clinical nephritis (e.g., resolution of proteinuria and hematuria, improvement of serum albumin, and preservation of serum creatinine).

After a median follow-up of 11 years, treatment with cyclophosphamide alone vs. combination with methylprednisolone was superior to treatment with methylprednisolone alone in terms of renal response and persistence of this response. Specifically, the study showed that combination therapy was less often associated with doubling of the serum creatinine as compared to cyclophosphamide alone (0 of 20 vs. 5 of 21 patients). Interestingly, the combination of cyclophosphamide and methylprednisolone was no more frequently associated with untoward events than the use of either alone. However, in March 2009 Genentech provided a press release that in the one year randomized placebo controlled LUNAR Trial the addition of rituximab to the standard of care with steroids and MMF was not associated with any significantly greater clinical response. Therefore, B cell depletion may not be of benefit in routine management of proliferative lupus nephritis but its role as rescue therapy or for subsets of patients needs clarification. Since only 25 or fewer patients were enrolled in each arm and the period of follow-up is still only 11 years, observation of larger numbers of patients over longer periods of time is necessary before the recommendation should be made that all the patients should receive treatment with the combination of cyclophosphamide and methylprednisolone. However, for patients with poor prognostic clinical scenarios, such as rapidly progressive crescentic lupus nephritis, lupus nephritis with recent, rapid deterioration of renal function, or, repeatedly, recurrent clinical nephritis, combination pulse treatment should be considered.

Mycophenolate mofetil (MMF), a purine antimetabolite that inhibits inosine mono-phosphate dehydrogenase, is being increasingly used to prevent posttransplantation rejection, and may be an alternative treatment for progressive or refractory lupus nephritis (5). In a small study, Dooley et al. found that four of five patients with diffuse proliferative glomerulonephritis refractory to cyclophosphamide responded to the administration of MMF, with concomitant clinical improvement (i.e., reduction in proteinuria). Subsequently, researchers found that 42 patients randomized to receive MMF plus prednisolone vs. oral cyclophosphamide for 6 months followed by oral azathioprine plus prednisolone achieved similar, high renal response rates (81% vs. 76%). Ginzler reported in the NEJM on a large series of 137 patients with active Classes III, IV, and V lupus nephritis randomized to conventional pulse cyclophosphamide or MMF, in addition to standard oral steroid doses. Both treatments again were associated with similar high response rates. In this study, MMF was less frequently associated with serious toxicity, such as sepsis. In fact, all the three deaths occurred in patients receiving cyclophosphamide. Furthermore, those patients randomized to cyclophosphamide were more likely to refuse treatment or to drop out. These data suggest that MMF is better tolerated than cyclophosphamide and, at least in the short term, is associated with similar efficacy. Investigators at the University of Miami performed a study in which patients after standard NIH induction with six monthly intravenous pulses of cyclo-phosphamide were randomized to quarterly cyclophosphamide infusions, oral azathio-prine or oral MMF (6). Both the cohorts receiving oral antimetabolites experienced lower rates of doubling of serum creatinine or death as compared to the group treated with continuation on the alkylating agent suggesting a "step down" to less toxic options after induction is a viable option. Finally, in the ongoing ambitious Aspreva Lupus Management Study (ALMS), a two stage induction and maintenance trial employing a randomized open label comparison of MMF with intravenous cyclophosphamide for the first 6 months, followed by a double-blind comparison of MMF to azathioprine for 3 years, induction responses with cyclophosphamide (98/185, 53%) as compared to MMF (104/185, 56%) were similar, further supporting view that for some patients ini-tial treatment with the purine antagonist is reasonable.

Rituximab, a monoclonal antibody directed against the B cell antigen CD 20, has been FDA approved for the treatment of non-Hodgkin's B cell lymphomas and rheumatoid arthritis. Though prolonged periods of B cell depletion have been seen in lymphoma patients treated with rituximab, this reduction in B cell volume is not associated with what might be an expected dramatic increase in infections. As reported at the 2002 American College of Rheumatology Meeting in New Orleans, groups in Philadelphia and Rochester, NY, observed that escalating doses between 100, 375, and 500 mg of rituximab were generally well tolerated in patients with lupus. In addition, researchers reported on six patients with lupus who received two weekly 500 mg doses of rituximab. Treatment was associated with B cell depletion and an absence of any significant increase in risk of infection, but with improvement in clinical measures of lupus disease activity (7). Specifically anemia, arthritis, and serositis responded particularly well to this protocol. In addition, of the six patients with nephritis their proteinuria improved. Subsequently, several open label studies have been published reporting efficacy in the treatment of both renal and extrarenal lupus. On the other hand, the Genetech EXPLORER Trial investigated in a randomized trial the benefit of 1,000 mg rituximab on day 1 and 15 as compared to placebo infusion in combination with mycophenolate for management of nonrenal lupus flare and did not demonstrate superiority. The LUNAR Trial studying the efficacy in patients with lupus nephritis is still unpublished.

There are multiple ongoing industry sponsored trials attempting to identify future novel options for treatment of lupus. For example, investigators completed a phase III trial with the B cell tolerogen, LIP 394/Abetimus, or Riquent in November of 2002. Two hundred and ninety-eight patients were randomized to either 100 mg of Riquent vs. placebo intravenously weekly. Patients enrolled in the study had persistent elevated anti-dsDNA antibodies and active nephritis within the prior 4 years to enrollment. The primary endpoint was time to next renal flare. Although the primary outcome did not achieve statistical significance, there was a reduction in the mean time to renal flare from 123 to 89 months and a reduction in treatment vs. placebo in the number of renal flares from 24 of 153 to 17 of 145 patients on placebo vs. experimental drug, respectively. Furthermore, the study identified that the major risk for renal flare was persistence of elevated anti-dsDNA antibodies. For patients in whom there was a persistent reduction in anti-dsDNA antibodies, the relative risk of renal flare was statistically lower than for those patients in whom DNA reductions did not occur or were not consistently maintained. The administration of LIP 394 was very strongly statistically related to a reduction in anti-dsDNA antibodies as compared to placebo ($p < 0.001$). More recent studies demonstrate that higher doses of Abetimus of 300 and 600 mg are well tolerated and associated with higher prevalence of significant reductions in anti-dsDNA. Another Phase III study comparing 100, 300, and 600 mg doses has been completed. A La Jolla Pharmaecuetical press release in February, 2009 reported that even the higher doses of abetimus did not significantly increase the time to flare in patients randomized due to presistently elevated anti-dsDNA levels. Additional novel therapies that are either in Phase I, II, or III studies include the use of belilumab, a monoclonal antibody to BLyS (B Lymphocyte Stimulator), abatacept, or CTLA-4 which is a receptor blocker of T and B cell costimulator pathways that is approved for treatment of rheumatoid arthritis, atacicept, or TACI-Ig, monoclonal antibodies to Type 1 interferon, monoclonal antibodies to C5 (which prevent generation of C5b and C5b-9), C5a receptor antagonists, and heteropolymers consisting of antibody to DNA and monoclonal antibodies to erythrocyte CR1. Future studies will determine if any of these treatments achieve safety and efficacy outcomes to justify their clinical use.

Case 2

A 17-year-old African-American female presented through the emergency room with severe chest pain accompanied by nausea. Three months prior to the emergency room visit, the patient complains of fatigue, malaise, anorexia, accompanied by 35-lb weight loss, intermittent fevers with a maximum of 102°F, and generalized myalgia and arthralgia. Evaluation by a local physician identified anemia prompting treatment with iron, a possible urinary tract infection resulting in treatment with co-trimoxazole, as well as HIV testing and psychiatric evaluation for anorexia nervosa. The presence of generalized lymphadenopathy led to an outpatient fine needle aspirate of a right supraclavicular lymph node which demonstrated nonspecific reactive hyperplasia. The patient presented to the emergency room with intense chest pain accompanied by nauseousness. On examining, she was normotensive, mildly tachycardic, and tachypneic. Skin exam did not reveal any malar rash or chronic, scarring, cutaneous lupus. The lungs were clear to auscultation without rub. The cardiac exam was without murmur or rub. The abdomen was soft and nontender without organomegaly. Extremity exam failed to reveal any pitting, pedal edema. There is no active synovitis. Although there is diffuse muscle tenderness, neurologic exam revealed no focal weakness.

Laboratory Data

Positive ANA at 1:320 with a homogenous pattern, a positive anti-dsDNA at 60 I.U. by ELISA, a normocytic anemia with hemoglobin of 8.6, hematocrit of 25.8, white blood cell count 4,600, a platelet count of 115,000, sedimentation rate of 46, normal prothrombin time, PTT slightly prolonged at 45 s, U/A with 100 mg/dl protein, large dipstick blood, 10–20 RBCs per high power field, 10–20 WBCs per high power field, C3 48 mg/dl (normal 75–130), C4 10 mg/dl (normal 16–35 mg/dl) albumin 2.9, 24-h protein collection with 2,000 mg 1 mg of protein, cholesterol 269, positive lupus anticoagulant with prolonged dilute Russell Viper Venom time which did not correct with a mixing study, positive anticardiolipin antibodies with 68 GPL units and 30 APL units, a biological false positive VDRL with RPR positive and 1:4, but negative FTA-ABS. Serum CPK and troponin are elevated. Serial EKGs without Q waves, but echocardiogram revealed inferior wall hypokinesis.

Working Diagnosis

A 17-year-old African-American female with new onset SLE with prominent cardiac involvement.

Differential Diagnosis

1. SLE with myocarditis
2. SLE with pulmonary embolus
3. SLE with pulmonary hypertension

4. SLE with myocardial ischemia due to coronary vasculitis
5. SLE with myocardial ischemia due to coronary vasospasm
6. SLE with secondary antiphospholipid antibody syndrome and coronary thrombosis

Additional Data

Cardiac catheterization via right femoral artery revealed total occlusion of the left anterior descending artery, distal total occlusion of D1 small vessel, total occlusion of distal circumflex, luminal irregularities of midright coronary artery with maximal obstruction of 30%, ejection fraction of 45%, and hypokinetic inferior and apical wall.

Diagnosis

SLE manifest by constitutional features with fever, musculoskeletal features with myalgia, glomerulonephritis with proteinuria and hematuria, positive ANA, positive DNA, positive antiphospholipid antibodies, and secondary APS with myocardial ischemia secondary to coronary artery thrombosis. This diagnosis is supported by the laboratory findings and the diagnostic cardiac catheterization. The echocardiogram makes pericarditis and myocarditis less likely. A spiral CT scan excluded pulmonary embolus. The echocardiogram also did not suggest evidence of pulmonary hypertension. The appearance on catheterization with abrupt interruption of blood flow in association with high titer antiphospholipid antibodies argues against coronary vasculitis, which although described in the literature is extremely uncommon, or vasospasm.

Discussion

Minor or low-grade chronic coagulation abnormalities are not infrequently observed among patients with active SLE, but disseminated thrombosis rarely occurs in SLE except in association with circulating antiphospholipid antibodies. Thromboembolic events are estimated to occur in about 30% of SLE patients with antiphospholipid antibodies and are considered to be related to the level of the antibody, the isotype (IgG) present, and probably, the length of time these antibodies have been present. The APS has a myriad of diverse clinical manifestations, all of which are attributable to a common pathophysiologic process, namely, large- and/or small-vessel, recurrent, arterial, and/or venous thromboses. Although the pathogenesis of thrombosis in APS is not completely understood, it appears to involve several different and complex mechanisms of interactions between the clotting system, antiphospholipid antibodies, vascular endothelium, and antiendothelial cell antibodies (AECA). Pulmonary hypertension is another important thromboembolic complication of SLE. Of interest, patients with SLE complicated by pulmonary hypertension demonstrated a marked elevation of IgG and IgM AECA compared with SLE patients without pulmonary hypertension. Evidence of episodic recurrence is a histopathologic hallmark of thromboembolic disease in SLE with APS.

The presence of antibodies to negatively charged phospholipids is associated with recurrent arterial and venous thrombosis, thrombocytopenia, and fetal wastage. The APS requires the demonstration of an antiphospholipid antibody (e.g., biologic false positive VDRL, lupus anticoagulant, anticardiolipin antibodies) and thrombotic phenomena. It is known that the presence in serum of this family of autoantibodies, perhaps operating through cofactors (e.g., beta2 glycoprotein 1 or prothrombin) can generate a thrombotic diathesis. The mechanism for this antibody-mediated hypercoagulable state has not yet been fully understood, although it appears to involve interactions between the antibodies to anionic phospholipid–protein complexes and antigen targets on platelets, endothelial cells, or components of the coagulation cascade. Experimental evidence exists suggesting that increased platelet aggregation, altered endothelial cell function (e.g., decreased prostacyclin or increased thrombomodulin production), or disturbed function of clotting factors (e.g., decreased protein C activation by thrombomodulin, decreased protein S function, as well as decreased prekallikrein and fibrinolytic activity) may explain the predisposition to thrombosis. The role of cytokines in the primary APS or APS secondary to SLE requires clarification.

Large- and small-vessel, venous and/or arterial thrombosis in SLE may be either limited to an end organ or widely disseminated, and occur as either an isolated event or in association with other manifestations of APS, such as Libman–Sacks endocarditis and recurrent miscarriages. Rarely, multisystem arterial and venous thrombosis results in what has been dubbed "the catastrophic APS" (CAPS) that may eventually prove fatal. The clinical and pathological profiles of APS-related thromboembolism are the same for APS associated with SLE as well as primary APS.

Larger-vessel arterial and/or venous occlusions in SLE with APS have been known to cause limb ischemia and gangrene; myocardial, bowel, and hepatic infarction; renovascular hypertension; and cerebral ischemia. Cerebrovascular occlusive disease is another common expression of thrombotic microangiopathy in SLE with APS. Rarely, ARDS, pulmonary hemorrhage, and recurrent microvascular thrombosis have been observed in SLE and APS. Cutaneous manifestations of SLE with APS include purpuric eruptions, livedo reticularis, and skin ulceration, all of which may be attributed to microvascular thrombosis rather than small-vessel vasculitis.

It has been stressed that the vasculopathy associated with the APS is generally noninflammatory. This is in contradistinction to the inflammatory lesions in SLE, which typically involve small blood vessels in the form of polyarteritis-type necrotizing vasculitis or leukothrombosis. This nonvasculitic nature of the APS is seen particularly in the vasculopathy associated with the CAPS, in which capillaries and small arterioles and venules are occluded with thrombi. A report of pulmonary capillaritis in two of the three patients without SLE but with antiphospholipid antibodies, however, suggests that some immunologically mediated vascular injury may occur in the primary APS.

The cardiac manifestation of the APS include valvulitis, myocarditis, presumably from diffuse multiple small vessel thrombi, intracardiac thrombosis, and as occurred in this case, myocardial ischemia or infarction due to an epicardial thrombosis (8).

Questions

1. A 22-year-old Caucasian female presents with a 1-year history of debilitating fatigue accompanied by intense generalized myalgia. Examination fails to reveal any skin changes and joint examination is without evidence of synovitis as on musculoskeletal examination, there are no warm, tender, or swollen joints. Multiple tender points are present. Laboratory tests revealed a positive ANA at 1:160 with a homogenous pattern. The anti-dsDNA, anti-Ro, anti-La, anti-Sm, anti-RNP, anticardiolipin antibodies, lupus anticoagulant, C3, and C4 are normal. The most appropriate treatment to prescribe is as follows:

   (a) Nonsteroid anti-inflammatory drug
   (b) Hydroxychloroquine
   (c) Prednisone
   (d) Hydroxychloroquine and prednisone
   (e) Duloxetine

ANA testing is very nonspecific as it is positive in 95–99% of all patients with lupus, but also positive in upward of 10% of all healthy females without the condition and the prevalence of lupus is only.1:2,000 Caucasian females. Therefore, many, healthy women or women whose symptoms and physical findings are not the result of lupus have false positive and nonpathogenic ANA results. Based on the prevalence of lupus (1:2,000) and prevalence of false positive ANA results (1:10 or 200:2,000) for every one-women with a positive ANA attributable to lupus, there are 200 women with a positive ANA that do not have the condition. To be diagnosed with lupus the, American College of Rheumatology requires the presence of at least four of the following 11 criteria: malar rash, photosensitivity, discoid rash, oral ulcers, arthritis with two or more joints demonstrating the cardinal features of inflammation (e.g., warmth, erythema, swelling, and tenderness), serositis, nephritis, neurological events, abnormalities of the hematologic system (e.g., autoimmune hemolytic anemia, autoimmune thrombocytopenia, leukopenia), positive result for the aforementioned ANA attributable to lupus, and additional evidence of specific serologic abnormality characteristic of lupus (e.g., positive dsDNA, positive antiphospholipid antibodies, etc.). The correct answer is duloxetine as the patient who meets criteria for fibromyalgia (e.g., chronic widespread nonarticular musculoskeletal pain with positive tender points) has a false positive ANA without any further history, physical examination, or laboratory findings to support a diagnosis of lupus, and the two drugs FDA approved for the treatment of this condition are the duel SNRI, duloxetine, and pregabalin.

2. A 30-year-old African-American female with lupus and biopsy proven membranous nephropathy is treated with 1 mg/kg of prednisone per day for 4 weeks with a subsequent taper. Treatment initially is associated with a reduction in 24-h protein excretion from 6.5 to 1.2 g per day. However, when the steroids are reduced to 5 mg a day, the 24-h protein excretion is 5.3 mg per day. The most appropriate treatment is as follows:

   (a) Add an ACE inhibitor or angiotensin receptor blocker
   (b) Resume prednisone at a dose of 1 mg/kg per day
   (c) Start treatment with monthly intravenous pulse doses of methylprednisolone
   (d) Start treatment with cyclophosphamide intravenous pulses
   (e) Start treatment with cyclosporine with 3 mg/kg per day

Class V membranous lupus nephritis is often treated at the outset with 1 mg/kg/day of prednisone or equivalent for 6–12 weeks. Regardless of response, glucocorticoids are usually then discontinued. Cyclophosphamide is generally reserved for those patients who have a concurrent proliferative component with the membranous lupus nephritis and continue to have clinical features of activity that typically includes not only proteinuria but either an active urinary sediment, persistent high anti-DNA antibody titer, or hypocomplementemia. Therefore, patients with membranous lupus nephropathy and persistent nephrotic syndrome, who have a component of proliferative nephritis, are considered for cytotoxic therapy. Patients with pure membranous nephritis and incessant nephrotic syndrome are candidates for therapy with cyclosporine (9). The cyclosporin dosage is typically 3.5–5 mg/kg per day and close monitoring of blood pressure and serum creatinine levels is required; paradoxical increases in serum creatinine levels can occur because of the potential nephrotoxic effects of this agent.

3. A 32-year-old Asian female with a history of lupus and Class IV diffuse proliferative glomerulonephritis is treated initially with a course of prednisone, a course of MMF when the disease relapses and ten treatments of cyclophosphamide when she develops an additional relapse with an abnormal urine sediment, proteinuria, and doubling at the time of the serum creatinine to 1.4 mg/dl. For persistent evidence of ongoing lupus disease activity appropriate treatment is as follows:

   (a) Referral to a nephrologist for vascular access in anticipation of hemodialysis
   (b) Referral to a transplant enter for renal transplant
   (c) Monthly intravenous pulses of methylprednisolone
   (d) Rituximab
   (e) Continued combination treatment with methylprednisolone and cyclophosphamide

The initial treatment of Classes III (focal) and IV (diffuse) proliferative nephritis is controversial. Many clinicians, including the author, recommend therapy of the first episode with prednisone 1 mg/kg per day (or equivalent) for 4–12 weeks. For those patients who have a significant response with reduction in proteinuria, leucocyturia, hematuria, and anti-DNA antibody levels and resolution of hypocomplementemia, glucocorticoids are tapered at 1- to 2-week intervals by initially 10 and then 5 mg increments. In the absence of ongoing active renal disease, these patients are monitored for recurrence of active lupus renal disease. For late and infrequent relapses, attempts at remission with additional courses of prednisone are considered. For an incomplete response as well as early or frequent relapses, cyclophosphamide is initiated.

Justifying the use of prednisone as first-line therapy of Classes III and IV disease is the observation that long-term remissions of proliferative nephritis have been observed with such an approach. Additionally, treating with prednisone alone allows reproductive function to be preserved, such that pregnancies can be completed in intervals before relapsed disease requires cyclophosphamide treatment. It is also notable that the efficacy of cyclophosphamide is best established in patients previously treated for their renal disease with glucocorticoids. For example, in the NIH studies comparing prednisone with cyclophosphamide therapy, patient enrolment occurred only after a mean of 22 months of treatment with glucocorticoids for nephritis and 3 years for SLE. The benefits of intravenous cyclophosphamide were achieved in groups of patients failing to respond to prednisone, establishing cyclophosphamide as salvage or rescue therapy for patients who are unresponsive to glucocorticoids. The major argument against using glucocorticoids alone for proliferative nephritis, especially Class IV, is concern that any delay in initiating treatment with cyclophosphamide will permit renal scarring, which may be underestimated by monitoring serum creatinine levels and creatinine clearance. Therefore, treatment should be individualized accounting for the prognostic information available from the clinical or biopsy data and the relative risks of treatment in the specific circumstance.

Some clinicians recommend cyclophosphamide contemporaneously with prednisone for Class III or Class IV disease, especially in the presence of moderate-to-high activity and elevated chronicity biopsy scores. Cyclophosphamide is administered intravenously at a dosage of between 0.5 and 1 g/m^2 monthly for 6 months. Each subsequent dose is titrated upward or downward by 10–25% to achieve a nadir white blood cell count at 10–14 days of approximately 3,500 per mm^3. Cyclophosphamide is typically administered with 4–24 h of intravenous hydration to avoid hemorrhagic cystitis. Those treatment centers that use abbreviated intravenous hydration often use 2 mercaptoethylamine sulfonate sodium (MESNA) to further minimize the risk of bladder toxicity. Ondansetron or granisetron can be used as an antiemetic to reduce nausea and vomiting.

Once initiated, the duration of cyclophosphamide therapy should be individualized. For patients with a less prognostically severe biopsy and an early clinical response, cyclophosphamide can be limited to the 6 month induction course of treatment. Recognizing, however, that studies have established that patients with a longer course of cyclophosphamide (i.e., 14 treatments over 30 months) had a lower incidence of relapse of nephritis, maintenance therapy consisting of cyclophosphamide administered every 3 months for an additional 1–2 years is indicated for patients with prognostically severe biopsies.

Prednisone and cyclophosphamide therapy of proliferative lupus nephritis is usually effective in between 60 and 90% of patients. However, there will be patients who will prove refractory [defined as either failing to respond, or relapsing with reappearance of a nephrotic syndrome or nephritic component (e.g., hypertension and active urinary sediment) sometimes even with loss of renal function] and will require intensification of therapy. The combination of methylprednisolone and cyclophosphamide on a monthly basis in these patients may prove effective. Therefore, answer (e) is correct as it is premature to consider dialysis or transplantation and ritixumab remains of uncertain benefit and should remain the option of last resort after all other standards of care have been utilized or until the LUNAR Trial is published demonstrating safety and efficacy.

4. A 26-year-old female with a history of lupus and secondary APS manifest by two episodes of deep venous thrombophlebitis with the last complicated by a pulmonary embolus is on chronic warfarin to maintain an INR of 2 and presents to the office 2 weeks pregnant. The most appropriate treatment is follows:

   (a) Continue warfarin
   (b) Add aspirin 81 mg per day
   (c) Add prednisone at 1 mg/kg per day
   (d) Switch the patient to low molecular weight heparin

There is no evidence-based answer to this question as no randomized controlled trials have investigated the management of APS in pregnancy. Open labeled trials have been published reporting benefits with aspirin, aspirin plus prednisone, IVGG, unfractionated heparin, and LMWH in patients with recurrent miscarriage and positive antiphospholipid antibodies. Since warfarin alone or in combination is contraindicated in pregnancy due to the significant risk of teratogenicity and bleeding answers (a)–(c) are incorrect. As this patient would be at risk for both a maternal thrombotic event as well as for a placental thrombosis, during gestation the best option provided would be a LMWH (10). This is preferable to unfractionated heparin as dosing is weight based and more straightforward. The major risk of course is for maternal or fetal bleeding and osteoporosis. Coordinated care with high risk obstetrician and maternal fetal expert is also appropriate.

5. A 41-year-old Caucasian female with a 6-year history of lupus manifest by episodes of photosensitivity, acute cutaneous lupus manifest as malar rash, polyarthritis, recurrent episodes of pruritus, and leukopenia has been managed on chronic hydroxychloroquine and short courses of low-dose tapering prednisone. The patient presents with 2 weeks of fever, pedal edema 2+ on the right with calf tenderness, and vision loss in the right eye. The most likely diagnosis is:

   1. Catastrophic antiphospholipid syndrome (CAPS)
   2. SLE with active renal disease producing nephrotic syndrome and periorbital edema

3. SLE with Raynaud's and ocular migraine
4. SLE with hydroxychloroquine neuromyopathy
5. SLE with cutaneous and retinal vasculitis

On examination, this patient has evidence for possible deep venous thrombophlebitis and central retinal artery occlusion supporting the diagnosis of CAPS. The syndrome of multiple vascular occlusions associated with high titer antiphospholipid antibodies (aPL) is known as CAPS (11). Although APS is typically characterized by thrombotic events that either occur singly or, when recurrent, are seen many months or even years apart, some patients with this syndrome may develop widespread, noninflammatory vascular occlusions (Table 19.3).

The first reports of patients with multiple noninflammatory vascular occlusions appeared in 1974. However, it was not until Greisman reported in 1991 on two patients with "acute, catastrophic, widespread non-inflammatory visceral vascular occlusions associated with high titer antiphospholipid antibodies" that the full spectrum of clinical features associated with aPL became appreciated. It is now recognized that aPL may be "asymptomatic" and observed in patients free of thrombosis or associated with one or two episodes of thrombosis typically involving only one artery or vein at a time with long periods (months to years) free of occlusive events. Alternatively, aPL may confer a risk for an ominous disorder characterized by multiple, typically three or more, wide-spread thrombotic occlusions often with marked ischemic changes in the extremities, livido reticularis, as well as renal, cerebral, myocardial, pulmonary, and other visceral organ thrombotic vasculopathy. Asherson, describing ten such patients in an article published in 1992, first proposed the term catastrophic APS.

Table 19.3 Criteria for the classification of catastrophic antiphospholipid antibody syndrome

Criteria for the classification of catastrophic antiphospholipid antibody syndrome
Evidence of involvement of three or more organs, systems, or issues
Development of manifestations simultaneously or in less than a week
Confirmation by histopathology of small vessel occlusion in at least one organ or tissue?
Laboratory confirmation of the presence of aPL (lupus anticoagulant or aCL)
Definite catastrophic antiphospholipid antibody syndrome
All four criteria
Probable catastrophic antiphospholipid antibody syndrome
All four criteria, except only two organs; systems, or tissues are involved
All four criteria, except for the absence of laboratory confirmation at least 6 weeks apart because of the early death of a patient never previously tested for aPL before the catastrophic event
Criteria 1, 2, and 4 antiphospholipid
Criteria 1, 3, and 4, and the development of a third event in more than a week, but less than a month, despite anticoagulation

Usually, clinical evidence of vessel occlusions, confirmed by imaging techniques when appropriate. Renal involvement is defined by a 50% rise in serum creatinine. Severe systemic hypertension (greater than 190/110 mmHg), proteinuria (greater than 500 mg/24 h). For histopathologic confirmation, significant evidence of thrombosis must be present, although vasculitis may coexist occasionally. If the patient has not been previously diagnosed as having AP.S, the laboratory confirmation requires that the presence of aPL must be detected on two or more occasions at least 6 weeks apart (not necessarily at the time of the event), according to the proposed clinical criteria for the classification of definite APS

In CAPS, the most characteristic involvement is of renal, pulmonary, cerebral, gastrointestinal, and cerebral vessels: In contrast to the noncatastrophic APS, DVT is uncommon. However; atypical occlusive events such as of adrenal, pancreatic, splenic, testicular, and cutaneous vessels typify CAPS.

In the absence of randomized controlled trials, optimal therapy for patients with CAPS is uncertain. In contrast to the experience with APS where Khamashta reviewed retrospectively, in 147 patients, the efficacy of warfarin, low-dose aspirin, or both in the secondary prevention of thrombosis, no single center, large series of patients with CAPS exists. A more recent prospective randomized trial of 114 APS patients suggested that more moderate-intensity warfarin anticoagulation was no less effective in preventing thrombotic recurrences as compared to high intensity (12). Treatment is therefore empiric. Because CAPS is a thrombophilic disorder characterized by wide-spread microvasculopathy, the rationale of treatment is to prevent thrombosis by anticoagulation, to prevent the production and circulation of mediators (i.e., aPL, cytokines, complement degradation products, anti-endothelial cell antibodies, etc.) which generate the hypercoagulable state, or to prevent both. In other words, treatment may consist of anticoagulation, immunosuppressives, such as corticosteroids or cytotoxics, or plasmapheresis. The role of antiplatelet agents, prostacyclin, intravenous immunoglobulin, ancrod, defibrotide, and other fibrinolytic treatment is less certain.

Patients treated with the combination of anticoagulation in addition to steroids plus a therapy which can, achieve a prompt reduction in APL titer, either plasmapheresis or intravenous gammaglobulin, had the highest survival rate of almost 70%. A role for cyclophosphamide is suggested by its use in many of the most severe cases, CAPS accompanying SLE, and knowledge it prevents the rebound production of pathogenic autoantibodies by autoaggressive lymphocytes. Patients have received ancrod, purified fraction of' Malayan snake pit viper venom, as well as defibrotide and fibrinolytics, such as streptokinase with uncertain benefit. There is an ongoing study with rituximab for patients with refractory APLS.

Answers

Question 1: Answer (e)
Question 2: Answer (e)
Question 3: Answer (e)
Question 4: Answer (d)
Question 5: Answer (a)

References

1. Wallace D. The clinical presentation of systemic lupus erythematosus. In: Wallace D and Hahn B, Eds. Dubois' Lupus Erythematosus, Lippincott Williams & Wilkins, Hagerstown, MD, 2006, pp. 621–628.

2. Belmont HM, Abramson S, Lie JT. Pathology and pathogenesis of vascular injury in systemic lupus erythematosus. Arthritis Rheum 1996, **39**:9–23.
3. Betsias G, Ioannidis J, Boletis J, et al. EULAR recommendations for the management of systemic lupus erythematosus. Report task for the EULAR standing committee for international clinical studies including therapeutics. Ann Rheum Dis 2008, **67**:195–205.
4. Illei GG, Austin HA, Crane M, et al. Combination therapy with pulse cyclophosphamide plus pulse methylprednisolone improves long-term renal outcome without adding toxicity in patients with lupus nephritis. Ann Int Med 2001, **135**(4):248–257.
5. Mok, C. Therapeutic options for resistant Lupus Nephritis Semin. Arthritis Rheum 2006, **36**:71–81.
6. Contreras G, Pardo V, Leclercq B, et al. Sequential therapies for proliferative lupus nephritis. N Engl J Med 2004, **350**:971–980.
7. Waldman M, Appel GB. Update on the treatment of lupus nephritis. Kidney Int 2006, **70**(8):1403–1412.
8. Tenedios F, Erkan D, Lockshin MD. Cardiac manifestations in the antiphospholipid syndrome. Rheum Dis Clin North Am 2006, **32**(3):491–507.
9. Austin HA, Illei GG. Membranous lupus nephritis. Lupus 2005, **14**(1):65–71.
10. Tincani A, Bazzani C, Zingarelli S, et al. Lupus and the antiphospholipid syndrome in pregnancy and obstetrics: clinical characteristics, diagnosis, pathogenesis, and treatment. Semin Thromb Hemost 2008, **34**(3):267–273.
11. Belmont HM. Catastrophic antiphospholipid syndrome. In: Khamashta M and Hughes G, Eds. Hughes Syndrome, 2006, pp. 152–161, Springer-Verlag London.
12. Crowther MA, Gisnberg JS, Julian J, et al. A comparison of two intensities of warfarin for the prevention of recurrent thrombosis in patients with the antiphospholipid antibody syndrome. N Engl J Med 2003, **349**:1133–1138.

Chapter 20
Immunodeficiency

Aymeric Louit and Pedro C. Avila

Abstract In this chapter, we will describe two cases involving human immune deficiency. One case involves a unique complication while the other case involves an atypical presentation. The first case describes a pregnant woman with recurrent sinusitis and neutropenias who developed pleural and pericardial empyemas. The second case is of a woman who presented with recurrent liver abscesses. Some of the related differential diagnoses are also discussed.

Keywords Common variable immunodeficiency • Chronic granulomatous disease • Liver abscess • Empyema

Case 1

A 38-year-old female was 22 weeks pregnant at the time of presentation to the outpatient clinic with complaints of recurrent sinusitis. She reported that her first sinus infection occurred 18 months earlier and was treated to resolution with amoxicillin. She subsequently had a sinus infection 5 months prior to presentation treated with amoxicillin, but without complete resolution, requiring further antibiotic therapy with amoxicillin/clavulanic acid 3 months prior to presentation. However, while on amoxicillin/clavulanic acid, the patient developed fevers and chills. She sought care from her obstetrician and primary care provider at 11 weeks gestation and was found to be neutropenic (WBC 900 cells/μl - normal range: 3,500–10,500 cells/μl with 300 neutrophils/μl - normal range: 1,500–8,000 neutrophils/μl) and hypokalemic (2.7 mEq/L - normal range: 3.5–5.0 mEq/L) for which she was referred to the emergency room, where she was found to also be hypotensive

A. Louit and P.C. Avila (✉)
Division of Allergy-Immunology, Northwestern University Feinberg School
of Medicine, 676 North Saint Clair Street, Rm 14-018, Chicago, IL 60611, USA
e-mail: pa@northwestern.edu

M. Mahmoudi (ed.), *Challenging Cases in Allergy and Immunology,*
DOI: 10.1007/978-1-60327-443-2_20,
© Humana Press, a part of Springer Science+Business Media, LLC 2009

with a blood pressure of 80/50 mmHg. The patient was admitted to the intensive care unit, given intravenous fluids, and started on broad spectrum antibiotics for neutropenic fever. The patient's blood culture grew out *Pseudomonas aeruginosa* for which her antibiotic coverage was adjusted and she was discharged 4 days later on 2 weeks of intravenous antibiotics. Her neutropenia was felt to be related to sepsis or a viral infection.

Two months prior to presentation, while traveling out of state, the patient again developed sinusitis symptoms and started another course of amoxicillin/clavulanic acid. Soon after treatment began, she was again found to be leukopenic (WBC 600 cells/μl – normal range: 3,500–10,500 cells/μl) with neutropenia (data not available) and admitted to a local hospital's intensive care unit. The patient's neutropenia resolved with filgastrim and she was discharged home. Her neutropenia was felt to be related to the administration of amoxicillin/clavulanic acid. However, a hematological evaluation revealed her to also be both lymphopenic and profoundly hypogammaglobulinemic (IgG < 33 mg/dl, IgA < 7 mg/dl, IgM < 4 mg/dl – normal ranges: IgG: 750–1,700 mg/dl, IgA: 82–400 mg/dl, IgM: 46–304 mg/dl) for which she was referred to our Allergy and Immunology clinic. Two weeks prior to presentation to our clinic, she again developed sinusitis symptoms confirmed by computed tomogram (CT) of the sinuses, which revealed pansinusitis and osteomeatal unit opacification (Fig. 20.1). She was treated with azithromycin and prednisone.

Past Medical History

At presentation, she denied any history of pneumonia, gastrointestinal infection, skin infection, or fungal infection. She did report postpartum perineal condylomata after term delivery via C-section of her first child, and a Staphylococcal infection of her nares (not MRSA) about 10 years prior. As a young adult, she had chronic idiopathic urticaria. The patient is an attorney and lives in a new condominium with

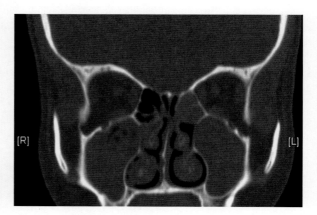

Fig. 20.1 Sinus CT demonstrating subtotal opacification of maxillary and left ethmoidal paranasal sinuses

her husband and 19-month-old son. She denied tobacco, alcohol, or illicit drug use. She denied any international travel. There was no family history of oncologic, hematologic, or immunologic disorders.

Outpatient Physical Examination

Her physical exam revealed persistent clear nasal drainage and cough productive of clear sputum. She was afebrile and normotensive, but was tachycardic with a pulse of 124. Her nares were patent with edematous turbinates bilaterally and no polyps. Her oropharynx was clear. Her lungs were clear to auscultation bilaterally. Her cardiac exam revealed normal heart sounds and a regular tachycardia. The patient had a gravid abdomen consistent with a 22-week gestation. She had an unremarkable skin exam.

Outpatient Laboratory Evaluation

Her laboratory tests revealed anemia and agammaglobulinemia (Table 20.1).

Imaging

See Fig. 20.1.

Impression and Differential Diagnoses

Immunodeficiency is the unifying feature for this patient's presentation given her recurrent infections and undetectable gammaglobulins. However, her quantitative immunoglobulin profile excludes her from diagnoses such as IgG subclass

Table 20.1 Outpatient laboratory evaluation

White blood cell count	8,500 cells/μl	Normal range (3,500–10,500)	Neutrophils	94%	(34–73)
Hemoglobin	9.1 g/dl	(11.6–15.4)	Lymphocytes	3%	(15–50)
Hematocrit	26.5%	(34–45)	Monocytes	3%	(5–15)
Platelets	367,000	(140–390)	IgG	<33 mg/dl	(750–1,700)
			IgA	<7 mg/dl	(82–400)
			IgM	<4 mg/dl	(46–304)

deficiency (IGGSD), hyper-IgM syndrome (HIM), and selective antibody deficiency with normal immunoglobulin (SADNI). Although her female sex, the phenomenon of lyonization and the possibility of autosomal variants do not preclude her from having X-linked agammaglobulinemia (XLA) and X-linked lymphoproliferative disease (XLP). However, her age and lack of evidence for hepatitis or Epstein Barr virus infection do not support these diagnoses. Furthermore, secondary causes of hypogammaglobulinemia due to malignancy, medication, or infection are not corroborated by her history. HIV was later eliminated by history and polymerase chain reaction (PCR) testing.

Because of her recurrent sinusitis and hypogammaglobulinemia she was started on intravenous immunoglobulin (IVIG) therapy the following day.

Clinical Course

Two days later, she was admitted to the hospital from her obstetrician's office due to 2 days of chest tightness, progressive dyspnea, and intrauterine fetal demise. A CT scan of her chest revealed a right-sided loculated pleural effusion and a large pericardial effusion with tamponade physiology, but no pulmonary embolus (Fig. 20.2). The patient underwent successful pericardiocentesis, video-assisted thorascopic surgery with chest tube placements, and fetal delivery. Both the pleural and pericardial collections grew *Streptococcus pneumoniae* for which the patient received broad spectrum antibiotics. The patient also received nine further IVIG doses during her 3-week hospitalization for persistent hypogammaglobulinemia (IgG range from <33 to 747 mg/dl).

Inpatient Physical Examination

Prior to draining effusions, the patient was afebrile and normotensive. She had a regular pulse at 158 bpm and was mildly dyspneic sitting up in bed. She had mildly edematous nasal turbinates without polyps. Her lung exam revealed decreased breath sounds bibasally without wheeze. Her cardiac exam revealed normal heart sounds and a regular tachycardia. Her abdomen was gravid and her skin exam was unremarkable. Her lower extremities revealed mild bilateral pitting edema.

Inpatient Laboratory Evaluation

Her laboratory tests revealed anemia, neutrophilia, and lymphopenia (Table 20.2). Her CT of chest and abdomen revealed right-sided loculated empyema and a large pericardial empyema (Fig. 20.2).

Table 20.2 Inpatient laboratory evaluation

White blood cell count	24,900 cells/μl	Normal range (3,500–10,500)	Neutrophils	97%	(34–73)
Hemoglobin	8.9 g/dl	(11.6–15.4)	Lymphocytes	3%	(15–50)
Hematocrit	26.3%	(34–45)			
Platelets	284,000	(140–390)			

Fig. 20.2 CT of the chest frontal (**a**) and cross-sectional (**b**) demonstrate large, loculated right-sided pleural empyema and a large pericardial empyema

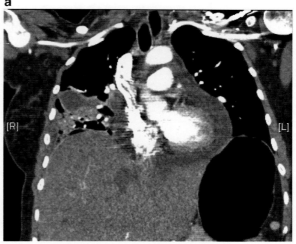

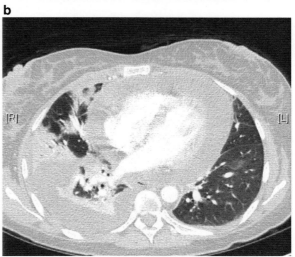

Imaging

See Fig. 20.2.

Follow-Up

She subsequently received IVIG therapy monthly and has had no further episodes of neutropenia or hospitalizations.

Discussion

Humoral immune deficiency represents the large majority of primary immunodeficiencies accounting for almost 65% of cases. Multiple diagnoses are included in this classification and although each is distinct, there is a discernable spectrum of disease with overlap in clinical and laboratory manifestations (1). We will discuss several of the humoral immune deficiencies here.

Selective IgA Deficiency

Selective IgA deficiency (IGAD) is the most common primary immunodeficiency with an incidence of up to 1:300 based on samples from blood bank donors, yet it is often clinically silent. When symptomatic, it resembles common variable immune deficiency (CVID) in its clinical presentation and molecular origins as they share some of the same mutations and major histocompatibility complex (MHC) haplotypes as discussed in CVID below. Like in CVID, patients with IGAD have a higher incidence of respiratory bacterial infections, but unlike CVID, patients with IGAD often experience genitourinary infections and have a higher incidence of respiratory and food allergies, suggesting a role of IgA in tolerance or prevention of sensitization.

Patients with IGAD also have an increased incidence of malignancy, especially involving the gastrointestinal tract. These patients have an increased incidence of clinically significant autoimmune disease such as rheumatoid arthritis (RA), immune thrombocytopenic purpura (ITP), and systemic lupus erythematosus (SLE) with anti-DNA antibodies present in many patients. Of interest, patients with IGAD may possess antibodies against IgA, which is the mechanism thought to explain anaphylactic reactions to blood product infusions that contain some IgA. For the same reason, IGAD patients are at risk of developing anaphylaxis to IVIG and this therapy should be avoided unless a concomitant IgG deficiency is also present. Reversible and sometimes permanent IGAD have been reported after treatment with certain medications including phenytoin, sulfasalazine, plaquenil, and penicillamine.

The four defining criteria for IGAD are an IgA level <7.0 mg/dl, normal levels of IgG and IgM, normal cell mediated immunity, and normal antibody production. Although B cell numbers are usually within the normal range, they express an immature phenotype (IgM$^+$/IgD$^+$/IgA$^+$) and they have an impaired ability to synthesize new IgA. IGAD is linked to IGGSD particularly of IgG2 and IgG4, which can also be clinically silent. Measurement of IgG subclasses or of the secretory IgA has not been completely proven to be of clinical utility.

Management is mostly expectant if identified incidentally. However, early treatment with antibiotics at the first signs of infection may be appropriate.

IgG Subclass Deficiency

IGGSD is another humoral immune deficiency state on the same clinical spectrum as CVID and IGAD. Overall, individuals with IGGSD are clinically asymptomatic including some with complete absence of a subclass, yet a relationship between IGGSD and an increase in sinopulmonary infections has been noted. IgG3 is the most common subclass deficiency in adults, and IgG2 deficiency is most often seen in pediatric populations. There are differences in the biologic roles of the various subclasses such as the response to polysaccharide vaccine antigen (i.e., *Haemophilus influenzae*), which is predominantly of IgG2 subclass in adults. Children of such patients have been found to mount polysaccharide antigen response via IgG1 suggesting that one subclass can assume the biologic role of another one, and in doing so, can render most IgG subclass-deficient individuals asymptomatic.

The defining laboratory finding is a deficiency in any of the IgG subclasses of greater than two standard deviations below the age-appropriate mean. Complicating the evaluation of IGGSD is that there is little consensus as to the actual clinically relevant cutoff values of the various IgG subclasses or to the method used to measure them. Therapy is aimed toward management of infections with antibiotics. There is no current indication for IVIG unless there is a concurrent specific antibody deficiency, that is, poor rise in specific antibody titers to vaccine antigens (i.e., Pneumovax).

Specific Antibody Deficiency with Normal Immunoglobulins

SADNI is a clinical entity that is characterized by poor response to vaccinations or infections, despite normal numbers of circulating B cells, T cells, and serum levels of immunoglobulins, including IgG subclasses. Most patients present in early childhood by demonstrating a poor response to polysaccharide antigens present in their scheduled vaccinations. It can also be identified in adulthood. It is known that infants do not respond well to neumococcal polysaccharide antigens without adjuvants, which suggests that this early childhood prevalence may actually represent a delay in immune maturation rather than a lifelong disease. Those with the true immune deficiency may experience recurrent and sometimes severe infections. Therapy is initially based on antibiotic prophylaxis and early treatment of infections, but persistent symptoms should warrant an early conversion to regular, periodic parenteral Ig therapy despite normal immunoglobulin levels as these patients are unable to respond to antigen challenge by producing a specific antibody response.

Transient Hypogammaglobulinemia of Infancy

It is well established that newborns are born with reduced ability to produce immunoglobulins compared with adults. Immunoglobulin levels rise after birth and reach full adult levels by adolescence. Some children have been identified retrospectively as having a more profound hypogammaglobulinemic period compared with their age-matched peers that resolves by 4 years of age. These children are at increased risk for sinopulmonary infections and may have poor response to antigen as well. Patients with recurrent or severe infections would likely benefit from therapy with IVIG or SCIG. Transient hypogammaglobulinemia of infancy (THI) can be distinguished from SADNI based on normal serum immunoglobulin levels and from CVID, IGAD, IGGSD, and XLA based on the eventual return to normal immunoglobulin levels identified retrospectively and in the absence of further parenteral Ig treatments.

X-Linked (or Bruton's) Agammaglobulinemia

XLA represents the most common immune deficiency identified in boys after 6 months of age when the maternal IgG is no longer detectable in the serum. It was first described in 1952 as the congenital inability to form antibodies (2). A small proportion of these patients, however, will be diagnosed with THI retrospectively. In 1993, the cause of XLA was found to be the absence of the Bruton's Tyrosine Kinase (BTK) enzyme located on Xq22. BTK is responsible for B cell receptor (BCR) signaling and B cell differentiation from pre-B cell to mature B cell. The diagnosis is definitively done by genetic testing looking for the absence of BTK. In its absence, patients with XLA have almost no mature B cells, which is demonstrated by the absence of circulating cells with mature B cell surface markers (CD19, CD20, and/or CD21) using flow cytometry. In addition, pathology shows absence of germinal centers in lymphoid tissues, which are atrophic, and serum immunoglobulins are absent. There are normal and sometimes increased numbers of functional T cells.

XLA patients have increased susceptibility to bacterial infections and have relatively normal antiviral activity. In addition, they are also susceptible to severe infections caused by *Ureaplasma*, *Mycoplasma*, and to meningoencephalitis caused by enteroviruses such as ECHO viruses, Coxsackie virus, and vaccine-associated poliomyelitis. There are autosomal recessive defects that have been identified that mimic the XLA phenotype and can be found in male and female patients as well (autosomal recessive agammaglobulinemia or ARA). These include defects in the IgM heavy chain, the Surrogate light chain $\lambda5/14.1$, the Igα chain of BCR, and the signal transducer B cell linker protein (BLNK). There are reports of patients diagnosed with XLA as adults, necessitating clinical vigilance for patients of all ages with recurrent infections. There is ongoing discussion in the literature as to whether all adult males with hypogammaglobulinemia and especially those with few to absent B cells should undergo genetic testing for XLA. XLA is also managed with chronic Ig replacement therapy and aggressive antibacterial therapy.

Hyper-IgM Syndrome

HIM is an entity often diagnosed within the first 2 years of life that is classified as both a humoral deficiency (autosomal recessive) and a combined humoral and cellular deficiency (X-linked) depending on the site of the defect. All five types identified (Type 1, X-linked; Types 2–5, autosomal recessive) are characterized by impaired isotype class switching with consequent laboratory findings of low levels of IgG, IgA, and IgE, but with normal to elevated levels of IgM. HIM Type 1 is the consequence of T cells not being able to produce functional CD40L (CD154), a critical factor on activated T cells involved in B cell class switching, the formation of memory B cells, and proper T cell function. As such, type 1 represents a predominantly cellular immune deficiency with associated early onset susceptibility to *Pneumocystis jiroveci*, cryptosporidia, candidiasis, and *Histoplasma* in young males. Neutropenia, sometimes severe, is a common finding in over half of patients and a higher incidence of malignancy is also reported.

An autosomal recessive inheritance pattern later discovered in females accounts for the remaining types of HIM, which manifests predominantly as a humoral immunodeficiency. Types 2 and 4 are associated with defects in the activation-induced deaminase (AID) gene. Type 3 is characterized by deficiency of functional CD40 on B cells. Type 5, with a defect in functional Uracil N-glycosylase (UNG), is phenotypically related to types 2 and 4. AID and UNG are both necessary enzymes involved in the somatic hypermutation process of isotype class switching in B cells. Among these types, neutropenia is less common and T cell function is clinically normal while hepatosplenomegaly and lymphadenopathy are prevalent.

HIM is managed with replacement Ig therapy, aggressive antibacterial therapy such as Pneumocystis prophylaxis, and if needed for neutropenia, granulocyte colony stimulating factor (G-CSF). Ig therapy does not correct the T cell defect of HIM type 1. In few cases of HIM type 1 with severe T cell deficiency, HLA-matched bone marrow transplantation has successfully reconstituted cellular immunity.

Common Variable Immune Deficiency

CVID is a common primary immunodeficiency affecting mostly adults with a prevalence of up to 1:25,000 among Europeans. It is a heterogeneous disorder which primarily affects the B cell compartment, but almost 50% have impaired T cell function, particularly in advanced cases. It is characterized by low serum IgG and IgA and/or IgM, and recurrent bacterial infections at sinopulmonary sites. This case was diagnosed as CVID and it illustrates how complex the infectious manifestations can be in this disease. Patients with CVID have a high incidence of chronic lung disease with bronchiectasis, autoimmune disease such as sicca syndrome, rheumatoid arthritis, and SLE, which all contribute to the ongoing morbidity with the passage of time. Patients also experience an increased incidence of malignancies and include non-Hodgkin's lymphoma and gastrointestinal cancers. Other findings include B cell hyperplasia and enlargement of secondary lymphoid organs such as enlarged tonsils, nodular lymphoid hyperplasia of the gastrointestinal tract, and splenomegaly; the latter is present in almost 30% of patients.

Although it can present in childhood, most cases are diagnosed in the second through fourth decades of life with a delay from disease onset to diagnosis of approximately 4–8 years. Patients with CVID have a reduced 20-year life expectancy, likely related to the comorbid conditions mentioned above rather than to infections (3). CVID can occur in families or cluster with other immune disorders such as IgA deficiency in a heritable fashion, but for many years a genetic association could not be identified. A study of multiple families revealed a predominance of two MHC haplotypes suggesting both a location for a susceptibility gene and the genetic similarity of CVID and IGAD on the humoral immune deficiency spectrum.

Molecular Defects in CVID

Recent advances have begun to shed light on the disease with the discovery of genetic mutations in five different genes: TACI, BAFF-R, ICOS, CD19, and MSH5. Mutations in TACI (transmembrane activator and calcium-modulator cyclophilin ligand interactor) were found in unrelated patients with CVID and IGAD, which may explain a molecular mechanism of disease via impaired immunoglobulin class switching. The B cells still express TACI, but are unable to class switch to produce IgG and IgA in response to a proliferation-inducing ligand (APRIL), one of the TACI ligands (Fig. 20.3.).

B cell activating factor receptor (BAFF-R), like TACI, is also a B cell receptor that binds to BAFF and promotes B cell survival and isotype switching. Only one CVID patient has been described with BAFF-R mutation. It remains to be seen if further molecules related to this signaling pathway including B cell maturation

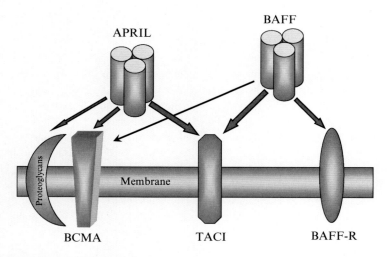

Fig. 20.3 BAFF and APRIL Receptors

antigen (BCMA), a third transmembrane activator receptor that binds to BAFF, can contribute to the CVID phenotype.

Another recently identified genetic defect found among CVID patients is inducible costimulator (ICOS). ICOS is expressed on activated T cells and transmits activating signals that lead to the production of IL-4, IL-10, and to the stimulation of previously differentiated effector T cells. IL-10 is involved in the terminal differentiation of B cells to memory and plasma cells. Homozygous ICOS deficiency expresses a phenotype indistinguishable from CVID with hypogammaglobulinemia, bacterial infections, splenomegaly, nodular lymphoid hyperplasia of the intestine, and increased incidence of malignancy and autoimmune disease. These patients have normal T cell numbers and normal T cell function, but the defect lies in the T cell interaction with B cells and class switching.

CD19 is a B cell receptor (BCR) coreceptor molecule that heightens B cell signaling after antigen challenge. CVID patients with deficiency of CD19 on B cells have normal overall B cell numbers, but are deficient in the maturation and differentiation of B cells from germinal centers. Consequently, patients who have one of the various CD19 mutations have impaired immunoglobulin production in response to antigenic stimuli.

MSH5 is an *Escherichia coli* homolog protein of MutS and is found in the MHC III region. It functions as a mismatch repair protein and contributes to class switch recombination and has more recently been associated with CVID.

Although very exciting work is still ongoing involving these five molecules, they likely represent a small portion of CVID defects as they are only present in ~10–15% of all CVID patients. We can therefore look forward to the identification of more factors yet to be discovered.

Classification

In 2008, a European consortium published a new classification system for CVID to help clarify the heterogeneity of the disease. It involves three groupings based on switched memory (sm) B cell phenotype assessed by flow cytometry. Indeed, certain features of CVID such as bronchiectasis, granulomas, lymphadenopathy, or splenomegaly can be linked to a defect at a specific stage of B cell development. For example, patients who are severely deficient in smB (CD27+) cells are more likely to have bronchiectasis and autoimmune disease.

Taken together, these represent important advances over the past decade in a disease for which an underlying molecular mechanism has eluded researchers since it was first recognized in 1953.

Therapy

The mainstay of therapy for over 25 years is periodic administration of immunoglobulin. In addition, aggressive anti-infectious therapy is initiated early to treat infections. Immunoglobulin (Ig) therapy was formerly administered intramuscularly, but once additives (sugar or amino acids) were introduced to prevent IgG aggregation, it became feasible to administer large and more efficacious doses by intravenous (IVIG) and subcutaneous (SCIG) routes (4). Each parenteral Ig lot is manufactured from pooled plasma product from 3,000 to 10,000 donors. It replenishes IgG levels but not IgA or IgM because it contains only trace amounts of IgA and IgM immunoglobulins. The typical therapeutic dose is 400–600 mg/kg per month given every 2–4 weeks in order to maintain the IgG trough levels greater than 500 mg/dl, a value recommended by the most recent JCAAI Practice Parameters (5). Some groups, however, find improved clinical results with higher trough levels up to 700 mg/dl, or using doses of 600 mg/kg per month (6). Ig therapy prevents infections and chronic lung disease, and is used in high doses for autoimmune thrombocytopenia. Unfortunately, Ig therapy is not effective for the comorbidities of CVID such as bronchiectasis, granulomatous disease, or malignancy. Chronic lung disease may benefit from aggressive therapy including corticosteroids, bronchodilators, and pulmonary rehabilitation. Effective therapies for these comorbidities such as immunomodulators or stem cell transplantation are under investigation since they likely contribute to the reduced 20-year life expectancy of CVID patients (Table 20.3).

Case 2

This is the case of a 46-year-old woman with a clinical presentation of sepsis who required evaluation and management of a recurrent hepatic abscess (7). She had a documented streptococcal liver abscess 18 months prior to presentation that was managed by surgical drainage and intravenous antibiotics. She developed recurrence of clinical symptoms of right upper quadrant abdominal pain and fever. An abdominal CT exam demonstrated a large liver abscess. Laparoscopic drainage was performed, but she subsequently developed subcapsular hepatic bleeding (Fig. 20.4).

Past Medical History

She denied history of pneumonia or sinus infections, but did report lifelong problems with refractory gingivitis. Her childhood was unremarkable for atopy, or severe and opportunistic infections. Her family history was remarkable for a brother who died of bilateral Nocardia pneumonia and a sister with gingivitis. She had another sister who was otherwise well. The patient was a dental hygienist, lived with her husband and was without children. She denied prior hematologic, oncologic, or immunologic disorders.

Table 20.3 Summary table of humoral immune deficiencies

Disease	Molecular defect(s)	Characteristic findings	Diagnosis	IVIG indicated?
CVID	TACI,BAFF-R, CD19, ICOS, MHC5	Sinopulmonary infections, autoimmunity, chronic lung disease	Low Immunoglobulins, esp. IgG, can also have low IgA and/or IgM	Yes. Lifelong therapy
IGAD	TACI	Sinopulmonary infections, autoimmunity, malignancy, increased frequency of allergic disorders.	IgA < 7.0 mg/dl, normal IgG + IgM, normal Ab production, normal cell-mediated immunity	No
IGGSD	Unknown	Sinopulmonary infections, autoimmunity, malignancy	Any one of the IgG subclasses 2 SD below the age-appropriate mean	Occasionally
SADNI	Unknown	Sinopulmonary infections	Poor response to vaccine with normal immunoglobulin levels	Yes, if aggressive anti bacterial therapies fail
THI	Unknown	Sinopulmonary infections	Decreased immunoglobulin levels that resolve with time	Yes, transiently
XLA/AR-A	BTK/IgM heavy chain, Surrogate light chain λ5/14.1, Igα chain of BCR, BLNK	Affects mostly males. Infections. Absence of mature B cells, no lymphoid tissue. Infections with ureaplasma, mycoplasma, vaccine-related poliomyelitis	Flow cytometry, genetic testing for BTK	Yes
XHIM/ AR-HIM	CD40L/AID, UNG, CD40	Infections, pneumocystis (XHIM), neutropenias.	Low IgG and IgA, normal or elevated IgM	Yes (with G-CSF for XHIM)

Fig. 20.4 Abdominal CT showing 9.1 × 7.5 cm heterogeneous lesion in right lobe of the liver consistent with an abscess (*white arrow*) and a large subcapsular hepatic hematoma (*black arrow*), probably a surgical complication of surgical drainage of the hepatic abscess. Reproduced with permission from (7)

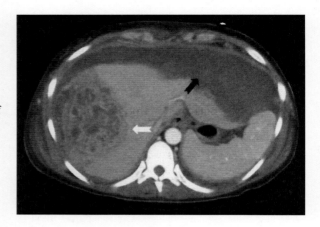

Physical Examination

She was afebrile, normotensive, and slightly tachycardic with a pulse of 102 bpm. There was no evidence of sinus disease or lymphadenopathy. She did have erythematous gingivae. She had tense, right upper quadrant discomfort without rebound or guarding. Cardiovascular exam revealed normal heart sounds and a regular tachycardia. Pulmonary, dermatologic, and neurological examinations were unremarkable.

Laboratory Evaluation

Drainage fluid from the liver grew *Streptococcus mitis* that was sensitive to penicillin. Quantitative immunoglobulins and complement levels were normal. HIV testing was negative. CBC showed neutrophilia and blood smear showed no giant granules in neutrophils ruling out Chédiak-Higashi syndrome (Table 20.4).

Impression and Differential Diagnoses

The recurrent severe internal abscesses again suggest that an immune deficiency is the underlying problem for this patient. The appropriate leukocytosis and normal immunoglobulin levels suggest that she has normal function of her cellular and humoral immune systems. Given the unusual recurrent infections with absecesses, the chronic

Table 20.4 Laboratory evaluation

White Blood Cells	22,600 cells/µl	Normal range (3500–10,500)	Platelets	542,000
Hemoglobin	9.8 g/dl	(11.6–15.4)	Neutrophils	85%
Hematocrit	29.2%	(34–45)	Lymphocytes	6%

Reproduced with permission from (7)

mucosal infection, and the Nocardiosis of her brother, a defect of innate immunity could be suspected. However, such defects are overwhelmingly diagnoses of childhood. Among these, Chronic Granulomatous Disease (CGD) given the abscesses and Leukocyte Adhesion Deficiency (LAD) given the periodontitis would be in the differential diagnoses, although both are usually childhood diagnoses.

Further Studies

Her neutrophil oxidative index was 4 consistent with defective oxidative function (Fig. 20.5). Furthermore, flow cytometry to detect the main four components of nicotinamide adenine dinucleotide phosphate (NADPH) oxidase system, gp91, p67, p47, and p22, revealed an absence of the p47 subunit (Fig. 20.5). Genotyping in the patient, in the sister with gingivitis, and in paraffin-embedded postmortem samples from her deceased brother; all revealed a classic GT deletion in exon 2 and a G784A mutation (Gly 262 change to Ser) in exon 8. The healthy sister had no mutations.

What Is Your Diagnosis and Why?

With these results a diagnosis of CGD was made. She began therapy with interferon-γ and prophylactic antibiotic treatment with trimethoprim-sulfamethoxazole and itraconazole. The patient recovered from her hepatic abscess after drainage and intravenous antibiotic therapy. There have only been a few case reports of CGD in adults reported in the literature as it is far more likely to be diagnosed in the first few years of life.

Discussion

Phagocytic cell disorders represent approximately 10–15% of all immune deficiencies. This arm of the immune system acts in a crucial role to support host defenses of which the predominant cellular actors are neutrophils and macrophages, but also include monocytes and eosinophils. We will discuss two different classes of phagocyte disorders here: defective oxygen burst and deficiency in adhesion molecules.

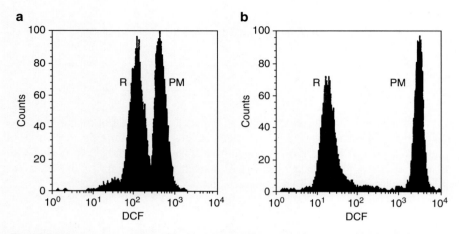

Fig. 20.5 Flow cytometry evaluation of patient and control subjects. Neutrophil oxidative index. Oxidative bursts of neutrophils from the patient (**a**) and from a control subject (**b**) were examined by flow cytometry using the dye 2,7-dichlorofluorescein diacetate (DCF), which becomes fluorescent upon exposure to reactive oxygen species produced by phagocytes. Neutrophils were examined at rest (R) and after stimulation with phorbol myristate acetate (PM). Compared with the control neutrophils, those from the patient showed a smaller increase in oxidative burst after stimulation (4× vs. 126×) and decreased maximum oxidative burst, indicating a deficiency in superoxide production. Reproduced with permission from (7)

Chronic Granulomatous Disease

CGD is a heterogeneous disorder characterized by recurrent infections due to the impaired ability of the nicotinamide adenine dinucleotide phosphate (NADPH) oxidase system to produce reactive oxygen intermediates in microbial killing. The NADPH oxidase complex consists of five subunits in which defects of any of these can cause clinical CGD (Fig. 20.6). Up to 70% of cases are X-linked due to the gene location of the largest subunit, membrane-bound gp91 in which over 300 mutations have been identified. The cytochrome b558 molecule is made up of the gp91 and p22 subunits. The remaining cases are autosomal recessive due to mutations in the other four subunits p47, RAC2, p22, and p67. Of these, mutations in p47 are the most common, representing over 20% of all CGD cases but with only one highly conserved mutation identified. Almost all cases are diagnosed by 5 years of age, however, a few cases, as illustrated above, are diagnosed in adulthood.

Most infections common to CGD patients are from catalase-positive organisms that can break down their own endogenous production of hydrogen peroxide, thereby preventing the defective CGD complex from utilizing the organism's own hydrogen peroxide against itself. The common pathogens include *Burkholderia cepacia, Serratia marcescens, Staphylococcus aureus, Salmonella,*

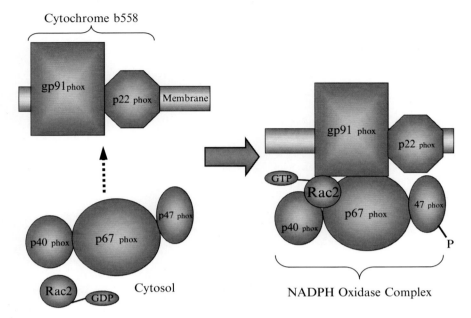

Fig. 20.6 NADPH oxidase complex

Chromobacterium, Candida, and *Aspergillus* species but there are many others that contribute to significant morbidity. These various species cause a variety of severe sinopulmonary infections, abscesses of the liver and the spleen, skin infections, and osteomyelitis. Patients with CGD also develop granulomas of the skin, gastrointestinal, or genitourinary tracts. Another feature of CGD is hypergammaglobulinemia from frequent infections.

Formerly, the nitroblue tetrazolium (NBT) test was the technique used to identify CGD patients. However, with increased prevalence of and expertise in using flow cytometry, the dihydrorhodamine (DHR) test has become the standard manner to identify CGD patients and CGD carriers. DHR emits fluorescence when it reacts with hydrogen peroxide, identifying normal granulocytes.

Prior to the advances made in understanding the pathogenesis of CGD, most patients died of infections within the first decade of life. Currently, life expectancy is improved into middle age with aggressive antibacterial and antifungal prophylaxis with trimethoprim-sulfamethoxazole and antifungal agents. In addition, interferon-γ therapy stimulates neutrophil microbial killing and reduces risk of serious infections in X-linked and autosomal recessive forms of CGD. Comorbid granulomatous disease can be successfully managed with systemic corticosteroid therapy, particularly in cases of obstruction by compressing tubular structures. Finally, in the past decade, stem cell transplant has also been shown to be effective for severe cases. It is performed when patients are infection free.

Leukocyte Adhesion Deficiency

LAD is another important group of phagocyte deficiencies characterized by abnormally functioning adhesion molecules that interfere with proper diapedesis of leukocytes. In LAD type 1 (LAD-1), the defect is in the CD18 (integrin β2) component of an integrin protein called lymphocyte function-associated antigen 1 (LFA-1; heterodimer of CD11 and CD18), an adhesion molecule important in neutrophil extravasation from the peripheral circulation to sites of infection. Clinically, this results in recurrent infections and delayed separation of the umbilical cord. Neutrophils are unable to leave the intra-vascular compartment and reach the affected tissue to mediate an appropriate inflam-matory response, thus preventing diapedesis and suppuration of active infections. This also results in increased neutrophil blood counts as high as 100,000 cells/μl during infections. Neutrophil counts can remain elevated during sterile intervals as well. Severe LAD-1 is seen in patients with <3% of functional CD18 and can lead to death in the first few months of life without medical intervention. Diagnosis is made by flow cytometric evaluation of circulating phagocytes.

In LAD type 2 (LAD-2), the defect lies in an abnormal GDP-fucose transporter important for glycosylation of protein in the Golgi apparatus, which subsequently does not produce a functional sialyl-Lewis-X protein, the ligand for E-selectin. Without it, leukocytes are unable to attach to vascular endothelium, the first step for extravasation into the tissue. These patients have similar manifestations to those of LAD1 namely, recurrent infections. However, LAD-2 also causes mental retardation, small stature, and abnormal facies.

A third form of LAD, designated as LAD-3, involves a mutation in the Rap-1 molecule, an important molecule involved in integrin activation. The clinical fea-tures in LAD-3 are similar to those of LAD-1 as these patients also have poor leukocyte transmigration into affected tissue. In addition, they have the propensity to bleed secondary to significant platelet aggregation defects.

As with other immune deficiencies reviewed here, management of LAD is by way of aggressive antibiotic therapy, but bone marrow transplantation has proven effective and is the current standard of care for the more severe phenotype. In addition, for patients with LAD-2, fucose supplementation has been used with reported success in reducing neutrophil levels back to within normal limits, decreasing frequency of infections, and improving psychomotor development.

Summary

The two cases presented in this chapter illustrate the breadth of the various primary immune deficiencies that are currently described. The rare prevalence of these diagnoses and the many others not discussed here make the case that no definitive "classic" phenotype can be put forth and that increased mindfulness on the part of the physician is needed to consider the divergence from "typical" presentations of immune system disorders.

Questions

1. Among patients with CGD, the most commonly affected protein subunit of the NADPH oxidase is:

   (a) p47
   (b) p91
   (c) RAC2
   (d) p22
   (e) p67

2. The main laboratory findings in IGAD are:

   (a) IgG < 500, IgA, < 100, IgM < 7
   (b) IgG normal, IgA normal, IgM normal
   (c) IgG normal, IgA < 7, IgM normal
   (d) IgG > 1,500, IgA < 7, IgM < 70
   (e) IgG < 500, IgA < 7, IgM < 70

3. IVIG therapy is appropriate therapy in all of the following EXCEPT:

   (a) CVID
   (b) XLA
   (c) X-HIM
   (d) IGAD
   (e) SADNI

4. Which clinical finding is more consistent with LAD-2 than LAD-1 or LAD-3?

   (a) Failure of umbilical cord detachment after birth
   (b) Retention of primary dentition
   (c) Recurrent purulent bacterial infections
   (d) Mental retardation
   (e) Bleeding disorder

5. Why is neutrophilia a common feature of LAD while neutropenia is more common among other immunodeficiencies?

   (a) Neutrophil leukemia is a common feature of LAD-1 and LAD-2
   (b) Impaired integrin and selectin function prevents neutrophils from leaving the bone marrow
   (c) Impaired integrin and selectin function prevents neutrophil diapedesis into affected tissue
   (d) Bleeding is commonly associated with neutrophilia in LAD-3
   (e) The defects in LAD prevent neutrophil apoptosis after stimulation and migration to inflammatory sites

Answers:

1. (b)
2. (c)
3. (d)
4. (d)
5. (c)

References

1. Avila, P.C. (2007) Primary immunodeficiencies. Mahmoudi M. (ed). Allergy and Asthma. Practical Diagnosis and Management, 1st Edition, McGraw Hill, New York, NY, pp. 266–290.
2. Winkelstein, J.A. et al. (2006) X-linked aggamaglobulinemia: Report on a United States registry of 201 patients. *Medicine (Baltimore)* **85**, 193–202.
3. Cunningham-Rundles, C., Bodian, C. (1999) Common variable immunodeficiency: Clinical and immunological features of 248 patients. *Clin Immunol* **92**, 34–48.
4. Berger, M. (2008) Principles and advances in immunoglobulin replacement therapy for primary immunodeficiency. *Immunol Allergy Clin NA* **28**, 413–437.
5. Bonilla, F. et al. (2005) Practice parameter for the diagnosis and management of primary immunodeficiency. *Ann Allergy Asthma Immunol* **94**, S1–S63.
6. Yong, P.F.K. et al. (2008) Common variable immunodeficiency: An update on etiology and management. *Immunol Allergy Clin NA* **28**, 367–386.
7. Lo, R., Rae, J., Noack, D, Curnutte, J.T., Avila, P.C. (2005) Recurrent streptococcal hepatic abscesses in a 46-year-old woman. *Ann Allergy Asthma Immunol* **95**, 325–329.

Index